KATINA I. MAKRIS, CCH, CIH

AUTOIMMUNE ILLNESS AND LYME DISEASE RECOVERY GUIDE

Mending the Body, Mind, and Spirit

Foreword by
MEREDITH YOUNG-SOWERS, D.DIV

Helios press

Skyhorse Publishing books may be purchased in bulk at special discounts for sales promotion, corporate gifts, fund-raising, or educational purposes. Special editions can also be created to specifications. For details, contact the Special Sales Department, Helios Press, 307 West 36th Street, 11th Floor, New York, NY 10018 or info@skyhorsepublishing.com.

Helios Press is an imprint of Skyhorse Publishing. Skyhorse® and Skyhorse Publishing® are registered trademarks of Skyhorse Publishing, Inc.®, a Delaware corporation.

Visit our website at www.skyhorsepublishing.com.

10 9 8 7 6 5 4 3 2

Library of Congress Cataloging-in-Publication Data is available on file.

Cover design by Jenny Zemanek
Cover photo courtesy of Thinkstock/PeterHermesFurian

Print ISBN: 978-1-63220-444-8
Ebook ISBN: 978-1-63220-757-9

Printed in the United States of America

Dedication

For Jake,

because you help me reach for the stars.

"Divine love has met and will always meet every human need."

—Mary Baker Eddy, *Science of Mind*

CONTENTS

Acknowledgments xi
Foreword xv
Introduction xviii

Part I Health and Healing 1
What Is My Role in My Recovery? 3
The Bigger Picture 7
The Importance of a Paradigm Shift in Medicine 19
The Wise Counselor 29
Defining Health 33
What is Dis-ease? 39
Why Do We Get Sick? 43
Predispositions and Constitutional Types: Why Some of Us Fall Ill 49
How to Work with Symptoms 55
Laws of Cure 59
Dashboard Light Doctor 63
Historical Overview of Medicine in the United States 69
Holistic Model of Health: The Philosophy of Natural Medicine 75
What is Mending? 83
The Mind-Body Connection 87
Resiliency 93

The Power to Heal 99
Epigenetics 100
Will 101
Rest 102
Support Systems 102
Self-Love 102
Faith and Positive Thinking 103
What Is My Role in My Illness? 105

Part II Overview of Autoimmune Illnesses and Lyme Disease 109
Overview of Autoimmune Illnesses and Lyme Disease 111
Chronic Fatigue Syndrome (CFS) 113
Crohn's Disease/Irritable Bowel Syndrome/Colitis 119
Fibromyalgia 125
The Adrenal Glands 127
Thyroid 128
Gluten 128
Molds 129
Yeast Overgrowth 129
Magnesium 129
Vitamin D 130
Liver Stagnation 130
Interstitial Cystitis 133
Lupus 137
Antibody Blood Tests 137
Other Blood Tests 139
Complement 139
C-Reactive Protein (CRP) 140

Erythrocyte Sedimentation Rate (ESR or "SED" Rate) 140
Blood-Clotting-Time Tests 140
Urine Tests 141
Multiple Sclerosis 147
Rheumatoid Arthritis 151
Thyroid: Graves' Disease and Hashimoto's Thyroiditis 155
The Lyme Disease Autoimmune Illness Crossover 159
Lyme Disease Basics 167
Lyme Disease Laboratory Testing 177
Tick-Borne Coinfections 183

Part III Healing Disciplines 191
What Is Naturopathic Medicine? 193
What Is Homeopathic Medicine? 199
What Is Acupuncture? 207
What Is Clinical Nutrition? 211
What Is Integrative/Functional Medicine? 215
What Is Metaphysical Healing? 221

Part IV Recovery Guide 229
Causes of Inflammation and Autoimmune Toxins 231
Role of the Adrenal Glands 237
Reducing Inflammation 247
Food 255
Foods to Eliminate 257
Paleo Diet 265
Good Fats Versus Bad Fats 267
Going Organic: Read the Labels 273
Amazing Amino Acids: Brain Chemistry and More 279

The Problem with Plastics 283
Electromagnetic Fields 287
Molds 291
The Need for Detoxification 295
The Role of Exercise in Mending 301
Cultivating Harmony: Your Sacred Space 305
The Influence of Thoughts 309
Our Own Inner Healing Pathway 313

Part V The Map 317
The Map 319

Part VI Mind-Spirit 327
Mind-Spirit 329
The Inner Tools We Bear 330
Suffering and Rebirth 333
Chakra 1 (Root Chakra): The Act of Being 337
Chakra 1 Exercise: "Basket of Gifts" 342
Chakra 2 (Sacral Chakra): Cycles of Change 345
Chakra 2 Exercises: "The Art of Letting Go" and "Bulbs of Spring" 351
Chakra 3 (Solar Plexis Chakra): Will and Intention 355
Chakra 3 Exercise: Moving with Intention 359
Chakra 4 (Heart Chakra): The Heart's Desire 363
Chakra 4 Exercise: Cupped Hands 367
Chakra 5 (Throat Chakra): Authenticity 371
Chakra 5 Exercise: Breathwork 377
Chakra 6 (Third Eye Chakra): Openness 379
Chakra 6 Exercises: Meditation 385

Chakra 7 (Crown Chakra): Crown of Divinity 387

Chakra 7 Exercise: Prayer 395

In Closing 397

The Seeker 399

Your Gift 403

Patient Case Stories 407

Rheumatoid Arthritis, Fibromyalgia, CFS Exposed 407

Twenty-Six Years of Chronic Illness: Lyme Disease in Tennessee ... 413

The Great Surrender: Death, Rebirth, and Creativity 416

Healing from Chronic Disease on the Spiritual Level: A Healing Journal 420

Our Life Purpose 426

Appendix 1: Lyme Disease Symptom Chart 429

Lyme Disease Symptom Questionnaire Checklist of Symptomology 430

Appendix 2: Pain Management & Antimicrobials for Autoimmune & Lyme Diseases 439

Common Herbals 440

Appendix 3: Autoimmune & Lyme Disease-Related Resources 447

Complementary Medicine Resources 448

Autoimmune Illness Resources 449

Additional Resources 451

Index 452

ACKNOWLEDGMENTS

Books like this do not get written overnight and a lot happens behind the scenes as well. Besides distilling my thirty years of practice and experience into words and a healing model, I feel the need to honor some very important individuals who helped *Autoimmune Illness and Lyme Disease Recovery Guide* reach its final form.

A handful of great medical masters provided me with their decades of clinical know-how and selfless attention to my work, in the critical hours I needed you the most—those final edits on content.

Thank you, brilliant Richard Horowitz, M.D, my twin aquarians with vivid spiritual understanding of these diseases, those extra hours you gave to me on your precious weekend time helped us all understand the crossover between the myriad of illnesses. Explaining so acutely how blebs do actually interfere with immune function is incredible!

Kenneth Liegner, M.D., I can always count on you. I reach out my hand and you are there, helping to guide me through a twisting path. Thank you for your immense kindness and professional collaboration. You shine in the history books and in my heart.

Mara Williams, LPN, my recent guest host at Lyme Light Radio, and such a dear friend and integrative medicine colleague, the autoimmune and lyme disease sections of this book would not be as accurate without your help. Thank you for your wise insights as you work so tirelessly in the deep trenches with thousands afflicted with these illnesses. Your dedication to those who suffer is as big as your heart is mighty.

Jeffrey Sullender, PhD, twenty-five years of friendship and colleagues for decades—besides saving my life ten years ago, we have traversed incredible literal and metaphoric mountain paths together. Your genius mind, our endless conversations, and our creative synergy helped me to write this very timely book! Thank you for our deep wellspring of collaborative vision and proofing, too!

Three years ago the universe aligned me to cutting edge, innovative Michael Arata, M.D., and how thankful I am for your support and kindness in the final read-through at the last days pre-press, as well as our mutual allegiance to facing the chronic disease crisis of our culture. You are a gem!

My editor Abigail Gehring, since that late summer day we sat in the coffee house in Brattleboro and I shared the layout of this book, you believed in my desire to help others and have been so supportive of helping me bring *Spirit* back into healing and our daily lives. Thank you for your gentleness and your commitment to my work.

Dede Cummings, my agent, you *rock*! Securing a two-book agreement and helping cement my pathway as an author and speaker was supreme! Thank you, wonder-woman.

My "guiding star," Suzanne Kingsbury, is a magnificent author, editor, Salon leader, soul sister, and creative genius who literally kept me alive post-op when I underwent dire major surgery as well as during the intense months of creating this book. Without your perspective and love, this book would still be inside me and not in written word. Bless you, Baby! You make me Dream Big.

Without a shadow of a doubt, my life as a writer would not exist without my incredible literary assistant Arianna Meehan. Thank you, beautiful lady, for the endless months typing, talking, assessing, caretaking, petsitting, and helping me create my work. I could not share all this knowledge without your patience and steadiness. I still see you on the beach at Frost Pond, the waters shimmering around you, our spirits laughing in play amid the heaving demands to glean words and metaphors. I am honored to have you by my side.

Lovely Autumn Kent, you are a treasure I cherish. Though I am gifted with Big Picture vision, I am a disaster with detail management. You, however, are the glue that keeps my office running, my schedule intact, my social media fresh, my clients and abundant creative energy in check!

Thank you from my true heart for all the oddball items you manage so effortlessly and the true generosity you share with me and my family.

Fearless Nell Conkright, you are my Artemis, jumping in to type complex work, when wicked pressures eclipsed reason. Thank you for your talent and exceptional savvy and for being brave when I faced very daunting life challenges in the midst of professional demands. My allegiance to our sisterhood spans beyond eons. Bless you!

To all my fellow writers at Gateless Gate Writing Salon in Vermont, your exceptional minds and rarified writing skills made me "write up." On those thigh deep snow clad nights we brewed together in syncopation as I birthed these chapters and you insisted I keep working, though my confidence was shaky. Thank you, elegant friends, for your love and devotion to the magic of words and our shared acceptance of intuitive forces plus discipline.

Ann Stokes, the pristine magic of Welcome Hill Studios is a precious balm to any artist at work. The many weeks I spent on your sacred land and in your studio cottage opened my channel to higher source. The richest pieces of this book were created in that hallowed vortex. Thank you for the encouragement and such amiable friendship.

The incredible guests on my program "Lyme Light Radio with Katina" educated me on so many salient pieces of what occurs within our body when tick borne organism infections set up camp inside us. I can not list you all, but let me offer you thanks for your tireless clinical work, lab studies, frontier edge thinking, and willingness to come on air with me and educate the world on an exploding public health care crisis called Lyme disease and its cross-over ramifications to autoimmune disorders. How honored I am to be in connection with so many great individuals and organizations.

Extra thanks to the three patient cases in this book; Gregg Kirk from Ticked Off Music Fests, Bethany, and Bonnie Huntsinger. You are very courageous individuals who have battled illnesses for way too long—decades in some cases—because our world did not understand or accept tick borne diseases as real or how devastating they can be to our bodily systems. Thank you for being honest enough to share your journeys with the world, you give depth and meaning to my messages here.

My friends and family are my bedrock. Being an author is not for the feint of mind or heart. Commitment, fortitude, discipline, sacrifice, and frenetic bursts of creative power or obsessed mindset are all givens. What is such a blindsiding agent is the toll completing a fully edited manuscript takes on the author and those close to us. Midnight hours, locked into deadlines, chewing on passages, we emotionally and energetically gain momentum and yet also afflict turmoil on those near us. Thank you, Jake, Vangie, Barbie, Joannie, Melanie, Lonny, Carlo, John, Nancy, Judy, Wendy, and all the others who have waited for me to come out of seclusion at the studio or when locked up in my own writing mind, and back out to you and my ability to play and dance and nurture our time together. Your understanding of my creative process and support means the world to me!

And, to the communities, health centers, rallies, fundraising events, and support groups around the country who I have worked with, visited, and shared my story and synergy with, thank you truly! So many brave and selfless souls are out there holding together broken hearts and families, because they care so purely about the suffering and hardships autoimmune illnesses and Lyme disease wreak in too many endless ways. Your collaboration of spirit has helped me muster the inner strength to write this book for the millions in need. My admiration for your work is steadfast.

Last and not least, Meredith Young-Sowers, D.Div., my mentor and sage, thank you for teaching me to love my life enough that I can take risk and challenge and marry it with faith and knowledge in such a way that healing wisdoms move through me and to others. I have grown so much as a healer because of you. Your Stillpoint Model invokes such truth and inner power. I am honored you have allowed me to share its enormous potentials in these pages. My gratitude to you is eternal.

With blessings,
Katina I. Makris, CCH, CIH

FOREWORD

When we pick up a book that has the power to change our lives, we feel it because of its integrity, its clarity, and its connection to our innermost thoughts and needs.

Autoimmune Illness and Lyme Disease Recovery Guide is that kind of book—a book for you to treasure, to learn from, and to become your guide to healing both from active disease and as a tool of prevention.

I've known Katina for more than twenty years and right from the beginning I was impressed with her potential as an intuitive healer. Today she is a heart-centered teacher who is forging a path into the *new medicine*.

The *new medicine* is more than mind-body connection, even more than mind-body-spirit alignment. The *new medicine* is a merger of the old ways of sensing and diagnosing disease as well as the new ways of integrating the biology of the physical body's processes with the emotional and spiritual awareness that our bodies are alive, vibrant, intelligent, and capable of great change and adjustment.

While we may already believe that the mind influences the body, it's been my experience from thirty-five years of practice that the body reads the mind's intention, consciously and unconsciously. No one wants to get sick or worse incapacitated by disease and yet these unwanted conditions can fill a need that we have to make change, or reevaluate a relationship or life path. When those adjustments are made and an inner direction accepted, then there is little need for the disease to persist.

Disease, whether tumor, autoimmune distress, or simple everyday ailment, offers a way to make something useful happen in our lives. Disease is a call for a response, not just from seeking to remove something, but in understanding why a condition exists and what need it has filled that can now be filled differently.

If we need a time-out in how to earn a living or deliver our unique contribution, for example, we may well find ourselves with chronic fatigue and fibromyalgia. If we have Lyme disease, we benefit from how we can bring more heart-centered effort and intention into our work.

In these pages, Katina gives readers a complete understanding of this *new medicine*—the workings of the body and mind and also the deep-hearted opening that is possible, even necessary in healing.

One of the things I most admire about Katina is her desire to learn, to heal herself, and to share what she's learned. I first met her when she was living in a nearby town and was the columnist at a local newspaper as a homeopath and also expert in natural medicine. Her column was widely read and appreciated. Years later when she was battling Lyme disease, we would talk about her condition and what was behind it. She had patience, even staying calm when she had to retreat to her couch for weeks and months with no let-up in symptoms, or seeking guidance from her own true inner self on ways to use the *new medicine.*

I have a picture in my mind of her tenacious spirit when she was a student at my Stillpoint School of Integrative Life Healing and she was so sick she had to lie on an air mattress in the back of the room. Yet she was there because she wanted to learn and to heal and to deepen her spirituality. She realized that healing personally would deepen her understanding of how to assist others on their healing journey.

This book will inspire you and give you what you need to turn the corner of a present illness and/or to assist others who are in need. It is also for the healers and healthcare providers who have been longing for a complete look at the intuitive body, mind and emotions, and spiritual direction for healing.

I am especially excited for Katina to *share* with you the very core of the Stillpoint work she learned that is the basis of Part V: Mind-Spirit, because it is a framework upon which to arrange the body's physical systems, the emotional beliefs and attitudes that correspond to each system, and the spiritual opportunities and possibilities that align with each of the seven primary energy centers or chakras. This model has helped thousands of people to shift into a healing mode, so through this book, it is my hope that many thousands more will find comfort, understanding, and healing from applying the information.

This book is written with the reader in mind. It is down-to-earth and at the same time stimulating and inspirational. No one can read of Katina's physical healing journey and remain untouched. You will know that she has been through what many readers are going through. She also has a significant standing in the world of natural medicine that will speak to everyone who hungers for more useful and quality information on healing and mending.

It is my delight to highly recommend this book to you. Keep it in your library, read and reread it, apply its principles and suggestions, and take into your very being the essence of life force that is offered here.

Healing is one part physical pursuit, another part emotional rewiring, and the final part is spiritual intention through union with the innermost aspect of you that is Divinity itself.

Meredith Young-Sowers, D.Div

Author of *Agartha*, *Spiritual Crisis*, *Angelic Messenger Cards*, *Wisdom Bowls*, and *Spirit Heals*

Co-Founder and Director of the *Stillpoint School of Integrative Life Healing*

Walpole, NH

March 2015

INTRODUCTION

Chronic healthcare problems have begun to surface at an alarming rate in recent decades. The spectrum of autoimmune illnesses has been in my lens since I first fell seriously ill in the summer of 2000, with what was initially deemed to be a sinus infection, then probable walking pneumonia, and finally labeled as chronic fatigue syndrome and chronic migraine headaches. Five years later, totally bedridden, broken, and newly divorced, I learned that actually I was maimed and struggling with several "hidden" infections. The primary misdiagnosed culprit was *Borrelia burgdorferi*, the bacteria that causes Lyme disease. I also hosted Epstein-Barr virus at frighteningly high levels, a parasite called babesia, and a whopping overgrowth of fungi. My lovely home in the New Hampshire countryside was mold infested and my immune system was spinning out of control with raging inflammation and multiple allergies, plus all sorts of depletions. With a shiny, bright, eight-year-old son under my wing, could I ever live to see him grown or be well enough to go to his Little League games?

After endless visits to specialists and renowned hospitals in New England with scant success of recovery, good fortune finally appeared in the able hands of a sterling clinical nutritionist colleague of mine who knew how to handle these runaway infectious "bugs" and, more importantly, how to restore the malfunctions of my failing body. We worked on detoxifying me from all sorts of externally and internally created toxins, rebuilding my fatigued adrenal glands and thyroid, helping my mitochondria create fuel again, and balancing out all sorts of neurotransmitters and blood sugar swings. It took me five years of devoted adherence to lifestyle, dietary, and emotional changes, and it worked! I mended 100 percent.

Even as a holistic healthcare practitioner myself, I had to examine my life and what made me fall so ill and vulnerable to these microbes, and to allow myself the time and process to embrace transformation on all planes—physically, emotionally, mentally, and spiritually. As a homeopath, I thought I was versed in helping others heal. This experience asked me to learn even more.

The great good of this journey is that I have spent the last fifteen years learning about the crossover currents of the exploding public healthcare crisis of Lyme disease (and other tick-borne diseases) and the relationship to autoimmune diseases. Though there is obvious linkage between them all, science has not yet pieced together the entire jigsaw puzzle. Some brilliant researchers and very talented and courageous practitioners are forging the way. My instincts tell me that when all the "dots" are finally connected, we will fully understand how these assorted microbes can trigger and mimic lupus and MS and Alzheimer's and more. Right now, though, what I can offer are the invaluable lessons of my own journey, which translates beyond the personal to the multiple millions who walk in the same shoes I did.

Chronic disease in the autoimmune and Lyme disease spectrum presents an individual with multiple challenges. Facing the realization that you are seeking talent and sources outside yourself to find wellness again is daunting and at times extremely frustrating. The endless days of pain, fatigue, solitude, dependency, and confusion seem endless. Many of us experience loss and despair. And yet, we also want to feel hope—hope for bright, happy times and relief from our suffering. Also, hope that someone will know how to cure us!

In these pages I share my understanding of what mending involves. Mending literally refers to the actual repair work and knitting together of a fracture or tear. Metaphorically, mending means so much to us on the inside of illness. When we fall ill to chronic disease we fracture in a certain way. Things are never quite the same. There is a sense of displacement or that you just do not feel quite right and that you want to correct it all. What I suggest is that something rather grand is being asked of you in this time of disorder. You are being asked to reflect upon your life status—your behaviors and choices and your habits. And then, you are being asked to make some changes in order to mend.

This book provides a toolbox of assorted options to consider. We explore a great deal of what encompasses health and healing and why we get sick. Also, we look at the role of various key factors that create the terrain for autoimmune illness and Lyme disease to blossom. Why do some of us fall ill to these conditions but not others? And, most importantly, how can I mend from the disease and reclaim my well-being and vitality?

The great arc presiding over the entire journey for me, however, has been the enormous breadth and depth of spirituality's presence. Serious states, like these diseases present, ultimately bring us into concert with energy beyond the simple self. We are entering the domain of personal transformation and what in modern times is akin to a quest—a quest for higher knowledge, for inner strength, and for assistance in the darkest of times. This journey asks for faith and guidance and an unfurling of the miraculous connection we innately bear between our mind and our body and our spirit. For we are marvelous and miraculous beings. We just need to learn how to stitch it all together.

I wrote this book for the all too many who feel at odds with themselves while ill or are perhaps a caregiver of someone in need. We bear enormous internal gifts. However, many of us have not been taught how to "turn on" the healing codes, or we have forgotten. Mending helps us find our inner compass, to recalibrate during a time of lost navigation and to set our sights on a positive outcome. Like any worthy voyage, not every day is a smooth passage. But you can still reach your destination! Optimal health seems attainable even in a stormy crossing. What I present is a fresh look at healing tools to apply. Not all these modalities will work for you, but they are worth examining.

In deepest respect I need to honor my very wise and gifted spiritual teacher and mentor, Dr. Meredith Young-Sowers, who trained me to become an intuitive healer and teacher. The metaphysical model I work with in this book is springboarded from her thirty-five years of knowledge and experience. The Stillpoint School of Integrative Life Healing and her model focus on the Seven Energy Chakras and correlating bodily systems and emotional couplings we all house. My own healing work with individuals and groups grew from her model. We will look at autoimmune illnesses, Lyme disease, and how to promote healing. These skills I share worked for me and many others.

My professional healing work with Lyme disease and autoimmune illnesses after thirty years in practice as a classical homeopath brings another lens into these conditions. In totality you will discover a multidimensional approach to recovery, one that incorporates natural medicine, orthodox pragmatics, and metaphysics. Most specifically we will chart a course together through the pivotal domain of personal transformation. For true healing happens on the inside.

Namaste,
Katina I. Makris, CCH, CIH
New Hampshire
Spring 2015

Medical Disclaimer

Please note that I am trained and certified as a classical homeopath (CCH) and spiritual healer (CIH). Even though I have worked with individuals in assorted forms of distress and illness, I am not permitted to make a medical diagnosis, perform a physical exam, or administer pharmaceuticals.

My orientation and work has always been to help support and reinforce the person and his or her natural bodily function, and not treat the disease, through the use of homeopathics and spiritual energy healing.

Throughout the pages of this book I refer to particular disease states and syndromes, and additionally I recommend integrative medicine doctors as well as allopathic physicians and naturopaths, acupuncturists, chiropractors, clinical nutritionists, homeopaths, and other healers. My message is that many of these chronic illnesses require more than one specific system of approach in order to mend and achieve a more optimal level of health, and ultimately move into remission or even cure.

Please note, however, that I do not attempt to treat or cure any of these conditions throughout these pages, but offer you suggestions and guidelines to seek out the properly trained and licensed professionals to work with you individually in your case.

My goal is to help initiate a stronger utilization of an integrated healthcare system in the USA and for people to realize they can obtain much more inner healing power than they ever dreamed. The information provided here is for your self-help and education.

The author and publisher do not attempt to offer a cure for any particular disease.

Katina I. Makris, CCH, CIH

Helios Press, an imprint of Skyhorse Publishing

PART I

Health and Healing

WHAT IS MY ROLE IN MY RECOVERY?

All individuals with autoimmune illness and Lyme disease are being asked to take a "time out" from life. Like a monk in his cave or the person who spends thousands of dollars to go on an idyllic yoga retreat, you are being asked at the level of body, mind, and spirit to take a retreat from your way of living and your acts of doing.

This illness shines the light on you. The persistence, the discomfort, the "foreign" feelings are real. They are wake-up calls to you that you can no longer run this template any more. It is not working for you, as your body and psyche have reacted strongly enough that you cannot ignore or push through matters any longer. No drug will make the symptoms go away and stay away. The anti-inflammatories, analgesics, mood enhancers, or antibiotics are only temporary fixes.

The real truth is that physically, your adrenal glands likely are being depleted and have tipped your entire endocrine system off-gear. Or the inflammation cascade is running out of control. Or maybe your body pH is too acidic, and microbes and fungi are overpopulating you internally. Perhaps food sensitivities exist, or heavy metals and chemicals burden you with toxins. There is an assortment of nutrient deficiencies, leading to your genetic "flaws" being triggered and showcased. Or, most intrinsically, you are doing something that goes "against your grain" and does not meet your heart's desire. Spiritually you are in crisis, because who knows how to mend a broken spirit?

In mending from chronic disease, the emotional and spiritual sides of the condition need as much attention as the physical. No being is one-dimensional; we are intricate, elastic, and always searching for homeostasis, or balance. Most importantly, our heart bears desire, and listening within to its callings is central for recovery.

Now I reach out my hand to you. Please take it. I am here to help. Let me guide you. We will walk together, now. You do not have to do this alone. I have been in your shoes. I know the ropes and can lead you out safely. I am here to bring you solace, to inspire you to try some new paths to wholeness. Besides offering you some tools and insights, I bring you hope. Because, if I went from bedridden and wheelchair-bound with CFS/ME for a decade, to vibrant and healthy and swimming a mile with ease, so can you!

The human being is amazingly resilient and adaptive when we provide it with the proper measures in the right environment. There are many wonderful books available on autoimmune disorders. However, this is the first book you will read that brings you in concert with your inner healing powers. You will not be sorry you read this book.

Some of you will say this sounds too simple to be effective, others will trust only the highest-pedigreed medical professionals, and others of you will say, "This book has given me my life back." You may have all of these reactions or others entirely. Ultimately, I share this knowledge because I care. I care about you, and anyone who has become ill and lost their way. Being alone or sick or scared is an awful feeling. Tragedy occurs much too often, in too many lives. Still, we can heal and grow and bloom anew with the right support.

These pages lay out some very essential aspects regarding health, illness, healing, and wellness. We look at the autoimmune and Lyme disease spectrum. We come to understand why these conditions have likely surfaced in you. I am helping to empower you. For you are responsible for taking an active role in your recovery. You can reclaim your health and well-being.

But, you must make a commitment. That commitment is to yourself, because you need the care, the attention, and the peace in order to get well. I will ask you to make some changes in your daily life, and encourage you to try some different options in lifestyle and healthcare. I do not have all the answers. My wisdom tells me you are eager to heal and curious about options. Most specifically, you want to gain control over these runaway symptoms. You feel like your body is out of your control, hijacked. And, in some ways, that is true.

What is also true is that you have access to inner reserves, which will shift your energy around, so that we can harness some of it for mending, and free the rest of it up for your healthier future.

Your role in recovery is to start paying attention to yourself and your lifestyle in new ways. Following the trends of our unhealthy, chemically laden food industry, pharmaceutical-based medical system, and electromagnetically saturated daily life is not supportive to the delicate workings of the endocrine, immune, and nervous systems. Twenty, thirty, forty years of GMO food in our grocery stores, too many chemical additives in cosmetics and leached from plastic bottles, and cling wrap have accumulated in your body.

Making conscious choices to eat organic foods (especially animal products—dairy, meat, poultry, fish) is important. So is removing the microwave, the cordless and cell phones, and the electronics from your bedroom. Your role in recovery involves becoming conscious about how harmful these associated influences become when tallied up.

Additionally, seeking out a top-rate, certified clinical nutritionist (CCN), naturopathic physician (ND), and/or integrative or functional medicine doctor is essential, for these type of practitioners will know what specialty labs to use for assessing your associated depletions, as well as how to remove heavy metals with chelation, and microbes such as *Borrelia burgdorferi* (Lyme disease), parasites, fungi, and the too common CFS/fibromyalgia/MS viruses of EBV, cytomeglia, etc.

Most essentially, following the healing exercises outlined in Part V of this book is crucial. Entering the domain of personal transformation and using the simple, yet powerful inner healing tools I teach you can be truly effective. I would not have made a complete recovery if I did not delve so deeply and consistently into these practices. They have been sacred, used for generations, and "forgotten" somehow in the last fifty years, just as these autoimmune-style illnesses started surfacing.

The time has come for you to gain control of your body, emotions, and mind. The mind is your most valuable asset. Using it wisely is critical. Part of my job in these pages is to help you hone your mind to turn on the healing pathway. You are capable of this. In fact, the promise for attaining these skills is very exciting.

Be positive. Recognize the opportunity. Do not be afraid or leery; these emotions will only limit or block your success. Open yourself up to discovery and embrace change, for anything is possible in your lifetime. You can create your healthier future. Physicians do not hold all the tools. More than half of the resources for healing exist inside you.

Honor your Self. Say, "Thank you, I am still alive." Look at what you do have; even if it is not very much, it is a starting place. Be grateful for the moment that is now, for this is an awakening and every day, every breath, every thought is a new opportunity. And, you can kindle new cell growth, new energy, a new future. Your ability to shift your thoughts will ignite the mind-body healing pathway. Together we will make strides.

I believe in you. You are strong and brave and beautiful. If no one has told you that in a while, I am reminding you now. The fact that you are reading this book illustrates this. Let us honor your healing journey. Keep a notebook or journal if it helps you, or use the blank pages at the end of this book. This guide is meant to help you keep pace with your recovery. You can run free again, beyond the pain and suffering and weakness. Have hope and trust in your future, and yourself. Believe.

THE BIGGER PICTURE

Think of a time period, or even just a day in your life, when you were in perfect health, filled with energy, happy, radiant, and enthused or inspired. Is the image of you one of your youth, as a child or teenager, a college-aged student? Or older perhaps, thriving in your twenties, thirties, forties, or later yet, your fifties or sixties? Close your eyes, glean this image of yourself. See your surroundings, the expression on your face, what you were doing, and were you alone or with others? Can you feel the weather, sense the lighting, see what you were wearing? Capture this time and place and essence of you right now.

Give credence to the enormous vitality, love, and beauty you embodied and actually still do, even if now you are encumbered with health issues, symptoms of discomfort, or emotional strife. That image we just retrieved—that time and place and true essence of you—is real and alive and what you were born to be and thrive as. Your spirit, your body, your emotional being is alive, or you would not be reading these words. Remember that image in your mind's eye; we will visit it daily from now on.

We are unique, wondrous, capable, and amazingly resilient beings. We have a very mighty organ called the brain, filled with enormous abilities and powers. The body we were genetically given is complex and essentially "self-righting," always trying to recalibrate and return to balance or homeostasis when moved into different environments or climactic conditions or when exposed to toxins, chemicals, microbes, and the energies of emotions. We often forget just how miraculous the human being is; sensing, adjusting, defending, and all internal systems working in complex synchronicity to maintain health and well-being. I marvel at our tremendous skills.

The human body alone is miraculous! The typical person is comprised of 206 bones, more than 600 skeletal muscles, five vital organs, six quarts of blood, roughly ninety pounds of water/fluids, twenty-eight feet of intestines, approximately 60,000 miles of blood vessels, forty-five miles of nerves, ten trillion cells, and energy states of so many mutable forms. If we could measure us in "wattage," like a forty- or hundred-watt lightbulb, we could better assess ourselves than merely by considering our looks, our health status, our career success.

Take a quick assessment of yourself and sense the energetic difference of feeling depressed and the dim energy wattage you express versus the brilliant glare of a brainstorming, creative moment when you are on high-beam energy output of a hundred-plus watts. They are quite different, aren't they?

Our emotional feelings obviously possess energy. Again, I ask you to sense within yourself for a few minutes. Close your eyes and recall yourself feeling sad. I see myself lying on my green floral print living room sofa, limp and lethargic, sadness weighing me down, tears on my eyelashes. I feel weak and deflated, with little energy and a depression setting in. My heart is broken. In fact, energetically I feel like I am lying on the bottom of the ocean floor or way down deep at the base of a well. I have very little energy output. I don't even want to lift my arm. My breathing feels tiring. I am withdrawn.

I contrast this to another energy state—anger. Anger may not be the most desirable emotion, and we know it can create destructive forces or propel us to outbursts. Anger has an energy form and when we do not stifle it, but express it, there is intense output; motion and even heat associated. Some people yell, others kick and throw things. Uncontrolled, impulsive anger can induce a brawl or act of violence.

If an unsuspecting person walks into a room where an angry person stands, even if they are still, you can perceive the energy of their anger. It may make you suddenly feel tense, frightened, super alert. This is very different than the flaccid energy of sadness. Anger is taut and high wattage.

I want to have you journey inside one more time now—let's seek out love. Close your eyes if it helps. Put your hand over your heart, take a few deep breaths, quiet your thinking. Recall yourself in love. Are you young and enamored of someone beautiful in your opinion? Or is it your newborn child you are enthralled with? Are you entwined in the roaring emotional and sexual chemistry of a mate or partner you cannot stay away from, racing to their side at any opportunity?

Love is so very powerful. See and feel that being who you opened your heart so fully to. How do you feel when you draw up this image of yourself? Love fills us, it empowers us, it makes us expand and extend beyond our selves; overflowing and bathed in an aura of magic.

The baby's tiny wiggling fingers, your mate's sunny smile, the warmth of your lover's breath on your neck. We feel good in these moments and we never want the feelings to stop. Our energy state glows like that hundred-watt lightbulb in full-spectrum glory!

I have asked you to visit these energy states for a reason. The reason is that as human beings (as part of the mammal kingdom), we are able to generate and express emotions. Our emotional fabric is real, valid, and entwined with our physical body; that phenomenal structure of bones and organs and cells.

Sometime in the 1900s, Western medicine decided to study and treat symptoms and illnesses in a methodology called science. The emotional and physical interplay of our whole person/being was actually disregarded and in certain decades ridiculed. Doctoring became a practice of focusing merely on physical symptoms, their constellation patterns labeled as disease diagnosis. Each generation to follow became more and more disconnected from the profound wellspring of our inner healing powers and actually relinquished self-ability and turned their body over to a physician at the mere commencement of symptoms, to be "fixed" with an externally applied modality; pharmaceuticals, surgery, "expert opinion."

The norm for mid- to late-century 1900s USA came to regard medical physicians as very knowing, powerful people whom we seek at great expense to help us when distressed. Centuries prior, the clergy held such status. In the Renaissance, artists were revered with gifts and powers. Indigenous cultures and BC tribes valued shamans and magi with their ability to move energy states and cull visions. Centuries revolve and societies morph. Now in the early phase of the twenty-first century, we are a Western world population of chronically "ill" people.

The average American fills twelve to fifteen drug prescriptions annually. Our country had a retail over-the-counter pharmaceutical trade of $96 billion in 2012 and, according to *Time* magazine statistics from 2009, we have begun seeking the use of alternative medicine to the tune of $40 billion annually. On the world health order status, the USA ranks the lowest amongst the eleven richest nations, lagging behind other countries such as England, Switzerland, and Sweden, and with small countries such as Malta and Singapore in top rankings.

Many factors coalesce, crippling modern America with massive case numbers of chronic disease and autoimmune illness. Since the 1950s we have witnessed a frightening spike in MS, lupus, Crohn's disease, food allergies, and autism in children, and the raging infectious illness epidemic of Lyme disease.

Some sectors chalk it up to lack of awareness fifty years ago, yet most of us instinctively know an amalgam of factors that have induced the maelstrom of suffering that more than 50 percent of adults age thirty and older are afflicted with. The disturbing reality is that we are less healthy than our parents and grandparents born prior to World War II who smoked, drank, and ate fats liberally. They were reared prior to processed foods and were rarely vaccinated. Smallpox was the only vaccine injected into their bloodstreams. They did not intake hydrogenated oils daily until the 1950s.

These generations ate fruits and vegetables typically "in season," consumed an heirloom non-GMO wheat, were electric-magnetic field-free, and didn't live in the radius of a nuclear power plant until they were adults. With one- (or no-) car households, their pace of living was radically slower, meaning their adrenal glands (fight-or-flight stress mechanism) did not have to sprint routinely during freeway high-speed commutes, multitask to dual-career households, or fret over "dropped" mobile business calls in mid-sentence.

So, the lard and the bourbon and the cigars may have "taxed" their bodies, but not nearly as intensely as the 112 additives consumed daily in foods, soft drinks, and fluoridated water that our kids also absorb. Once we stir in the emotional energy states highlighted a few pages ago, a picture is being painted—we have a physically overpolluted body, which swims with often very potent negative energy states. Our jobs, our relationships, and our lifestyles commonly are peppered with stress, whiplash pace, soaring demands, and unresolved conflicts.

The chapters to come will illustrate the very obvious correlation between both extreme emotional feeling states or prolonged emotional feeling states, as relates to illness and symptomology. We are not divided up into parts, but woven together in a cohesive tapestry. We are beautiful, creative, sensitive creatures who thrive when love, compassion, support, cooperation, and freedoms are provided. Our creative output, our health and well-being, and states of love and joy have been radically compromised.

Though as dour as this scenario sounds, there is hope! We can be healthy and vibrant and even recover from a panoply of symptoms and conditions. Remember—you are capable of resiliency! We manufacture new cells every day of our lives. The older, toxic ones can be replaced with fresh, healthier newbies. Your organs and glands can be nourished and replenished from their depletions. Damages can even be corrected in many instances.

The good news in the gateway of this twenty-first century is that we now have terrific restorative supplements available to us from high-quality sources. The synergistic healing properties of natural plants and their centuries-old effectiveness are returning to healthcare. A strong movement toward organic, non-processed food is resurfacing, and most precious to each and every one of us is the truth that we bear innate healing powers. That glorious brain I noted houses a true gift—your mind. And, we can access its enormous healing prowess.

As a young girl, and even as a tragically bedridden adult (maimed by advanced neurological Lyme disease/CFS/migraines in my forties), my profoundly wise father had a message he would deliver to me often: "God gave you a mind. It is your job to use it. And use it properly. Do not waste it on negative thoughts or greedy desires. If you focus your mind and use it wisely, you can achieve anything in this lifetime. Healing is in your hands, not another's."

Left for dead in the minefields of the Philippines in World War II, my father was a survivor, a thriver actually, and would go on to defy the odds numerous other times in his life, overcoming catastrophic car accidents, eighteen pulmonary embolisms, bankruptcy, and more. Always, always, I witnessed his mind-set, his belief system, and enormous willpower. By example he taught me invaluable life lessons. He was absolutely correct—the power of our minds and how we use them is stunning. We can use our minds to create our future. We can use them to help us heal.

The current-day coinage of rallying our inner healing skillsets involving the very capable workings of the mind-body healing pathway is called "epigenetic medicine." Over recent decades brilliant doctors, psychologists, spiritual healers such as Dr. Andrew Weil, Dr. Deepak Chopra, Carolyn Myss, Bruce Lipton, and Dr. Meredith Young-Sowers have illustrated to us in their teachings and books just how resourceful the human being is. They are reminding us that we are more than a system of bones and muscles, organs and glands. Few and far between, yet enormously popular and intimately accurate, these brilliant guides have shone a light in the darkened chambers of millions of peoples' life sufferings. They bring us insight and inspiration.

I am a natural healthcare practitioner of thirty years. My orientation has always revolved around supporting the human body and psyche with the aid of natural medicine and the somewhat eclectic modalities the masses refer to as non-scientific. Though not researched to the tune of millions of dollars in United States science processes, many of these modalities are centuries old, and broadly used with faith and success internationally.

Natural medicine practices are traditionally gentler, more ancient, and resonate more comfortably with a sensitive body and being. Not all of us are so fine-tuned. Some can be injected with radioactive dyes for CAT scans or down six beers without recourse. This does not mean these measures are good for you, but your system may be able to handle these toxins or elements and then recalibrate. But, more importantly—what are the long-term repercussions? Thirty years later will your assorted systems be collapsing? Will you experience kidney failure, hypertension, or pancreatic cancer from regular diet sodas or margarine? I am an intuitive, strongly sensing being. I follow my instincts and simultaneously pay keen attention to my body and psyche's reactions. If a drug or food or a person upsets or harms me, I choose to avoid this. This ability helps me avoid many conditions, and to regenerate as well.

The disassociation from self-care and body awareness in the twentieth century psychologically turned the United States into a society dependent on doctors as "fix-it" gurus, with much drug popping and mass merchandising of our food chain. We became out of tune with our inner guiding radar, and abandoned skills such as intention, belief, vision, affirmation, congruency, and contemplation.

We have become beings who seek support, satisfaction, reward, and resurrection from externally directed measures. We go binge shopping, buy snazzy cars, ramp up on more stimulation, gorge on larger meals, ingest whopping doses of sugar and drugs and random sex, expecting to feel better, have immediate gratification, or be cured from the gout, depression, or colitis more quickly by a pill or another human being.

Meanwhile, why have we relinquished our own powers? What happened to rest, playing a non-electric instrument, using your hands to create something tangible (like a bird feeder or a piece of clothing)? Why do the majority of us not know how to ignite our skills of perception or receive a message from Higher Knowledge (God, angels, Buddha, your divinity)? Do you know how to set an intention or make a prayer effective for healing?

We are all born to create, contribute in service to mankind, and ultimately are able to manifest resources for our basic human needs (money being one thread, intimacy and nourishment others). Willpower and love and hope are givens. Young children display these beautiful qualities effortlessly. They are not meant to be weaned out of our repertoire by left-brained, overly scholastic-based, didactic educational systems. These precious qualities are, conversely, meant to be honed and shared throughout our lives. Perception, imagination, artistry exist in us all, yet get jettisoned too early—unlike our Renaissance forebears, who cultivated these gifts like golden treasures.

Our attitude has become lopsided. We strive for success on a great deal of externally directed productive, yang (male) energy. The program has been emphasized to get an advanced academic education, climb the career ladder, work long hours (even on weekends), amass possessions, own a home, juggle a mortgage and loans, listen to the media frenzy, go fast, and live hard. And then we are exhausted, frazzled, bickering, and divorcing, raising children on electronic news feeds and synthesized foods. These youngsters rarely build tree forts, catch polliwogs, or bake a cake from scratch. Men are often impotent by age fifty-five and the United States is walloped with autoimmune illnesses to the tune of 50,000,000 individuals.[1]

---

[1] (AutoImmuneSummit.com)

Where is the other end of the seesaw, the inner reflection, the ability to receive affection, the act of being with yourself, savoring a quiet hour by a pond or meditating in silence, a candle your sole companion? Do you teach your children how to listen to their heart's calling or help them attune their sense of direction by the placement of the sun or stars in the sky?

Some of this sounds old-fashioned. Modern, forward-thinking, scientifically based stances are favored in general by every "next" generation. Progress and growth are, of course, valuable. Stagnation or reversal are typically not allies to a business, a body of water, or a relationship. But, in the instance of modern-day health, my experience shows me we are not getting healthier as a population, but instead reversing and becoming quite dis-eased, even spiritually stagnating.

Thirty years in private practice has enabled me to witness trends, shifts, positive developments, and also a disturbing reality—the youngest generation is more sickly than its grandparents.

Childhood obesity, diabetes, and mood disorders are rampant. These youngsters have too many hormonal disrupters in the foods, from petrochemical derivatives mimicking estrogen to additives fiddling with their neurochemistry. Additionally, they are cooped up with reduced recess and gym classes in their school day, and plugged in excessively, eyes glued to electromagnetic-radiating technology that we have somehow come to deem as "benign."

This is not a pretty picture I paint, but unless you live off the grid in rural Montana or Alaska, the majority of the USA's citizens are steeped in a mélange of chemicals, EMFs, and stress-inducing hormones, and are overworked, undervalued, and dependent on external "fixes" to boost their energy, their moods, and their conveniences.

Without a shadow of a doubt, we are in the throes of a societal health crisis. Though we may live longer than our forebears, into our eighties and nineties, these elder folks are littered with illness symptoms, very much in need of physical care, and rarely held in familial bonds. Most of us will die not at home, surrounded by loved ones, but in a hospital or assisted-living environment, surrounded by tubes.

We all must practice self-care and personal awareness, beginning in childhood. The more in sync one can be to their level of health and happiness, and understand how to recalibrate when the early symptoms of imbalance manifest, the greater the potential for a life of optimal wellness and fulfillment is. And, in the same breath, I tell you that it is never too late to start. Learning how to be self-aware is part of healing. Coming to understand the role of our emotions in relationship to chronic illness is enormous. Discovering how to process or move a particular emotional pattern can be life-changing.

Emotional states hold specific energy forms. Positive emotions resonate to higher vibrations, negative ones to lower frequencies. The human body and its intricate network of cells and symptoms prefer certain vibrational frequencies. Joyful, enthused, love-filled states are lighter, quicker, and induce the brain to release endorphins, the "feel-good" hormones that support good immune function.

Fear, animosity, and greed vibrate at deeper, lower rates. If these feelings are held for durations, the energy pattern will embed, in turn affecting associated organs and cellular function. Over time it is simple to see how the bitterness of disdain could breed stomach cancer or unresolved grief can induce recurrent bronchitis and asthma.

Not every disease is caused by emotional imbalances. But, coming to understand the interplay between our body and mind in relationship to sickness gives us a toolbox to work with. Healing is in your capacity.

I will take you on a journey, weaving body, mind, and spirit. You will come to discover the incredible workings of the endocrine system and how the delicate nuances within can induce all sorts of symptomology and heath disorders when it is out of balance.

I will guide you through the fascinating domain of our seven energy chakra sites, how they interface with the physiology of specific bodily systems, and even more artfully, the relationship of how certain emotions correlate to certain organs.

We are multidimensional beings and ever-evolving. Movement, expression, creativity, and contribution are our cornerstones. When these are in good order, health and well-being are more readily attained. When we lapse or ignore these foundational pieces, troubles brew, suffering mounts.

Mending is your personal process. No one can do it for you. Yes, there are gifted practitioners, therapists, doctors, friends, clergy, even animals that can prompt the support you require, or provide the catalyst you need, but ultimately healing is a journey, and one you can take as a quest or ignore as too treacherous or unworthy.

My hope is that you will seek the quest. For life's greatest lessons, deepest rewards, most sterling moments, are bred not from the externalized world of possessions and status, but instead from the inner riches gained from personal discovery and loving compassion.

You are too precious to ignore.

THE IMPORTANCE OF A PARADIGM SHIFT IN MEDICINE

"Serious illness is our spirit's calling for ultimate full-life change. All of our bodily systems, our spiritual and emotional fabric, are being asked to transform. We can no longer run on the old "grid." That pattern was not as healthy and productive as you maybe perceived it to be, even if aspects of your life felt rewarding or fulfilling."

Fourteen years ago I was living my dream life in a quaint New England township with a beautiful family and a handsome husband, a country home, throngs of friends, and a thriving practice as a classical homeopath. I sat on the national board and helped write the national homeopathic certification exam. My popular bi-monthly newspaper health column was clipped out and sent to friends around the globe by my devoted readers. I was a wife, a mom, a great friend, and a caring neighbor. I thought I was doing everything right and yet chronic fatigue syndrome, constant migraines, irritable bowel syndrome, horrid neck pains, apparent fibromyalgia, and hidden misdiagnosed Lyme disease took me down—way deep down—and forced me to change.

For five years I spiraled down a long funnel of darkness and despair as symptoms morphed. I bottomed out in a wheelchair, bed-bound and riddled with palsies, tremors, dementia, and pains clutching my heart. I was too weak to walk unassisted or shower alone. A good day was when I could make a sandwich. Some nights I felt I would die in my sleep and never see my darling seven-year-old son grow up. Dozens of prominent doctors and hospitals had no real answers for me other than another drug to try and too many thousands of out-of-pocket dollars spent. How could an athletic, ambitious, talented, vital person wither to such a pathetic state and no one in the medical kingdom have a method to help me heal? Even my beloved homeopathic masters were stumped, helping me gain a few weeks of renewed mental clarity or less body pain, only to slip back down the crevasse again into collapse. I was desperate, despondent, and near death.

A brilliant PhD clinical nutritionist colleague of mine was the savior who looked at the three negative Lyme disease tests I had as "inaccurate" and had me retested at two state-of-the-art tick-borne-disease specialty labs. He was certain my thyroid, adrenals, "gut," and liver were compromised and my body loaded with toxins and dormant viral infections "gone wild" from battling an aggressive bacteria for over five years. I sat in shock listening to this savvy practitioner relay how Lyme disease spirochete bacteria auger their way from bloodstream to tissues and organs en route to the brain, mimicking all sorts of disorders and diseases. The Infectious Disease Society of America had labeled this shape-shifting bacteria only as a short-term infectious illness of limited duration, leaving thousands of physicians in the dark as to the fact that "chronic" forms of the illness exist, akin to its cousin syphilis, and that I was not alone; hundreds of thousands were suffering as deplorably as me. Too many doctors are not aware of how Lyme bacteria can progress into chronic issues.

Ashen gray and weepy, I was struggling to hold my body still, the tremors jarring me in the chair as I absorbed this rather disturbing scenario. Sure enough, he was correct—three weeks later the two labs verified I was ultra positive on the *Borrelia burgdorferi* protein titer tests! All the commercial labs had missed it and cost me everything!

My successful career and savings were gone, my marriage destroyed, the family home sold, and my children bouncing between two households. Besides this horror, my emotional state was acutely fragile and my spirit clearly broken. How would I mend?

Empowered by receiving a proper diagnosis I was determined to beat back the bacterial infection and restore all the damages and depletions the organisms induced. I held great confidence in this talented practitioner and was now also in the good hands of an integrative medical doctor. We all knew it would take time and patience and more rest and deep restoration, as all my systems were next studied to discern what supplements and treatments I required. Detoxification, mineral loss, neurotransmitter imbalances, mitochondria failure, chronic inflammation, hormonal destruction, and much more were all factors. In totality, my healing recovery required five years of hard and devoted work. Every day I worked on healing. The first year I was still bedridden, and it took two more years before I could drive a car!

Ultimately, I was forced to change almost every aspect of how I lived my life—my healthcare management expanded beyond drug doctoring. I had to change my food choices, my sleep cycles, how I managed my intimate relationships, my multitasking, my self-care, the ability to nurture my dreams and to attune to my deep gifts of creativity. This all required my earnest attention. And unbeknownst to me, I eventually discovered that my spirit was crying out for care and expression. I was crippled because I could no longer function on the old model I had been reared on in post-WWII America. I had to refabricate my own grid.

Such illnesses are powerful "wake-up calls" and ask us to summon our own capacity for self-reflection and also to learn how to surrender. I had to surrender to the process of death and rebirth. I needed to let go of my many emblems of success in the United States, which I had built my life upon, and instead search within for what the inner me really needed in order to thrive. It was frightening to lose my career and income, husband, and health. I felt so insecure and alone and confused and daunted. Yet, a very gifted spiritual healer appeared on my horizon and her great insights and deep, nurturing belief in my future helped me find my North Star of divination and a pathway out of this trench of illness and heartache.

I learned how to listen within, to honor my instincts, to not be afraid to change, and in turn to trust that I would be guided and protected by God, or a universal force greater than the single earthling called "me." I was afraid and I also had nothing more to lose. I chose to live, and I chose to live with quest and commitment and belief. Everything has changed and today I am more alive and creative than ever! I healed fully and learned so very much along the way, fueling me to share my understandings with others in need. I also viscerally learned the hard way that a huge paradigm shift is necessary in our culture regarding illness, doctoring, and more profoundly, healing. And, blessedly, each of us bears great internal powers of resiliency and resurrection.

Our connection to the divine reaches us no matter what our circumstances, no matter how fixed we are in our lifestyle or defense postures. When it is time to change, our life steward presents the opportunity. This is more deeply understood as personal transformation. Personal transformation is a deep, soulful journey, akin to Persephone's descent into the underworld and hell fires of personal demons and treacherous obstacles, even what some call imprisonment. But, ultimately, if we listen within, if we learn how to let go so we can find faith, trust, balance, and self-love, we can recalibrate, receive higher guidance, and grow in vastness and depth. We return to the land of light and the living refreshed, resplendent, and graced with creative outpourings and ultimately an open channel to the Divine.

Like a mother who is willing to sacrifice her own self-need for her child's well-being, we too must accept the gesture of self-nurturance. This is not an easy task at first for most of us in modern Western society. We put others ahead of ourselves, including job demands, chores, partners, and our children. This is all acceptable, to a point. But where is the tipping point? That fulcrum of sacrifice and self-care? Serious illness, like the autoimmune spectrum and the crossover underpinnings of often hidden Lyme disease, puts a bright spotlight on this very intrinsic life-sustaining issue. Many equate this to a shamanic journey of deep cultivation.

Everyone, myself included, afflicted with chronic disease, needs to delve into her personal relationship with Self. What can be let go of? What do you now sacrifice in order to heal? How can I find my personal inner authority and place of sanctuary? The journey within is magical when we learn to embrace it and not just continuously rail against all we are not doing and what we are losing and how shrunken our world has become. These are hard lessons and very strident trials. And they are great teachers and help hone true character when we quit fighting the tide, the expectations, the shoulds and woulds and have nots. For your spirit is your greatest guide and when you can feed it, most anything is attainable, as long as greed and jealousy and ego are not in the mix. The journey inward is the most remarkable one I have taken, even though visiting the land of Brazil and the waters of the Caribbean are also enchanting! I will never regret the illness as a teacher, though I had to work hard to master the trappings of my emotions.

Most chronic disease and syndrome cases ask a being to enter the domain of retreat and solitude, to move inward and open to spirit's tappings. When we are seriously ill, the hamster wheel absolutely must stop! Immediately! No more multitasking, zooming, late hours, ignoring your time for quiet and serenity. You are being called to. Can you hear the whisper, the voice, the urge, the desire? It took me many years of tragic suffering until I was able to really understand that it was not all about symptoms and making them go away, or which doctor or medicine I had, or the exact yoga asana or the time I spent seeking answers from others. The illness was a train wreck and that wreck made me slow way down to a complete dead stop and to really look at my ways of doing and being in life. In the end I gained an entirely new paradigm on what healing truly entails and why our culture is so riddled with chronic disease.

We all have our own rhythms. These rhythms must be honored. Our culture is forgetting how to. All we do is push harder and faster. Breaking the pace is a push against the tide, but I promise you will be healthier for it. We have a lopsided healthcare system in the United States. The technology and science are brilliant and courageous. Yet, the element of self-care is scant and healing gestures somehow got dropped from medical school training. I truly admire the great minds who have mastered organ transplants, skillfully remove tumors, push the envelope on the stodgy pharmaceutical teepee and seek integrative medical training, as well as the compassionate, expansive minds who look at the big picture in illness, gleaning old truths and modern nanotechnology in a new expanding form of individual-practice management. We, however, need a massive paradigm shift regarding self-care, wellness thinking, and, though hard to admit, the big hospital bastions need to be "broken down," akin to the Wall Street and financial world collapse, and rebuilt from the ground up; keep the best of technology and weed out all the excesses.

I cannot provide all the answers, but the ones I recognize are feasible—a return to the small, private-practice family physician, a new form of health insurance that covers natural medicine treatments, a totally revamped food industry (bring back our private, organic, local farms with solid United States government incentives and support), really curtail the plastics industrialization, ban Roundup and cling wrap from the market, reinstate recess and daily gym class, teach doctors about chronic inflammation in medical school and the list of what induces this, and how to correct chronic conditions with lifestyle alterations. Let us create multidiscipline integrative healthcare centers in every town and every city.

Just as essential is the message that we need to slow it all down! How do you regain stillness? And how can small businesses and big corporations create beauty and fifteen-minute breaks to walk in the courtyard and garden or greenhouse for some balancing negative ions and spiritual food? How can you exercise your body's big, broad muscles faithfully?

There is much to tackle. Every day a better step can be taken in your own life. You have control over your body, your lifestyle choices, your mind, and your magnificent spirit. A shift is deeply critical if we want our lives to be healthier, less stressful, and more productive. The insane work hours, two working parents just trying to keep their heads above water, and their children reared by schoolteachers and poorly behaved peers, versus the wisdom of elders who have been relegated to assisted living, are burdening our daily communities. Older folks are valuable and America forgets this. Their experience and tough knocks shed perspective and "horse sense" our youngsters need in their daily lives. The Northern Hemisphere is spinning at a beyond acceptable rate. Our outer and inner habitats are out of sync. But we can influence the inner.

Like the revolving seasons of nature, we must honor the deep rest of winter, the creative juices of spring, the receptivity and growth of summer, and the hard work of harvesting our efforts in fall—only then to return again in cycle and rhythm to the deepening of drawing in and integration that winter provides.

I created this book because I want to urge an awareness transformation regarding illness and healing. I have devoted years to this project because I have been in many of your shoes and I made that frightening, death-call journey into Hades and back out into the light. I am hoping to teach you how to access potent self-healing skills, and to remind you that anything is possible!

I am graced to have a second chance in life, not by accident, but by hard work and willingness to help usher in change within myself, and with those I touch. I lend my energy and cross the ranks as we embrace personal transformation and the absolutely essential need for an evolution in the way we manage healthcare in the United States' medical system and also personally in our own daily life.

America needs an Integrative Health Care System that houses medical doctors and nurse practitioners under the same roof as clinical nutritionists, naturopaths, acupuncturists, homeopaths, reiki and cranial sacral therapists, and chiropractors and osteopaths. There are very talented, educated, tuned-in practitioners dotted all about our states who would better serve our weakening societal health if they could be united. The time to create a healthy doctor-patient relationship needs to be recreated. Care requires "connection," not just expertise. The wealth of first-class nutraceutical-grade supplements, herbals, and homeopathics available are wonderful additions to later twentieth-century healing, and yet they are not accessible unless you get to the correct practitioners.

Until we get an aware president or first lady in the White House who have utilized, and understand the value of, integrative medicine, we are left with an Eisenhower-era healthcare model. However, healing can happen at home, in your own body and mind, with the assistance of some well-sought-out practitioners and guidance here to help steer you. Most importantly, I want to remind you that you are not alone—50,000,000 people in the United States and 250,000,000 around the world suffer from autoimmune illnesses, and an estimated 20,000,000 have been afflicted with tick-borne diseases (some as crossover misdiagnoses to autoimmune) in the past four decades.

We can change the future of autoimmune illnesses and Lyme disease. Some very talented practitioners have a grasp in the underpinnings. I feel the awareness shifting, the call of hundreds of thousands of voices in dire need, pleading for help. We are no longer satisfied with multiple pharmaceuticals as our crutches, nor the fact that multiple symptoms manifesting in a checkerboard around our body and psyche are palliated and propped up by an array of different doctors and/or medications. We are seeking healing and wellness, not dependencies and mismanagement. Too many people are too smart to be strung along with no real answers on how to truly heal, but instead are forced to cope.

I believe in the power of the mind, the calling of our heart, and the mighty force of our will. When we can draw on these inner resources we can move mountains. We can effect change. We can heal ourselves, others, the planet.

Let us anoint our journey through these pages with the calling in of spiritual guidance and allow us individually and collectively to experience the universal power of love. If this sounds too "far out" for you, skip it, jump ahead to the next chapter. For those of you inclined now, please take a moment with me.

Intention

I would like to set a healing intention for all of those struggling with the many autoimmune diseases, as well as each of you who is afflicted with Lyme disease. Close your eyes if it helps. Put your hand over your heart. Take three long, slow, deep breaths, breathing way down into your belly, not just in your upper chest. Follow your breath with your mind's eye. Feel the pace of doing this slowly. Now, drop your awareness down into your heart. Feel its steady, knowing presence. It is wise and loving. It is from our hearts that we heal. Keep your focus on your heart center.

I speak these words of healing intention, with love and in hope. Hope for your healing, for the world's collective healing, and for an end to suffering. Here are my words of healing.

Read these words out loud now:

I believe in a healthy future for myself, for my loved ones, and those who suffer illness.

I trust that the right people, resources, and energies will align to arrest these epidemics and bring us clearer diagnostics and an integrative healthcare system with restorative facilities.

With my own personal will and intention I move forward into a happier, healthier, illness-free tomorrow.

May I be guided and protected.

Read these words to yourself daily until they are memorized. You are bringing grace and meaning into your spirit, and together we are weaving a power cord of intention and shift for the society. One droplet of rain feels like a mere nothing, but a million droplets of rain create a huge storm. We energetically can create that cleansing storm.

THE WISE COUNSELOR

"If we wish to see change for the better externally, we must first see change within ourselves."

—David Manners

Change is a constant force moving through us and the world. Though we see and feel constancy in the ever-reliable rhythm of the seasons, they in themselves represent change. We count on the return of springtime with the buds of new growth, or the wrinkled face of autumn as leaves shed and winds fly. Then the darkness and snows of winter drive us deeper into enclosure and all intrepid fortitude. In counterpoint, the ample beauty of summer skies and generous warmth ease us, bringing freedoms and laughter to build, achieve, and hold onto.

Many of us rely on routines, a relationship, and a paycheck to maintain a familiar lifestyle or level of comfort. This is helpful in itself; order and predictability assure less stress and a platform for us to grow with. Yet, around this tendency to hold on tightly to what we know or have created, wisdom asks us to recalibrate, and as the seasons vividly illustrate, change is always asked of us. Stagnation, uniform constancy, a monotone pattern suppresses the spirit, squelching dreams, we wither on the vine, our expansive heart energy cramps up, mood disorders ensue; autoimmune illnesses, heart disease occur.

However, there is constancy in the vital dance of change or transformation. This is known as Opportunity. We are blessed with an opportunity to have a life and an experience while inhabiting this magical planet in a giant universe of energy states. Many of us, however, are unconsciously skimming through the experience—occupying these precious years in a mundane status of idle shopping, gossiping, consuming, and polluting the environment or hectically trying to keep pace with all our chores and responsibilities. Distressed over oil prices, our natural environment being destroyed, not enough dollars in our pockets, or lost in addictions and time-bytes, a significant disconnect has occurred. What does such a heart speak of? Can we hear our inner self? Do we sit in quietude, tune in, and corral the greed or fury or fear? Is it possible to find peace in such a heart?

When we sustain our Self, let down the façade, put down the shield of defense or bravado or responsibility, what do we find inside? Each of us was born with a soft heart space—a gentle, open ability to receive affection, nurturance, and love from another. As infants, we gurgled with smiles, coos, and dewy curiosity. Through the years and the layered events of schooling, environment, and others' actions, many of us reflexed, reacted, and perhaps built up insecurities and protective behaviors. Inside there is still a tender heart. It may be buried. It may be seen only in the glimmer of romance or when a friend is in need. But that beautiful, loving heart is alive in each of us, to the very end.

If we wish to see change for the better—a safer school, a kinder spouse, a more peaceful world, a return of our health from sickness—well, first each of us must attune to the reality that we can initiate a momentum of change by beginning with internal work. We must attune to our heart. It is wise. It is loving. It is our own. And like our unique fingerprints, each heart shines in its special individual way. Love is its juice. A heart needs to be fed, or it will rust up, load with plaque, seize up, and die. A heart, even when filled with passion and purpose, also calls out for peace and beauty. For when we live in peace, we are more available to shape and in turn create healing within and without. We are open to the opportunity life presents us.

Try taking time to be alive in stillness, not doing anything other than appreciating a lovely sunset, the comfort of your armchair, or your steady breathing. Ignore the myriad of "to do" list items, the buzz of the electronic kingdom, the world issues in the media or on TV. Let go for a few minutes. Steady your mind and the tumbling thoughts. Be grateful. How does this moment feel?

Throughout the pages ahead we will be working with this wise counselor within—your heart. I will guide you into the treasure trove of profound internal healing tools we bear. My role as your guide is to help you access your personal powers. Together we will discover many riches and I will share my insights. My wish is that you gain a sense of strength, relief, and personal growth. Love is the ultimate healer and in these pages I share my appreciation of healing and my love for humanity.

I will help you in the chapters ahead to find that pearl of spiritual calling. It is actually residing in your heart space, waiting for you to claim it, and in turn nourish your self-intimacy. For only then, when we accept the ebbs and flows like moon cycles and nature's seasons, rather than fight the tide or push upstream, does our psyche, our spirit, and eventually our cells and body find balance or homeostasis and return to wellness. This journey is sacrificial. Like the lamb to slaughter, the shedding of autumn foliage, a mother's nurturance, we must let go!

Drugs, herbs, supplements, and healthy diets are wonderful externally applied tools offering support, a crutch for better systemic function. These are our helpmates on the material plane. We will explore these invaluable tools in these pages, too.

But, on the internal plane, at the metaphysical juncture, only you can make these shifts. Only you can create shifts of consciousness, only you can open to your higher source, only you can learn to honor your rhythms, love yourself, attune to nature, and in fact, it is you who can set deep healing in motion.

Right now I would like to take us all into a sacred place—our heart center. For those inclined, I will take us on a brief metaphysical exercise. It takes a mere few minutes. My intention is to have each of us glean what our heart is asking for regarding our healing and wellness. In the chapters to come you will learn how to activate power in our mind-body healing reservoirs and discover other skills that our culture glosses over but that have enormous potent healing effects.

Let us start by connecting to your very wise counselor—the heart. From our first breath to our last dying one, this powerful, patient organ keeps pace and rhythm and sustains our life force, and it bears deep omniscient insight. When we live from our heart and not our mind, our choices and resolutions and pathway are honest and giving. Right now I want you to say hello to your most treasured ally. Take a moment. Close your eyes. Put your hand over your heart. Draw your mind's eye down into your chest. Feel your heartbeat. Acknowledge this faithful organ and the steady, tireless work it does for you 24/7. Say thank you to your wondrous heart.

Next, ask yourself this question and listen within for a word, a thought, a feeling, and an image. This is a message of importance to you. Here is the question—read it, and then just receive.

"What do I need to embrace for my healing?"

Write this down. Hold this message. Your wise counselor has spoken. Remind yourself that this message came from your own internal power. Feel the essence. Choose to embrace this message. Read it every day. Your heart knows. Allow yourself to follow this change. The journey is beginning.

If we see change within ourselves, we can see change externally. It all begins with us. One individual at a time. As the seasons so faithfully remind us, we must ever evolve. Everyone has this internal opportunity for transformation and healing. Peace begins in the heart. Welcome to your future.

DEFINING HEALTH

Health is defined in Webster's Dictionary as "the absence of disease." These words assume that anything less profound than a disease is not a state of ill health. Some of us may feel ill before a disease is diagnosable via blood testing or other examination procedures. We are often told that there is nothing wrong with us, even when confusing symptoms exist. Discomforts certainly are not signs of optimal health and need to be accounted for, in some way. Typically these complaints signify imbalance in a system where cellular pathology has not yet manifested, but early symptomology does exist, and is real. If we pay attention to these early symptom pictures and remedy them promptly, we would end up doctoring from a less crisis-oriented posture to a more wellness-directed one instead.

A wellness approach happens to be natural medicine's (now more commonly referred to as functional or integrative medicine) strong suit. The philosophy of natural medicine is a holistic model, with three cornerstones to health. They are: balance and wellness on the physical, emotional, and mental planes. When all three facets of our being are functioning optimally, we resonate in harmony, exhibiting energy, enthusiasm, and fulfillment in our lives. If one corner becomes overtaxed or undernourished, we notice a dimming of our capabilities and functions. An example would be fatigue or back pain compromising our energy. Belabored for long periods, apathy replaces enthusiasm, or instead of feeling fulfilled and active, dissatisfaction may set in.

When we are able to identify what contributing factors have thwarted us and make corrections, health usually returns. If the situation is ignored and we push onward, assuming the discomforts will disappear, our organism is taxed even further. We can take only so much of this pattern. Eventually we weaken significantly, developing a more serious, diagnosable disease condition where cellular pathology and organ malfunction exist, and then are verified via lab tests, scans, and physicians' clinical diagnosis.

From the natural healthcare perspective, an individual's wellness is assessed on all three planes. Quite often an imbalance on one level may readily instigate an imbalance on another level. Like a three-legged stool, when one leg is wobbly, the whole balance of the stool suffers. Months of dissatisfaction in a stifling work environment may induce apathy. This apathy, in turn, can lead to weight gain due to craving serotonin-prompting carbohydrate foods, then prompt a sluggish lymph system, which in turn brings on repeated sore throats. The individual's apathy and job displeasure actually require more critical attention than the sore throats. Just hitting the throat pains with NyQuil or lozenges, or trying to diet off the weight, will not address the root cause. If these emotional concerns at the job situation are not addressed, the sore throats will most likely resurface with frequency, and a chronic pattern commences.

In our amazing wholeness as complete beings, our body was not so haphazardly designed that the various planes are not interrelated. When we understand the importance of these relationships, and approach healing from this perspective, our overall health status can be greatly enhanced. Instead of treating malfunctioning parts only (lupus, IBS, arthritic knee), the objective is to study the person's whole self and treat him/her and not the disease. This is how the term "(w)holistic" was coined; from the whole-person approach.

The natural healthcare methods rely predominantly on techniques that promote more optimal whole-being function. As the individual's weakened areas are supported there is no longer any reason for the illness to exist. We heal from our own inner abilities, which have been stimulated by herbs, homeopathic remedies, nutritional support, or bodywork. Allopathic medicine, which is the conventional system of medicine in the Western world, relies predominantly on drugs or surgical procedures to counteract or suppress a symptom. A decongestant would be taken to thwart the congestion of a head cold. A natural healthcare method would instead focus on improving sinus and lymphatic drainage function through aids such as a neti pot and herbals like slippery elm and echinacea to help the system complete its intentional healing efforts. If the imbalance is on the mental or emotional planes, there are natural healthcare tools to advance the redundant emotional "recording" along.

When a person's health condition is approached in this vein, the main emphasis is to enhance overall function and resiliency. Some life-threatening states, such as heart attack, require specialized medical treatment. Most importantly, chronic illness, especially those in the autoimmune and Lyme disease spectrum, benefit enormously when holistic or integrative medicine philosophies and techniques are used to support and nourish the imbalances and depletions, in turn helping a being to restore and heal from within. Quite often, it is more than just one "thing" that has allowed you to become ill, a conglomerate of factors.

Within the past decade, the United States has witnessed a resurgence in popularity of natural disciplines. Acupuncture, massage therapy, homeopathy, yoga, and naturopathy are being regularly sought out. During this upcoming decade, these methods should figure even more strongly into our healthcare system as the public asks for more availability, and some physicians are actually seeking complementary alternative medicine (CAM) training after "traditional" medical school.

When we are able to unite the two hands of healthcare—the diagnostic and pharmaceutical tools of allopathic medicine, with the restorative therapeutics of natural medicine—we will find true healing. For we all know two hands working together are better than one!

The United States is behind the times regarding integrative medicine. We are the only modern country I can think of that has a pharmaceutical-/procedure-only-based system of doctoring. All of Europe, Canada, South America, and Asia, for centuries, have had herbalists, homeopaths, naturopaths, bodyworkers, and even restorative healing spas (some are part of national healthcare systems) integrated in their healthcare practices. French, German, and Indian doctors are schooled in homeopathy. Canada pridefully claims wonderful naturopaths. Where would China be without the ancient art of acupuncture? Spirituality is blended into Japanese, Latin, and South American healing as normal.

If it takes an infectious disease epidemic and a crippling generation of baby boomers and their offspring to plead for integrative medicine and a return to wellness through the gifts of natural medicine and the wisdom of spiritual healers, then the tipping point has come.

Good health is our birthright, and finding that balance on the three-legged stool is essential, more than ever in our helter-skelter, overexternalized lifestyle of modernization. The hippies used to say "go hug a tree." As silly as this sounds, the truth is that slowing down, appreciating nature's bountiful gifts, and finding your own inner wellspring of resource is not a bad idea. For in our truest sense of Self, we touch our greatest strength—wisdom. Wisdom is an all-knowing guide and will surely bring you in concert with the right physician or healer or counselor, helping you find your return to health.

When your body or mind is presenting symptoms, please pay attention to your inner wisdom. Do you have a "sense" of why you are off balance? Seeking the aid of an appropriate physician or natural healthcare practitioner should be a partnership model, whereby your instincts are appreciated and their healing skills are supportive and restorative for you. Then regaining your wellness and "the absence of disease" will be truly rewarding for both of you on your journey to recovery.

WHAT IS DIS-EASE?

Too many people are struggling with syndromes, conditions, diseases, and sometimes constellations of symptoms with no frank diagnosis. Many of you may realize that your body is off balance, you are not feeling well and wondering just *what* is wrong with you. We seek the expert authority of a physician most commonly to help address our woes. Generations ago, self-doctoring, a local midwife, homeopath, or herbalist were a small village's or town's choice for medical woes. Since the 1920s doctors have become a mainstay as science has grown in fantastical proportions. We have gained a new industry—pharmaceutically created medicines for treatment of illness states. We have also learned vast amounts about the body when it "misfires" and as a result many diseases have names and can be diagnosed and treated.

The average American lifespan is almost double what is was 150 years ago. Modern medicine, sanitation systems, and more ample food supply (versus semi-starvation in winter months) help us live longer. And, sadly we have more dis-ease. I hyphenate this word for a reason, to illustrate its undertones.

Here are some salient pieces on disease from Wikipedia:

> A **disease** is a particular abnormal, pathological condition that affects part or all of an organism. It is often construed as

a **medical condition** associated with specific symptoms and signs. It may be caused by factors originally from an external source, such as infectious disease, or it may be caused by internal dysfunctions, such as autoimmune diseases. In humans, "disease" is often used more broadly to refer to any condition that causes pain, dysfunction, distress, social problems, or death to the person afflicted, or similar problems for those in contact with the person. In this broader sense, it sometimes includes injuries, disabilities, disorders, syndromes, infections, isolated symptoms, deviant behaviors, and atypical variations of structure and function, while in other contexts and for other purposes these may be considered distinguishable categories. Diseases usually affect people not only physically, but also emotionally, as contracting and living with a disease can alter one's perspective on life, and one's personality.

Death due to disease is called death by natural causes. There are four main types of disease: pathogenic disease, deficiency disease, hereditary disease, and physiological disease. Diseases can also be classified as communicable and non-communicable. The deadliest disease in humans is ischemic heart disease (blood flow obstruction), followed by cerebrovascular disease and lower respiratory infections respectively.

In medicine, a **disorder** is a functional abnormality or disturbance. Medical disorders can be categorized into mental disorders, physical disorders, genetic disorders, emotional and behavioral disorders, and functional disorders. The term *disorder* is often considered more value-neutral and less stigmatizing than the terms *disease* or *illness*, and therefore is a preferred terminology in some circumstances. In mental health, the term *mental disorder* is used as a way of acknowledging the complex interaction of biological, social, and psychological factors in psychiatric conditions. However, the term *disorder* is also used in many other areas of medicine, primarily to identify physical disorders that are not caused by infectious organisms, such as metabolic disorders.

A **syndrome** is the association of several medical signs, symptoms, and/or other characteristics that often occur together. Some syndromes, such as Down syndrome, have only one cause; others, such as Parkinsonian syndrome, have multiple possible causes. In other cases, the cause of the syndrome is unknown. A familiar syndrome name often remains in use even after an underlying cause has been found, or when there are a number of different possible primary causes.

Predisease is a type of disease creep or medicalization in which currently healthy people with risk factors for disease, but no evidence of actual disease, are told that they are sick. Prediabetes and prehypertension are common examples. Labeling a healthy person with predisease can result in overtreatment, such as taking drugs that only help people with severe disease, or in useful preventive measures, such as motivating the person to get a healthy amount of physical exercise.[2]

The term "dis-ease" is used as a substitute for the word *disease* by individuals and healing communities who are aligned with wellness. In stating this, it is their intent to place emphasis on the natural state of "ease" which has causally become imbalanced or disrupted, and desire to not give too much focus to a particular ailment. The mind-set is to return to comfort and good health and not be caught in the negative peril of a disease diagnosis, which sounds ominous and never-ending. Also, dis-ease asks us to examine just how or what made us tip out of balance into feeling so unwell.

A person who has been diagnosed with diabetes will say, "I am a diabetic." Wouldn't it be more resourceful and optimistic to say, "I am challenged with diabetes"? Please don't give your personal power over to a language or a dis-ease! Think about how you frame matters

2. Wikipedia contributors, "Disease," *Wikipedia, The Free Encyclopedia*, https://en.wikipedia.org/wiki/Disease, accessed June 26, 2015

by saying, "My MS," or, "My migraines are giving me such anxiety." The use of "my" associated with a condition really embeds the illness and its irregular vibrations deeply into your pscyhe. More and more people are discovering how the words we utter and write carry power and are altering their voices accordingly.

I recall the obvious stance I took when I would say, "The Lyme disease, or the chronic fatigue is acting up," instead of, "No, I can't go to the party because of my Lyme." Owning a disease does not feel like a very prideful or happy place to be in the big scheme of life. Owning vitality and creative purpose are so much more enlivening. Think about these concepts.

Essentially, disease is a medical term. That is *it*! You do not have to be it, you can be *you* and you can live with some symptoms and still function well or even help them go away. For centuries midwives, healers, doctors did not have disease diagnosis for everything. Look in the old homeopathic text from the 1800s—there are billions of symptoms that are worth tending to, but removing them was/is all possible without a diagnosis.

Now, let us move on to matters of healing.

WHY DO WE GET SICK?

If the human body is a self-regulating and self-healing organism, why do we get sick? Our bodies do an amazing job of thwarting infections and imbalances in spite of more bacteria being present in our systems than our own natural flora. We are brilliantly designed beings, able to adapt to constant exposure in our habitats and the new ones we travel to. Yet susceptibility is the critical link to how we can fall ill.

Identifying the factors that make one susceptible to illness can help us prevent further problems. There are seven major elements that factor in to set off an illness. If we are negligent in any one category, most of us manage. When our system becomes stressed in two or more categories, then our illness susceptibility heightens. Susceptibility is an interesting arena. Different individuals show susceptibility to manifesting certain conditions or illnesses. We often see trends in a family tree, i.e., obesity, heart disease, repeated infections, or migraines. Other conditions are not so consistent, yet susceptibility is a known factor.

Doctors and nurses working in hospitals filled with vicious germs like MRSA and staphylococcus seem to rarely contract the infection due to their developed passive immunity, yet a patient just operated on is very vulnerable. My best friend is extremely vulnerable to pneumonia and bronchitis, with dozens of bouts in her lifetime, while I have never had either infection. Meanwhile, my system is very prone to bladder infections. These are obvious examples of susceptibilities.

Constitutional predispositions are so-called "weak links" that demonstrate tendencies to certain illnesses surfacing. Theories abound as to why middle-aged women are prone to fibromyalgia, and matured men exhibit the highest rates of Parkinson's disease.

Susceptibilities in all individuals, no matter the illness, tie into the fundamental foundation stones of health. We need to tend to these essential elements consistently. Autoimmune illnesses or tick-borne diseases can more readily manifest when these foundation stones have wobbled. Let us look at what these factors are.

Nutritional Imbalance: Americans have developed food habits that do not support optimal physical or mental well-being. Each person must establish a well-balanced diet of protein, vegetables/fruits, complex carbohydrates, and healthy fats to be able to supply the body with proper energy for tissue maintenance, cell growth, and regeneration. Avoiding foods with preservatives, chemical additives, sugar, refined GMO grains, and saturated fats is important. Trying to eat as many unprocessed foods as possible is a must. The less a food looks like its original form, the less nutritious it is for you. Steamed broccoli looks much like it does when it comes out of your garden. Pasta bears little resemblance to the original grain it is derived from. The more a food is tampered with—ground down, blended, coated, or heated—the more its nutritive enzyme, vitamin, and mineral content is lost. Microwave cooking breaks down natural enzymes, as does high heat or barbecue grills. Slow, low-temperature cooking preserves the best nutrients and enzymes.

Structural: Optimal balance of our structural body is a key factor. The nervous system supplies critical information to every single cell of our body. The spinal column houses this vital master control network. Maintaining correct alignment and function of the spinal column, as well as muscle tone, is important. Regular exercise for stabilizing the musculature and good postural habits are not to be overlooked.

Ergonomics of a firm mattress, proper lumbar support in your chairs and car seat, and how you sit and stand need to be heeded. Hours at a computer or any repetitive motion create notable muscle tension and restriction of blood flow. Massage therapy, chiropractic work, yoga, movement therapy, and daily exercise all aid in achieving more stabilized structural balance and release spinal nerve impingements, as well as keep muscles and joints supple.

Circulation: We need movement and oxygenation in order to function well. The heart/lungs/circulatory/lymphatic systems require the stimulation of regular movement and exercise. Without this, the body's function will deteriorate from inadequate oxygen utilization and stagnant, dead blood cell debris. The development of stamina and flexibility in the body also enhances our capacity to deal with physical and emotional stress. Make sure to get at least twenty to thirty minutes of aerobic activity and ten to twenty minutes of stretching per day. We are so sedentary in today's lifestyle. Upright vacuum cleaners, drive-through windows, and other modern conveniences prevent us from regular walking, squatting, and the use of our large muscle groups, which we are designed to use daily. Fitness is key for wellness, and exercise is part of recovery.

Sleep: Cells generate most quickly while we sleep. Dreaming also allows us to process many emotional intricacies of the day. Our system needs to rest and slow down. Many of us lead chock-full lifestyles. When we need to grab an extra hour somewhere, many of us tend to shortchange ourselves on sleep. Instead of the seven to nine hours most healthy adults require, many folks are sleeping only five or six per night. Aging and illness occur more quickly with this pattern. We should be more protective of our sleep, turning off all electronics, even the WiFi, at bedtime. Keep TVs and computers out of the bedroom since they emit electromagnetic radiation.

Stress: Continual stress in life disturbs the body's routine performance. Over a period of time stress can lead to fatigue, pain, and decreased organ function. Learning skills that will eliminate stress and its negative effects is important. Relaxation techniques such as yoga, meditation, biofeedback, or gardening can help reduce the negative consequences and elevated inflammatory production of cortisol as relates to stress. It is close to impossible to avoid stress-inducing incidents completely. Learning how to manage and respond to them, however, is vital. Nutritive supplements supporting adrenal function and the nervous system are beneficial.

Toxins: Chemicals are everywhere in our environment, foods, and bodies in the modern era. One hundred years ago the big chemical companies and pharmacies were just emerging; DuPont, Johnson & Johnson, Merck, Monsanto. Now there are thousands, and they have saturated us with compounds that our body was not designed to handle. The liver and kidneys must work nonstop to identify and remove these toxins. Many of these chemical compounds are insoluble and difficult or impossible for these simple organs to remove. We end up with an internal toxin stew that eventually damages our weakest parts, inducing symptoms as plain as fatigue, or as complex as rheumatoid arthritis. Avoiding toxic elements, routinely eating antioxidant foods, and using cleansing herbs are very valuable in our times.

Fulfillment: All of us need to feel positive about ourselves in some significant aspect of our lives. When we feel satisfied or content about how we lend ourselves to a certain situation or role, we emit many positive chemical responses in our body. This fulfillment can come in a host of ways—through our parenting, work, marriage, community service, spirituality, friendships, and more. There are many programs any of us can become involved in, like Big Brothers/Big Sisters, CASA, the Red Cross or Salvation Army, Habitat for Humanity, environmental organizations, community suppers, volunteering in schools, churches, and humane societies, or creating something of your own, like healthy cooking classes, family meditation time, and so forth. (Visit VolunteerMatch.org or other sites to find where help is needed in your area.) This "food for the soul" goes a long way, and has not been liberally encouraged, with the enormous pressure so many of us have had to scramble to make ends meet, juggle home and career, and keep our children safe and on track. But neglecting this piece can leave us empty in a very critical way.

By following these steps to good health we can have some means of control over how well we stay. Self-awareness and self-responsibility are key elements in this equation. Wellness is not something another person can bestow upon you. It is a matter of taking care of yourself by monitoring key components and being attentive to how you live. From this level of more optimal health there is less chance that major illness will knock you down. For those of you scoured by chronic illness, take some time to think about these aspects highlighted. Are there areas you need assistance with, or obvious historical markers you recall that threw off a couple of these categories? Make some notes if it helps you outline your needs.

PREDISPOSITIONS AND CONSTITUTIONAL TYPES: WHY SOME OF US FALL ILL

Illness makes us weary. We feel so many assorted complaints—weakness, pain, sluggishness, or heavy thoughts and even bizarre symptoms or feelings that scare us, like your heart gripped in a vise clamp, or a pain in your belly so raw that not one sip of water can be tolerated.

Inflammation is a common denominator in all autoimmune disorders, including Lyme disease. Depending on the disease and the individual, the inflammation can rear its ugly head in a variety of ways. Each individual exhibits what I refer to as a Russian roulette of symptomology, dependent on their constitutional or genetic predispositions. We all have our so-called "weak links"; the type of illness states or symptom pictures we are prone to show when overtired, undernourished, toxic, poorly balanced, overextended, or infected.

I have never had pneumonia, bronchitis, strep, or an ear infection, as my genetics help me there. But, I broke several bones and my teeth twice in childhood accidents. Obviously, my predisposition involved my skeleton and teeth. Knowing what I know now as a healthcare practitioner, a vitamin D deficiency was likely apparent in my genetic roulette, especially considering that my father also had cervical and lumbar vertebrae broken in accidents!

When I was stricken with that odd, intense flu the summer of 2000, besides the vertigo, swollen glands, and flu-like symptoms, the most overwhelming and consistent ongoing issues for years were vicious meningitis-style migraines, maiming me for days on end. Migraines ran on my mother's side of the family; we chalked it up to a family "predisposition." I had seventeen neurologist visits before discovering the underlying cause!

Five years into the fiery debacle of the constant nerve inflammation I learned the real story, which was that the Lyme bacteria had colonized in the occipital nerve, with inflammation soaring out of control. Twelve hundred mg of Advil every three hours was merely skimming 10 percent off the pain. Opiates, ergot, morphine—nothing would stop the searing knives scissoring the left side of my brain. My suffering was profound.

Days and nights propped on ice packs, in a darkened bedroom, food tiptoed in on trays, my young son squirreling up close to me at bedtime for a snuggle, as Mommy was still too frail to walk down the hall to his room or venture down the oak stairway to the sun-splayed living room. Locked alone in isolation for years as these violent migraine attacks ransacked me nearly daily; the only fortifying agent in my world was to just "hold on," to pray it would all pass.

Forty-eight to seventy-two hours later the migraines would usually lift, and I would be trashed—exhausted, as wobbly as a newborn fawn, tenderly stepping outside onto our back lawn, sunglasses on, the fresh air and my radiant poppy beds so brilliant and glorious, yet also startlingly bold after three days chambered in dark and stillness. Each rebirth after a migraine siege felt like a window of glory to me, a miracle that the tsunami of pains was receding and a vivid natural kingdom lay at my doorstep—birdsong, squirrels scampering on high limbs, and my children's playful glee all ribbons of beauty! A new dawn for me again.

And still, I lived in constant fear and trepidation that the crippling pains would return, spiriting me away from the real world, the everyday world, the world my friends and family all moved through with ease and energy and nonchalance. Driving, grocery shopping, fluorescent lights, busy offices, airplanes—how effortlessly they handled it all pain-free! I, instead, would be hysterical or incapacitated or locked up at home on ice and drugs, in the dark.

I share this personal suffering not to induce sympathy, but to illustrate this is where the inflammation sat in my body. The microorganisms of infection also resided in my gut as irritable bowel syndrome. The cause was Lyme, but the symptoms were what they were because of my setup, my genetic Russian roulette, my constitutional predisposition, passed from the family lineage.

Aunt Joan, Papou Tom, and two maternal cousins were all prone to migraines, though far less extreme than mine. Dad had GI issues galore—he was always finessing his menu to raw and simple. Ultimately, in his eighties, he was diagnosed with celiac disease. The Lyme bugs found their home in my weak links. I was misdiagnosed for five years with chronic fatigue syndrome, irritable bowel syndrome, and a migraine/anxiety syndrome complex.

Your constitutional makeup may orient the organisms to set up camp in other body systems where your genetic weak links lie, such as the heart and its pericardium outer lining; or your joints and synovial lining, mimicking rheumatoid arthritis; the thyroid as Graves' disease or Hashimoto's thyroiditis; or maddeningly, the nervous system, with insomnia, depression, lupus, multiple sclerosis, ALS, or Tourette's syndrome surfacing. After all, did a relative suffer with mood swings or drink heavily from depression or dwindle with neuropathy? This could be your Russian roulette constellation.

From the lens of integrative medicine, we have learned a few key points about autoimmune disorders and the vulnerability certain individuals exhibit for chronic Lyme, tick-borne organisms, and viral infections to manifest as chronic disease, as well as the immune system to go "out of control," creating assorted autoimmune syndromes.

Several of the following contributing factors "set up" a person so that their body and psyche and autoimmune system lose their natural balance, and the body "turns" on itself mistaking our own bodily cells as foreign "invaders." This means too much inflammation causes corrosion of joints, destruction to glands, organs, nerves, fascia, and concurrently negative self-defeating behaviors such as obsessive-compulsive disorder, insomnia, depression, bulimia, binge eating, suicidal thinking, and alcoholism.

If multiple of these factors exist, you are especially vulnerable:

- Inadequate amount of antioxidant vitamins: A, B, C, D, E
- Deficiency of trace minerals: zinc, molybdenum, manganese, selenium
- Deficiency of minerals: magnesium, iodine, potassium
- Heavy metal toxic accumulation:
    - Mercury: the two most common forms: tuna or swordfish and dental fillings, plus additives in certain vaccines
    - Lead paint and pipes
    - Copper pipes
- Imbalanced gut flora, setting up yeast/candida overgrowth. This creates inflammation and "leaky gut syndrome" as well as not enough good bacteria to gobble up invasive organisms.
- Gluten intolerance or sensitivity
- Food allergies (corn, dairy, eggs, soy are very common)
- Mold sensitivity or damage
- Parasite infection (travel to foreign countries, raw fish or meat)
- Toxin overload (pesticides, plastic by-products that mimic estrogen, additives in processed foods and cosmetics)
- Infection of tick-borne diseases (Lyme, bartonella, babesia, mycoplasmas, Rocky Mountain spotted fever)
- Viral infections
    - Epstein-Barr
    - Cytomegalia

    - Coxsackie
    - C. pneumonia
- Consume sugar and/or coffee regularly
- Family history of autoimmune-style illness, allergies, mental illness
- Imbalanced pH
- You were born after 1960
- Multiple immunizations, especially after 1970
- Trauma in your history (physical, accidental, or emotional)
- Consistent stress or major stressful event(s)
- Electromagnetic energy overload
- History of cancer, diabetes

The good news is that all of these above categories are successfully dealt with, corrected, and healed with the good work of natural medicine doctors such as naturopaths (ND), clinical nutritionists (CNC), and integrative medicine or functional medicine doctors (CAM). Certain chiropractors (DC), or osteopaths (DO), are trained in the appropriate specialty testing, diagnostics, and treatment of these imbalances.

When you can detoxify the body, eliminate offending agents and microbes, rebuild depletions, and resurrect a nutrient-rich diet, along with exercise and the invaluable skills of mindfulness and spiritual reserve, then finding renewed health is possible. Overcoming chronic illness, such as the autoimmune disorders or chronic tick-borne infections, is very feasible. Much of this resurrection is controlled by you.

Nourishment is a significant theme in this book. Those of us born after 1960 are seriously "undernourished" due to depleted soils, GMO foods, major toxic loads in our food chain, and many chemically laced and processed foods. This is all correctable, however. The pages ahead spell out the road to recovery.

HOW TO WORK WITH SYMPTOMS

When we are healthy and vital we feel great! Boundless energy, restorative sleep, happy moods, expansive creativity radiates from within. We are not annoyed by rainy days or fettered by a physical complaint; a sense of well-being presides.

The majority of humans live into their twenties before they are lassoed by chronic physical or emotional symptoms—though people born after 1990 are more likely to suffer from peanut allergies, ADD, or asthma from the time they are young. The point here, however, is to understand our being's purpose of manifesting symptoms. Symptoms actually do have a reason other than just being annoying or painful.

The dictionary defines symptom as "manifestation, indication, indicator, sign, mark, feature, trait, medicine prodrome." I think of symptoms as helpmates. Just as the "check engine" light pops on in your car when there's a problem, a symptom is a warning, a clue. The "symptom clue" is to alert us that something is not running smoothly or adequately within.

In common acute woes or illness, such as a skinned knee or cold, the symptoms will usually clear in a matter of days as the body uses its natural pathways of cleansing and immune vigilance to make mucus or pus to flush out a microbe and pump inflammation to a site to cause surrounding tissues and vessels to swell and confine any foreign object or germs from invading deeper into our systems, thus keeping germs or infection localized.

We have several lines of first defense, all protective guardians to our deeper organs and life-sustaining systems. Most external is the skin, next the mucous membranes (sinus, throat, ears, eyes, rectum, vagina, urethra), and then the lymphatic system with tonsils and lymph nodes secreting white blood cells and fighter T and B cells ready to gobble up germs that have "slipped" past the skin or mucous membranes into the bloodstream.

A basic tenet of natural or integrative medicine is to not stop or suppress the symptoms of acute illness by using a decongestant or anti-inflammatory, but to let your body handle the cold or flu bug on its own with rest, fluids, and the aid of natural immune function supports like extra vitamin C, zinc, echinacea, and elderberry plants. This reasoning is based on the merits of allowing your immune function to run its "paces" a couple of times per year as the system and our resistance become stronger and make fresh antibodies each round. Plus, suppressing a body's natural detoxification pathways (runny nose, diarrhea) means you are actually driving the invader or toxin farther into the body to more vital organs like the lungs or small intestine. So, the numerous rounds of NyQuil given to a child can suppress the T-fighter-cell production, weaken their immune ability over time, and send a common cold into a deep chest cough, bronchitis, or even eventually breed asthma. Then, a respiratory predisposition sets in as a pattern.

We want to facilitate the swiftest, most productive activity of our first line of defense warfare, avoiding constant use of antibacterial soaps, cough suppressants, or steroidal creams. The better a body is at swift anti-germ warfare, with a solid defense system, the healthier states we maintain. So, homeopathics, herbs, nutritive supplements, probiotics, tonic teas (like soothing a sore throat with slippery elm) are helpmates in boosting immune support.

However, when these acute symptoms linger, well then we must heed their warning. The post-cold rattling chest cough, the knee pain three weeks after the marathon race, the recurrent headache on waking are expressing imbalance and distress within, demanding attention from you! Like that "check engine" light, this post-acute symptom is your warning light.

As homeopaths we have a phrase I like: "Let your symptoms be your guide," meaning we take a homeopathic remedy (or any medicine) not routinely, but only when the being expresses a need for it via symptoms. (A chapter on homeopathy lies ahead.) Medicating constantly was not nature's design. Propped up on mood-enhancing SSRIs need not be the new normal.

A worthy healthcare practitioner's best skill set is to be a keen observer, a top-notch listener and reliable "matchmaker." Naturopaths, homeopaths, acupuncturists, integrative medicine physicians, herbalists, and medical intuitives are trained more effectively than the average allopathic medical doctor to utilize these skills. This does not mean that MDs do not utilize these talents, but many are too rushed in seven-minute office visits, or dependent on merely prescribing meds for what I call glaringly obvious symptoms such as heart attack, hemorrhagic ulcer, kidney stones.

Observing and listening to a patient and connecting their symptom(s) to the physiology of the various organs, glands, and systems should help the practitioner "match up" where the root causative distress or imbalance lies within (e.g., bowel, blood sugar problem, thyroid?). From there, investigation may continue through physical, hands-on examination, laboratory testing, or some sort of more complex or invasive procedure if necessary (e.g., CAT scan, tumor biopsy).

Holistically thinking, however, we want to remember the goal with these symptom clues is to restore the being to optimal health and wellness via supportive aids and techniques, replenishing our imbalances and dysfunctions, not to make us drug-dependent, consigned to chronic illness or endless doctor-hopping.

Symptom(s) are a wake-up call, telling you that you need to pay attention, now! Your body or feelings are speaking to you and you must listen within. Just dashing off to the drug store for a palliative chemical, or to the doctor for an external fix-it medicine is not always successful. I am reminding you that it is your responsibility to care for your self. Your symptom(s) are asking you to get still, be quiet, tune in, and sense "just what" this ill health, pain, or anxiety is about. You know something within, energetically, emotionally, intuitively, that a doctor, scan, lab, or hospital may never pick up. Most of us are able to "sense" what is awry; the deeper truth to the symptom than "oh my knee hurts," or "the bloaty belly is so annoying," or "my weak legs are scaring me."

I am not suggesting you become your own doctor, nor that you ignore medical help. My intention is to help those of us struggling with autoimmune illness or other conditions to realize we do have some influence, ability, and power surrounding our conditions, symptoms, health, and well-being. The purpose of this book is to assist in reclaiming our Inner Healer and to find the access points to generating energy shifts and in turn promote healing energy. This can be achieved. Getting well is feasible! We are putting healing power back in your own hands to some degree, not merely looking for external resources to fix you. There is a duet at play here—you and your practitioner can harmonize, initiating a healing interplay.

LAWS OF CURE

As we work toward mending, our symptoms should lessen. If you are using homeopathics, acupuncture treatments, energy medicine like Reiki or cranial sacral therapy, and herbal protocols or quality nutritive supplements designed in a restoration fashion or for detoxification purposes, we should note signs of progress as you begin to heal. Practitioners are trained to observe and work with symptoms.

As you heal, you should begin to feel stronger, your energy return, mental clarity resume, and a sense of well-being ensue! Soon, there will be more spring in your step, greater enthusiasm for life, and your feelings of love and passion will replace despair and lack of hope.

As we are working with our symptoms with our practitioners, in regard to our long-term treatment, there are specific signs—called directions of cure—that they note. A model of these innate healing processes defined by a very talented and famous homeopathic physician in the early 1900s is known as "Hering's Law of Cure." This renowned physician's tenets are what homeopaths and many CAM practitioners still scrutinize in case management and are very worthy for you to remember in the progress of your own healing case. If your practitioner does not know of "Hering's Law of Cure," please print it out and show it to them.

The body is smart. Symptoms move from our most external lines of defense such as skin and mucous membranes and sinuses and lymph nodes, and progress deeper into organs, such as the lungs or digestive tract or the joints and ovaries. The more compromised we are and the less resistance we have to maintaining balance, the deeper the illness will drive. Many times someone starts out with a skin rash or eczema and if it is palliated or surprised with cortizone cream it is not uncommon to soon see respiratory allergies or asthma arise, as we have just driven the instability, and usually offending allergen, into a deeper organ like the lungs or our joints. Natural medicine sees the urinary, digestive, lymphatic, and skin as the major vehicles for elimination. You want to promote cleansing from an infectious or allergic substance, not squelch the natural methods and simultaneously drive the offending agent into deeper, more vital body parts.

Pay attention to Hering's directions of cure. They mean you're making progress:

1. The condition/symptoms move from a deeper organ to a more external organ, such as lungs to sinuses or joints to skin.
2. The symptoms progress from above downward—fibromyalgia or Lyme disease muscle pains that plague the upper body and then move to the lower body is a prime example. Or neck and shoulder pains instead move to the ankles or feet.
3. We heal in the reverse order of the symptoms' appearance. This is a very common one and wise to keep note of. If your initial symptoms were headaches and then you developed fatigue and after that you developed irritable bowel syndrome and eventually you manifested fibromyalgia, in following these "laws of cure," it would be obvious to a homeopath and other natural healthcare practitioner that most likely the fibromyalgia would start to mollify first, then the digestive issues would clear, and eventually your fatigue would start to go away. Probably the last symptom to clear would be the headaches, as that was the initial weak link. This would likely

happen over months and not necessarily be immediate. However, I have seen homeopathic remedies clear chronic cases in a couple of months' time when the exact right remedy at the right strength is found.

4. Symptoms move from the mental plane to the physical. Most of you may not realize that people with severe mental illness usually do not have a lot of physical complaints. Schizophrenia or OCD compulsions are examples of our most vital organ, the brain, being in trouble and imbalanced. There is a likelihood this individual had some physical complaints years prior, but they disappeared and then these clinical mental disorders surfaced. (I think of tick-borne diseases whenever I encounter a mental illness, by the way!) With Hering's guiding principles of cure, we would expect to see the OCD start to improve at the same time that the patient begins to manifest food allergies or back pain. The level of imbalance within their system has moved from the mental plane to the physical. As we support the physical with restorative aids, usually herbals and homeopathics or nutritional changes, the physical symptoms also begin to clear.

With these directions of cure in mind, you can begin to see how your healing is taking shape, rather than view your condition as a haphazard, confusing constellation of symptoms. It is like peeling away the layers of an onion. We remove each symptom as it appeared over time. Sometimes, as we work on addressing suppressed bodily functions, toxic overloads, microbial infections, or even just chronic symptoms, the assistance of the recalibrating supplements, homeopathics, and even antibiotic therapy for long-term infections can induce what we call a "healing crisis" or "herxheimer" reaction in an individual. This means your constellation of symptoms may actually spike in intensity for a few days or a couple of weeks, then bring on noted improvement. What has occurred is that the immune and detox pathways have been sparked into stepping up a notch and as they work more properly (via supportive measures), a major purge occurs, whereby you feel rather "flu-like" or a headache worsens or your fatigue deepens for a spell. Do not lose faith or think your new practitioner is poisoning you. This is likely your body recalibrating and working better. However, if you feel worried or the healing crisis lingers for more than two weeks please check in with your practitioner for fine-tuning and support. We welcome healing crisis as a good sign that your immune and detox systems are actually still vital enough to engage, but do not need you to suffer too long. Fine-tuning of dosages, etc. can be done.

The overall emphasis is to keep working with your practitioners and if progress is not being seen in six months or so, perhaps you need a better match in terms of a practitioner whom you can work with and who understands you emotionally as well as physically, and how to fine-tune your protocols. Healing is a journey and a helpful, seasoned guiding practitioner is worth her weight in gold.

DASHBOARD LIGHT DOCTOR

The American medical system has long been revered around the world, with Third World countries sending some of their most dire cases to our doctors for lifesaving procedures. Over the last century our scientific edge in research has been applauded; cardiovascular care, reconstructive surgery, and crisis management are our fortes. But, the United States healthcare system has lost its golden throne; Norway, Japan, and Canada have trumped us in our scientific breakthroughs. Far more innovative drugs are coming out of the Czech Republic and Germany.

Abysmally, our society's overall standard of health has plummeted to a weakly #38 on the World Health Organization statistics. Morocco and Malta exhibit a healthier population. Multitudes of factors contribute to America's healthcare demise. The list is long. Our food chain is polluted by GMOs and tainted by chemicals. The soils are leached and nuked with Roundup (glyphosate). Our children are overstimulated with growth hormones in their milk and animal products. The carbon footprints on our earth and skyscape are vast. Antibiotics have been doled out far too leniently, making microbes stronger and more resistant. Bottled vitamins are synthesized chemicals. Vaccinations are laced with mercury and toxins. We swim in a frightening swarm of escalating electromagnetic radiation fields, and sadly our physicians are trained merely in how to be "dashboard light doctors," angling to fix what is visibly broken or bleeding or seriously wounded.

Long gone is the family doctor with good "horse sense," able to lance a boil at the kitchen counter or ease a postpartum mother through the baby blues with an herbal tonic and a good homespun supply of moral support. The tickling cough versus the croupy cough called for horsehound syrup or a mustard plaster; now all coughs are suppressed with Robitussin PM.

Our science-minded medical schools produce marvelous surgeons and specialists attuned to weaseling out organ malfunction, but they are not good generalists. It is a rare American physician who practices non-pharmaceutical-based medicine. The pill-and-procedure is relied upon heavily, as each specialist trains his or her eye to the "dashboard light" symptom to alert him/her to malfunctions, just as a car-part error warns the driver via blinking notification.

Stroke, broken bones, appendicitis, hernia, miscarriage, traumatic injury, and brain tumors are glaring and obvious—our physicians' modern pharmaceuticals and procedures can tend to them lickety-split. For this we are grateful.

But, the mysterious symptoms—the migrating joint pains, the lunar migraines, the constellation of neck pain and bellyaches with insomnia and arrhythmias—befuddle our modern-day American doc because he has lost his/her "horse sense," the ability to corral several symptoms together and recognize inflammation as the root cause, or a food intolerance, or maybe a mineral deficiency. These simple, sensical pieces get glossed over since pharmacology is now the mainstay in medical schools. United States Americans are supposed to be healthy and able and robust. Nothing extra is assumed to be necessary for a human's proper health than our trans-fat-laced foods and fluoridated, chlorinated water, and encapsulated schoolrooms, bathing our children in an airless fluorescent light spectrum. Oh yes! This is what we now accept as normal and healthy.

Somehow, we aim to rear vibrant, inquisitive children this way, even with their thyroid function at half pace from fluoridation and their curious minds dulled down by dioxin fumes reeking from cleaning solvents in the hallways. Tally in the sugars and white flour, decreased gym classes for endorphin production and cardiovascular conditioning, and our children are allergy-riddled, diabetic, and learning-disabled in far greater proportions than their parents were at the same age.

Of course, the average adult American is thirty pounds overweight, dependent on coffee and sugar for energy, and living in a ceaseless frenzy of work, home, errands, and chores. The scenario is one of disharmony, imbalance, lack of nourishment, and a bleak future unless you choose to take personal control to change your lifestyle.

My grandparents lived to their late eighties and nineties, and they ate bacon and butter, drank whiskey, and smoked. Because they were born in the 1890s, they didn't consume hydrogenated oil until they were fifty years old, nor did they eat fruit out of season, sprayed with preservatives and ripening agents. They had homemade bread, cooked with lard, and played gin rummy and laughed like schoolkids every Sunday, enjoying life and family time, beach days, and a much slower pace of living. Smoking wasn't good for them, of course, but the carcinogens in the cigars they smoked were more easily handled because their nutrient levels were so much higher, due to the non-processed, local foods, and their stress quotient and cortisol regulation much more normalized. Their immune function was strong enough to handle a noxious agent or natural lipid from butter.

My mother was less healthy than her mom, and died of cancer at age sixty-eight. I battled chronic Lyme disease for a decade in my forties. I can't help but believe my grandmother would have had an easier time recovering than I did. I was a 1960s kid raised on DTD misting, fish sticks, and soda pop, and my Long Island neighborhood was on the nuclear power plant's radiation sweep. These vile chemicals, the lifestyle choices, and increasing smog levels likely killed my fine-boned, elegant mother too early, and junked up my liver and stressed my immune capabilities and adrenal glands enough so that when the aggressive *Borrelia burgdorferi* bacteria of Lyme disease entered my body, I was ill-equipped to defend myself from its invasive, multisystemic effects. My genetic predisposition tainted my mitochondria function to collapse into chronic fatigue syndrome. The infection depleted my essential fatty acids and induced neurological problems, while simultaneously inflaming my intestinal mucosal lining with irritable bowel syndrome. My fast-paced lifestyle threw fuel on the inflammatory, infectious fire. This was a far cry from my hardworking grandparents who worked twelve-hour days on their feet in the delicatessen and coffee shop, but also ate local produce and read the paper barefoot in their backyard every summer evening.

Dozens of "dashboard light" gastroenterologists, neurologists, and endocrinologists could not weave together my symptom constellation, and instead scoffed a formerly athletic, outdoorsy individual like me as "perimenopausal" and too anxious, prescribing an ever-more-pricey migraine drug. Rather than seeking a way to rebuild my system, they recommended Prednisone for my unending five years of IBS. All of this doctor-hopping was forlornly isolating and disappointing for a healthcare practitioner.

In a wheelchair and weeping at my seventeenth visit to my acclaimed neurologist, I pleaded for help; why was I too weak to walk or shampoo my hair unassisted, with foot-drop MS-like symptoms scaring me and these weekly migraine sieges torrential and incapacitating? How come every six months I was worsening and more weird symptoms were emerging? What could he do? Who could help me? I helped so many others get well; why could no one cure me?

"I have no clear answers for you, Katina. You do not have a neurological disease according to our tests. We should try an antiseizure medication for the migraines. Maybe that will help you?"

In shock, I did not want to take Topamax, with its numerous side effects, and be doped out in even deeper malaise than my malfunctioning brain and body already were. "Who can help me?" I beseeched. "Do you know another doctor who would understand why my body is failing at age forty-seven?"

The fancy-titled specialist peered at me behind fine-rimmed glasses. Perplexed by my years of decline, he kindly said, "Let's give you an antianxiety medication for a few weeks—Xanax. Perhaps a chronic fatigue specialist at another hospital could help you?"

Inside my core, I knew this man had no "horse sense." He could not connect the dots between my multisystemic mystery, and he was dismissing me. I nodded in sheer discouragement, feeling massively let down by this famed doctor and our medical system. My boyfriend wheelchaired me to the car and I cried trickling tears the entire ninety-minute ride home, my fogged mind layered in a gauzy film and my spirit plummeting down a funnel of despair.

How could a talented homeopath like me, with an 85 percent success rate in my office, helping over a thousand clients regain their health in twenty years of practice, gain absolutely no direction or relief from these world-class medical greats in their temples of technology and laboratories? I was crushed, and rightfully so. This experience left me devastated, and clearly at rock bottom.

I was not alone. My story is the story of millions of Americans. I was eventually "dumped" in the autoimmune illness bucket as you may have been. But like me, many of you can regain significant levels of wellness or even make a full recovery. The important step is looking beyond managing the symptoms with palliative medications to get to the underlying predisposing issues.

Are you an individual who carries a tick-borne disease infection (Lyme, babesia, etc.)? Do you have heavy metal accumulation? Could you have food sensitivities and be eating the aggravating ingredients to trigger soaring inflammation? Is your liver burdened and loaded with solvents like glyphosate or tetrahydrochloride (dry cleaning agent)? So many factors contribute to chronic fatigue syndrome, Bell's palsy, lupus, and many chronic diseases that can be worked with. Keep reading! We must understand that the United States has grown into a fast-paced, toxin-laden, chemically tainted culture with more increasing velocity every decade after World War II.

What we find in 2015 is a staggeringly illness-ridden populace, with a relatively small number of integrative medicine doctors and natural medicine practitioners available who understand the full scope of the dynamics of whole-being treatment. We have gotten way off-kilter. Thoreau and Emerson and Dr. Spock would be aghast.

Let's gain some perspective and help you regain some control over your own body and health. You have enormous inner healing resources to tap into. They are called resiliency, willpower, creativity, belief, devotion, and intention. The chapters to come in Part V discuss this in great depth.

HISTORICAL OVERVIEW OF MEDICINE IN THE UNITED STATES

As our medical system has taken form in the USA, many interesting pieces of the evolution are rather illuminating and put matters in perspective as to how we became focused as a primarily drug-directed management protocol. Here is a brief overview of healthcare in the United States over the last 150 years.

In the later decades of the 1800s, much of the basic healthcare in this country revolved around traditional herbal medicine passed down through the generations, primarily amongst women. Most mothers schooled their daughters on gathering wild herbs, roots, and seeds and on how to make teas, poultices, and tinctures for a variety of common ills. Wounds, fevers, stomach disorders, and chest complaints were all regularly treated at home. Additionally, many women, particularly those in frontier cabins and in covered wagons, carried and used herbal or homeopathic remedy kits.

When conditions did not respond to at-home measures, a physician may have been sought out, though many rural communities and small towns did not even claim a physician. Midwives were often the most skilled and experienced practitioners in a town, with a plethora of knowledge on herbs, homeopathy, birthing, and rudimentary medicine, including surgery. Times were very different. People lived close to the land and in relationship to the seasons. Conditions could be harsh. Many children died due to infectious illness, and only the toughest of the gene pool pulled through.

Physicians in those days may have been an eclectic physician similar to a naturopath, or a homeopath, or a medical doctor. Training as a physician was not nearly as extensive as it is now. In some cases people were "lay physicians," having learned on-the-scene nursing and doctoring skills during the emergency needs of the Civil War or at the knee of a physician father. The modern medicine of today is a far cry from those rather ragtag times. Not much regulation existed then, as patents were not yet required on medicinals. Consequently, circus sideshow vendors were hawking curative snake oils and potions. Traveling caravan healers professed the wondrous workings of miraculous elixirs. Many stores advertised herbal tonics, which were essentially 90 percent alcohol with a couple of herbs thrown in. It was a bit of a free-for-all. Dentists were still looked at skeptically. Instead, barbers pulled teeth. Aspirin emerged by the late 1890s.

Amid all this cacophony, some good healing work did exist. There were many competent physicians and famously successful hospitals. Homeopathic medicine was a very popular discipline in the 1800s, being that its remedies were more akin to herbs. Many people were inclined to stay with these gentle substances while slightly fearing the stronger allopathic medicines of the era, such as mercury, arsenic, and morphine. In fact, some of the prominent families of this time, such as the Rockefellers and Carnegies, relied on homeopaths as their family physicians. Throughout Europe and America, homeopathy showed stunning successes with the powerful diphtheria and typhoid epidemics, losing far fewer numbers than the allopathic world. Poor hygiene and unsanitary water spread microbes in fleet-moving epidemics. Towns and families experienced devastation regularly.

Meanwhile, death knocked regularly at most every family's door. Even in the early 1900s, children were still succumbing to dehydration during fevers, pneumonia claimed people in their youthful prime, tuberculosis was raging. Then, a phenomenal development occurred: antibiotics. Penicillin was truly a wonder drug at its inception. Blood poisoning, gangrene, and kidney infections were stopped dead in their tracks. Thousands of lives were saved. It is easy to fathom how people were so impressed by this modern medical miracle. By the 1930s, the tide started to turn. Instead of questioning medical practices and the drugs, people now felt that the herbs and homeopathic remedies were old-fashioned and too slow acting. They embraced the medical world and the growing pharmaceutical industry seemingly overnight.

During World War II, thousands of lives were saved from war injuries and infections that would have been tragedies twenty years prior. The pharmaceutical world was growing overnight with heavy funding from the very wealthy big corporations. Simultaneous to all this, the FDA had implemented the much-needed patenting laws, finally weeding out the falsely claimed curative substances of yore.

A man named Abraham Flexner was also appointed by the United States government as a "Quack Buster." His job was to eliminate the charlatans and snake oil salesmen as well as to condemn unsanitary hospitals and teaching facilities; some unfortunately were still managed under post-Civil War conditions. Flexner personally disrespected herbalists, homeopaths, mesmers (magnet therapy), and eclectic physicians. With his tremendous power he closed down all but one of the homeopathic medical schools, the Hahnemann College in Philadelphia, PA, and dozens of homeopathic hospitals were no longer eligible for government approval. Eclectic physicians and herbalists were fined or thrown in jail for practicing medicine without a license. Some kept their professions alive by quietly practicing in their basements, but practitioners of natural medicine became few and far between.

Fortunately, for homeopathy's sake, the FDA had approved homeopathic remedies as over-the-counter substances that followed patenting requirements to exact specifications. Because of this fortunate act of Congress, homeopathic remedies are still maintained in pharmacies that have been closely monitored by government standards since the 1920s. All remedies are approved and recognized as FDA over-the-counter status even now.

By the 1950s, the vaccines had wiped out many childhood epidemics. The modern doctor was now seriously schooled in pharmacology. Milk was pasteurized, babies were delivered in hospitals by doctors, not midwives, and breastfeeding was scorned as being "tribal." With the postwar economy boom and society riding high on the momentum of a blossoming technology, science entered all of our lives. The next five decades became modern scientific medicine's arena. Tremendous discoveries and advances were so plentiful, they catapulted us into an amazing world of discovery.

The twentieth century and now the dawn of the twenty-first century have really been allopathic medicine's shining glory as pertains to science and technology. We have learned astronomical amounts of information about the body, its physiology, details about disease processes, and, most remarkably, diagnostics. Today's advances in surgery and the miraculous vision of CAT, nuclear, PET, and MRI scans would astound our relatives from the late 1800s. It would be almost unimaginable for them to fathom that organs can be transplanted, that robots can perform surgery, and that babies can be created in vitro.

The medical world is now more open to accepting the knowledge and awareness of older, more traditional disciplines and natural modalities, too. Since Dr. Andrew Weil's breakthrough book, *Spontaneous Healing*, his illumination of the success of alternative medical practices with many illnesses has opened a pathway of consciousness for individuals, the medical world, and society at large. Consequently, we are witnessing prestigious medical schools like Harvard offering integrative medicine symposiums and in-house lectures; Mind-Body Consciousness, Stress Management Techniques, and The Awareness of Human Touch have entered the hospital and clinical settings. Many contemporary allopathic physicians are curious to investigate some of the more established methodologies of the alternatives. Look how far nutritional awareness and advice has come in the past two decades. Eating cruciferous vegetables to deter cancer was considered hogwash twenty years ago, but now is endorsed everywhere.

The best is yet to come in healthcare. The blending of the two worlds of allopathic and natural medicines creating a broad and resourceful tapestry of strength to rely on is manifesting in our lives. Hopefully, science will finally spend the time and money to unearth the actual workings of some of the alternative disciplines. Coupled with today's tremendous diagnostics and advanced nursing skills, we are on the brink of the most exciting time and promising vision for our health of tomorrow. I actually feel the tides turning in my thirty years of healthcare work.

Losing the family physician of the early and mid-1900s dissected our healthcare system into nonaligned parts, but my sense is that the burgeoning autoimmune illness and Lyme disease crisis will actually realign us to that "macro" lens of doctoring we all need. The early seismic quakes are happening. Tune in to Lyme Light Radio Wednesdays, 4 p.m. ET/1 p.m. PT, for a view into cutting-edge scientist and physician insights. Also, the radio show *Dead Doctors Don't Lie* by Dr. Joel Wallach consciously educates listeners on a daily basis about the nature of true healing and American medicine's need for transformation.

HOLISTIC MODEL OF HEALTH: THE PHILOSOPHY OF NATURAL MEDICINE

Natural medicine encompasses many healing disciplines of the world that aim at using substances or procedures that reinforce the body's natural healing pathways. These disciplines rely on the time-honored wisdom of ancient practices and, occasionally, more modern techniques. These methods do not normally include pharmaceutical drugs or surgery in their treatment protocols. Natural medicines are made from chemical-free, organic substances existing in nature. They are not man-made or synthesized. These plants, minerals, or animal products may need to be boiled, pounded, or extracted for consumption, but the substance itself has not been adulterated with additives.

Natural medicine disciplines are not taught to conventional doctors in American medical schools. Consequently, most practitioners of natural medicine are schooled in separate institutions and hold different licenses, such as naturopathic doctor (ND), doctor of chiropractic (DC), licensed acupuncturist (Lic. Ac.), or classical homeopath (CCH). Medical doctors (MD) who happen to be nutritionists, functional medicine doctors, or homeopaths receive their schooling, and their certification, outside of medical school. In Europe and other countries, medical schools may include natural (functional) medicine education as part of their curriculum. For instance, more than half of the medical doctors in France are also trained in homeopathy.

Sometimes the terms holistic, alternative, or integrative medicine are used interchangeably regarding natural medicine. Let us take a closer look at these terms, as there are points of delineation among them.

The term complementary or alternative medicine (CAM) means that one such modality may be used as a complement alongside conventional (allopathic) medicine. The individual's intention most often is not to replace the conventional protocol with a natural approach, but to use it in conjunction, as a facilitating measure. One good example of this is the use of herbs or acupuncture for nausea while undergoing chemotherapy treatments, or for pain relief while on RA treatments.

Alternative medicine is another term for complementary medicine. Some people choose to use an alternative discipline as a replacement for allopathic medicine; others will elect to integrate it as a complement. Using chiropractic to address back pain instead of an orthopedic physician is an example of relying on an alternative medical approach versus the mainstream approach. All natural medicine is essentially alternative or complementary in respect to conventional medicine, but not all of the disciplines are holistic.

Holistic medicine includes a variety of disciplines. They may employ differing methodologies but share a common philosophy. The philosophy is that the human being is a complete, or whole, being. His/her physical body and numerous parts are not separate from the emotional and mental planes, but instead are interrelated. The person's complaints are looked at in totality, giving the practitioner a "big picture" of what is going on. Particular symptoms are not treated individually, but as part of the whole. The recurrent kidney infections, tendency to wintertime bronchitis, insomnia episodes, chronic fatigue, and mild depression you may be experiencing are seen as pieces in one's personal health puzzle. This constellation of symptomology will guide the practitioner to a particular homeopathic remedy, acupuncture treatment, nutritive supplements, or herbal formula plan that will rebalance the system. Symptoms will disappear of their own accord as the inner homeostasis, or balance, is regained. Holistic practitioners do not treat diseases, but instead treat the person.

Almost all of the disciplines recognize that the being wants to heal. The body wants to return to homeostasis, wherein no symptoms or ill health are experienced. Our internal gyroscope is constantly trying to find our midline point. During acute episodes, our systems will rely on their own innate cleansing outlets to achieve this goal. The mucus discharge of a cold or allergy attack attempts to flush out the invading microbe. Fever aims at making the environment too hot for the microbe to survive in. Diarrhea purges the tainted food or foreign amoeba. Sunburn pulls us away from the more damaging UVA rays. The list goes on.

Natural approaches in healing choose to support the person during these processes. Instead of thwarting or arresting one of these natural bodily functions, we rely upon protocols that move the process along a bit more efficiently. The lobelia tea can help expectorate the rattling phlegm of a deep chest cough; the chiropractic adjustment will take the pressure off the pinched sciatic nerve.

Chronic conditions such as irritable bowel syndrome or fibromyalgia indicate that there is disturbance, weakness, or overactivity manifesting in the person. Again, the methodologies focus on supporting the person and his/her laboring areas. Symptoms are seen as clues for the practitioner as to where the system is struggling. We want to assist the body and mind with the process that is underway. If it could, the body would have already righted itself, and the picture would not be chronic. Because the complaint has become chronic, or cycles around in a recurrent pattern, the individual needs some support to settle the disharmony.

Acupuncture, aromatherapy, Ayurveda, chiropractic, Chinese herbal medicine, homeopathy, macrobiotics, bodywork, naturopathy, reflexology, and Reiki are some of the more commonly referenced disciplines in the domain of natural medicine. Many other seemingly esoteric practices exist too, such as magnet therapy, and Feldenkrais work. They too have their niche.

The United States uses a now staple form of medicine, called allopathy. Our physicians are schooled in symptom assessment and management of those symptoms by "stopping" them with an antagonistic agent. The primary focus of allopathic medicine is to address malfunctioning parts of the body by use of drugs or surgery, which counteract a symptom. It gained its bedrock of foundation here in the United States, with the advent of the pharmaceutical industry around the 1930s. Because there is no whole-body/person/being philosophy in its foundations, allopathic medicine does not broaden its lens and see the "big picture" of each complete being. Instead it focuses only on the broken parts. Thus, the focus is on counteracting all the varied bodily dysfunctions with the use of antibiotics, antihistamines, antispasmodics, antidepressants, anti-inflammatories, antitussives (cough suppressants), analgesics, and on and on.

Such applications are well suited to the self-limiting acutes, such as poison ivy, muscle spasms from overuse, or diarrhea from food poisoning—these ailments would pass on their own, but may be experienced in a more tolerable fashion with the aid of a drug. This protocol is also tremendously helpful during emergency situations such as heart attack, hemorrhage, or the galloping progression of sepsis (blood poisoning). Malfunctioning organs, like the pancreas and the insulin deficiency of diabetes, are directly addressed by such therapies. Surgery is the other mainstay of allopathic practice, relied upon when organs are so diseased they need to be removed, tumors must be excised, bones require setting, or clogged arteries need to be cleaned out.

Allopathic medicine is not holistic, but instead treats individual symptoms and individual parts. A different medication will be prescribed for each of the different symptoms. One will be given for the kidney infection, one for the Crohn's disease, another for the insomnia, and maybe a fourth for the depression. More importantly, the kidney infections are not typically addressed in a preventative fashion, only during their acute flare-ups. Allopathic medicine does not have the resources to support the body in such a restorative sense. The methodologies are well suited to firefighting the crises of acute conditions, emergency care, or some pathological disease processes, but they are not well versed in addressing pre-disease states and imbalances.

Many of you may have had the experience of visiting your MD with symptoms or complaints, to find that examination, blood work, and scans show no significant results. "All is fine," your MD says. "It is probably just stress; go home and rest." Some cases will clear on their own. Others may linger and become chronic. You are then left suspended in confusion and frustration, with no constructive steps to take. You do not feel right, yet have no idea what is possibly wrong, and no real grasp on what to do next. Fortunately, these situations of imbalance, of pre-disease pathology of autoimmune-style conditions, or chronic Lyme disease, often respond well to one of the avenues of natural medicine.

At this point you are curious to try a discipline of natural medicine, but you have some questions. First, should you try acupuncture, clinical nutrition, homeopathy, naturopathy, Ayurveda, or something else? Turn to the Recovery Guide on page 229 for more information on these different modalities. Secondly, insurance does not usually cover these expenses, so you must pay out-of-pocket. Will it be expensive? Thirdly, you may be wondering how to find a good practitioner in whatever discipline you choose to embrace. Here in the United States, we do not have integrated medicine in our primary healthcare system and medical insurance benefit programs, so we must step outside of the mainstream model and function independently of that structure. Americans spent $34 billion on alternative medicine in 2009. Our needs are changing. We seem to need more than just conventional allopathic medicine, and, apparently, are willing to pay for it, if it will help us. Finding a referral or contacting a national organization is probably the best method currently to locate a qualified practitioner.

Advocates of natural medicine tend to rely primarily on the natural methodologies for the bulk of their healthcare troubles, turning to allopathic measures when situations are life-threatening, in emergencies, when surgery is indicated, or when a natural approach has proven ineffective. Why do some people shy away from conventional allopathic medicine when there is a drug for most every common illness? A few reasons exist.

The first reason is that some people do not like putting chemicals in their bodies, especially strong ones like pharmaceuticals. These concentrated synthetic substances tax the liver significantly, as this organ is responsible for filtering out all impurities from our system—alcohol, fats, chemicals, drugs, and toxins. Drugs weaken the liver and other parts of the body over time. The more one ingests, the greater the cumulative effect.

Secondly, all the "anti" properties of most acutely directed allopathic drugs suppress the body's innate healing abilities. Such repeated practice eventually breeds a suppressed immune system, meaning even poorer response to offending bacteria, viruses, pollens, etc. This is particularly consequential with children. Antibiotics for every cold, cough, and ear infection prevents their developing immune system from running its paces, leaving a less mature immune system for adulthood, creating food allergies, and later in life, often, autoimmune illnesses.

Lastly is dependency. If your body has not learned how to make its own antibodies to particular bacteria or how to balance neurotransmitters, and instead relies on an outside antibiotic or mood-regulating drug, it does not have that antibody or mood-regulating drug in its arsenal for when that specific bacteria, or seasonal shift, reappears. So you are sick again, take an antibiotic, repeat the cycle, and create a dependency. Letting your body "do its thing" during simple acute illness, especially in childhood, breeds better health. You do not have to flounder through it, but can rely on natural supportive methods, if necessary.

Allopathic medicine has its strengths, which are wonderful and perfectly appropriate in many invaluable capacities. The enormous strides in diagnostics and surgical technologies during the 1900s cannot be replaced. Thousands succumbed to gangrene or pneumonia before antibiotics, so we know how valuable they can be, especially when deep internal organs are involved. The same holds true for certain heart medications. We live in a cleaner, less infested world in the Western Hemisphere because of these advances. I do not want to give the impression that I think one approach is all-encompassing or better than another. Each has its merits and weaknesses, and all should have their appropriate places in our healthcare system. Which brings us to the crux of our healthcare dilemma of recent years: choice.

In the United States there has not been much choice in healthcare during the last century. Most of us knew only of allopathic doctoring, as so many of the natural disciplines were disregarded or scorned by the American Medical Association (AMA), which became the dictating body in our culture regarding health practices. Availability of the alternative disciplines has been very scarce. Since the 1980s, some of the limitations of allopathic medicine have become too obvious to ignore, causing many unwell people, especially those with chronic illnesses, to start seeking out other options.

At this point most of us recognize the time has come for our healthcare system to broaden its scope. Preventative care, depletions, and pre-disease states are all beautifully addressed by many of the natural approaches. Doctors, hospitals, even HMOs are beginning to recognize this; the more progressive ones are now incorporating massage therapy, mindfulness techniques, acupuncture, and Reiki into their services, creating practices now labeled as "Integrative Medicine Clinics."

There is much to explore in your journey through the territory of natural medicine. Some of the practices are very structured in their schooling and certification/licensing procedures. Others have not yet achieved that level of organization or mass acceptance, which in turn necessitates formal standardization. Some areas of our country boast an array of available alternative practitioners, while in others not a soul is found. We must recognize we are the only modern Western country of the world that does not include natural medicine and clinical nutrition work in its primary healthcare system. England, France, Germany, Italy, Canada, Japan, India, and Argentina all incorporate these modalities.

What we aim to focus on here includes the blending of the best of traditional and complementary medicine, as well as highlighting the very important aspects of emotional and spiritual healing. When we overlook these areas, we are unable to become completely well.

We must not gloss over the significant power of emotions. Three potent emotions that factor in strongly during the healing process are acceptance, compassion, and love. Even when employing the most well-directed techniques, supplements, or drugs, the individual needs to tap into this emotional space as well. Some people do this instinctively, consequently making smooth recoveries. Others fight their own inner selves, or do not have awareness of this inner realm. It is a piece of medicine that doctors have ignored for decades, but are now realizing is integral to healing. Some medical schools are now teaching classes on communication and emotional interplay between doctors and their patients.

For our own sake, and that of others, we must acknowledge acceptance within ourselves. Acceptance that the bothersome condition has had a purpose in showing you and your practitioner where imbalance lies. Acceptance that there is a reason for this burden. Acceptance that one's being has the desire to heal. Alongside this is compassion. Compassion from the practitioners and caregivers who understand that someone is uncomfortable and in need. Compassion for their momentary vulnerability. Compassion within the individual, toward themselves, for their own personal struggles. And finally, love. The greatest power of all. Love for the person in need. Love for our wellspring of gifts and our powers of healing. Love for ourselves, even in the midst of trials, tribulations, and woe. Love for the majestic beauty of life.

WHAT IS MENDING?

The challenges life brings us take endless forms. Many of us know the heartbreak of losing a loved one, a marriage crumbling, or our child succumbing to drug addictions. We have tasted the bitterness of disappointments in promises unkept, job situations turned sour, or a friend ending up being a liar. The process of becoming conscious and present with your self through these life trials is so intrinsic in the process of mending.

Illness is a strident teacher. So many of its lessons ask us to face personal demons. More aptly we look fear, failure, loss, and the quagmire of sadness straight in the eye. Our inner resources are tested, we question mortality and faith, and we wonder where we fit in the scheme of this process called life.

The opportunity for personal transformation through the vehicle of illness should never be dismissed. Though we believe someone wiser and more educated, a particular potion, or a drug will cure us, instinctively most of us recognize somewhere, in our deepest heart of hearts, that mending from our travesties is actually in our own hands.

Yet we feel lost and alone and confused and afraid. This is vital! You are on the cusp of your awakening by allowing these feelings to be real. By accepting them as part of your life equation you are "waking up," or becoming conscious to your life path. This is the important first step.

However, when we dig our heels in, resist, stay locked in a spin cycle, the ability to allow our spirit room to expand and seek higher ground is thwarted. Permitting yourself the time and generosity to let go of these emotional trappings is an important next step in mending. The suffering is too heavy, too painful, and eclipses one's ability to live wholly in life, open and with love.

The art of mending is intricate and finely crafted, like a sacred journey, meant to be attuned to the present. Sickness forces us to extract ourselves from the outer world and so many functions. It asks us to become very Zen, to "Be Here, Be Now." Illness puts all the big life questions on the table for us and strips us to bare bones. All the excesses and props, the good and the bad, are up for examination.

No matter our socioeconomic level, career placement, relationship status, age, gender, or location on the globe, serious illness is a modern-day quest for the "holy grail," or your surrender at the high altar. If we look at the very conscious lifestyle of the Mennonites or Buddhist monks, we note a simple grace to their daily lives. Taking care of basic human survival needs—growing food, providing shelter, sharing in community, honoring honesty—comprise their rhythms and the excesses are purged.

This lifestyle may not be desirable or attainable for many of us, but the lessons are invaluable. For in the simpler habitat these folks reside in, they take care to mend the break in a pasture fence or a rip in an article of clothing or the miscommunication between two people. The cultivated attention to care is obvious.

I recall my very worldly father also so aptly teaching me how to mend. When my treasured bedtime stuffed animal, Bunny, had a ripped and dangling right arm from too much love and wear, Dad set up a surgical "suite" on his home office desk. We laid out a clean towel, got needle and thread, a standing magnifying glass, and extra desk lamps as he prepared to mend my treasured "Lovey," my security stuffed toy. Dad showed me compassion and care as I stood beside him handing him the scissors and thread on command. While Bunny was being mended, we showered love upon her.

I respect the warm feeling of knowing my father was helping restore my Lovey as good as new, and the palpable ministration we put into this process. As Dad looked into my eyes after the final closing stitch, proving that Bunny was now recovered, I felt in my heart that with true care and devotion anything or anyone could be "mended." I hugged that soft, floppy rabbit so tight to my chest, so very grateful to my dad. He patted me reassuringly on the shoulder. "Love her more than ever, sweetheart. Take good care of her and she will mend."

Dad taught me the value of tending our wounds and tears, and that love is such a powerful healer. Though his nimble fingers stitched the torn arm together, internally I sensed that it was our shared attention and loving care that could surmount any trial or tragedy. This tiny metaphor reminds me of what rings true for us all in our journey of recovery—love is the greatest healer and a very wise teacher.

We may mend a wound with stitches or a broken vase with glue, but mending ourselves when seriously ill asks us to embrace love in the truest of all ways. Self-love is not easily claimed. Our conditioning has angled us to love others and objects and escapades with more focus than our own spirits and bodies. These destructive autoimmune illnesses and the crossover components from tick-borne-disease infections do not allow any more slack time for an individual. You are on that desktop surgical table! You are now on a quest, and the destination is not a specific location, but your acceptance of awakening to consciousness, which is the path to enlightenment.

Lyme disease and autoimmune illness can be turned on their side, if you see this situation from a new perspective. Besides all the doctoring and necessary bodily supports, the other aspect of these illness challenges is to embrace the spiritual transformation you are presented with. The time has come for you to care for YOU.

The consistent theme in my personal story and the hundreds I have encountered who have made it to recovery, or what some coin as remission, is the ability to let go of the mental and emotional darkness in our lives, allowing it to be replaced with the eternal light of love and self-worth.

And in the same breath I acknowledge this is often very hard to achieve totally on your own. Do not be afraid to seek counsel from a therapist, spiritual healer, minister, empathic elder, shaman, or wise family member who can offer you support and guidance along the journey, just as my dad and I walked side by side in the triage office operating table, mending my torn Lovey.

You can mend, and please know that something very beautiful and grand awaits you on the other side. For the gifts born during the transformational process of mending are profound. The kindred spirits you meet, the creative energy you tap into, the new work you bring to the world is breathtaking and deeply meaningful. Allow grace the room to take form. Your new presence and life form is waiting to be born. Reach forward, let go of your fear, believe in your tomorrow. For even with rips and stitches and broken shards of your spirit, you can bring yourself back together again on a new level of consciousness. Mending is an act of beauty.

THE MIND-BODY CONNECTION

Everyone realizes that a little love goes a long way. When a child gives you a big smile, or a friend sends you a card because they are thinking of you, you feel good. How could you remain angry for long when you arrive home from work and your ever-happy dog is practically jumping out of his skin with joy to see you? There may be something more to these positive emotional interchanges than just their momentary worth.

Studies show the ill effects of negative emotional situations on our health. There is a higher incidence of heart attack in people who have recently lost a spouse. People who have never been married live a shorter lifespan than their counterparts who have shared permanent companionship. Those who live alone develop chronic illness more frequently. Obviously, loneliness and lack of daily one-on-one emotional interplay fit into the scheme regarding wellness.

Many therapists and doctors encourage the elderly who live alone to adopt a pet—a cat, a dog, or even a bird. The act of caring for another living being creates a healthier and more loving atmosphere. Animals can emit feelings of love and affection to their owners, which helps fill a void in these individuals' lives. Such positive emotions have a healthful effect on our physical body as well.

The immune system is an amazingly intricate network of glands, organs, nerves, and cells, continuously striving to keep our bodies in homeostatic balance by ridding invasive germs, toxins, rogue cancer cells, etc. We cannot identify one master switch to the immune system, as it is a combination of factors that keeps the human "machine" running effectively. We now understand that, interestingly, a huge core of it lies in the balance of "flora" and function of our GI tract! However, when the immune system weakens and our "defenses" are down, illness occurs.

The pituitary gland, located in the skull, is responsible for regulating the other glands of the body, instructing them when and how much of the specific hormones are to be released. Hormones are involved in a myriad of functions, some of which are directly responsible for keeping immune response high. An example is the thymus gland, which produces natural germ fighters, called T-cells. Studies have shown that AIDS and leukemia patients have reduced T-cell counts.

The brain controls the pituitary gland. Emotions such as loneliness, depression, or fear signal the brain to alter pituitary function, as the body senses that danger is at hand. The amygdala portion of the brain holds our emotions. What we see, hear, and feel are all carried by nerve receptors straight to the amygdala. Good and bad images and sensations get recorded and in turn trigger the pathway to our pituitary gland and other endocrine glands in an orchestration.

If we are depressed, the pituitary slows its pace, not cueing the other endocrine glands as promptly. If the other glands then are not secreting as many hormones, then various minor imbalances may occur, such as poor sleep, changes in menstrual cycle, or a weakened immune response (with fewer T-cells present to fight foreign invaders). If negative emotional states have been present for an extended period of time, this depressed immune system function could certainly be prime breeding ground for a chronic illness, such as asthma or MS, to develop.

Unfortunately, a vicious cycle may occur. When mired in chronic sickness, feelings of depression and fear naturally surface. More aggressive emotions, like anger or panic, are common too, and can induce the adrenal glands to produce adrenaline. This substance triggers several responses in the body, one of which is to heighten our reactionary self-protective skills and thinking clarity, another is to dial down the thymus gland, whereby barely any T-cells are being produced at all. The scenario is ugly—you are battling a serious illness, fearful for your future, angry about it, have a short supply of T-cells, and now you have shut down their production even more so while your mind is revved up! What do you do? Learning to work with our emotions and senses can be key helpmates.

Ignoring feelings is not effective for the long run. Finding ways to safely express feelings, without damaging others, helps in purging these immunity-repressing emotions. Writing, talking, punching pillows, and counseling are all possible outlets. So are trauma-release therapies like EFT, EMDR, and biofeedback.

Activating the parasympathetic branch of the nervous system is a central issue. This system encourages the glands and organs of the body to function with more consistency. This is the calmative branch of the nervous system. Soothing mental and physical activities will induce parasympathetic action, which in turn stimulates the hormone production of the thymus and other glands. Meditation, prayer, yoga, visualization, singing, and relaxation tapes are examples. Laughter, love, and companionship also fit into the picture. These positive emotions breed a more relaxed mental state, encouraging the parasympathetic nervous system to flourish, and ultimately a more hefty production of T-cells and other immunity constituents are released and the runaway adrenal gland pump is quieted.

Perhaps the lesson in all of this is to share our love and compassion with one another. Dwelling on negative feelings does not serve us well. Learning how to be in touch with these emotions and how to process them is a critical piece in balancing our total health picture. Introducing a soothing de-stressing component into your lifestyle is a healthful plus. The benefits of positive relationships go a long way. Living in balance, within our own body and mind, as well as in relationship to one another, is a lifestyle choice that will undoubtedly bring us increasing health.

When we are trapped alone at home in a sickbed for long spells, or do not have a spouse or mate or family around, isolation becomes a serious matter for the infirm. Being sick and in pain is awful, even if you live in a big household or have a supportive partner. But those who live alone can get caught in a vortex of despair and suffering quite easily. I was there. I know how desolate and hopeless some of you feel. Suicidal thinking is very common with chronic Lyme disease. The ability to hold on and believe you actually could be strong enough to dance or travel or play with your offspring can feel like an absolute impossibility for many of you.

These feelings are not farcical. They are real and you must learn how to engage the mind-body healing pathway in a new, positive direction to stimulate the pituitary, release the trauma from the amygdala, and jump-start the immune function and induce the production of the "feel-good" neurotransmitters serotonin and dopamine.

We all recall Norman Vincent Peale and his laughter therapy. I recall my bedridden father rehabilitating himself from paralyzed vocal cords and serious cardiovascular damage by watching Marx Brothers movies for days in a row! After eighteen embolisms post-op nearly took his life (he was declared dead—flatline heart monitor and out-of-body experience), he came home and watched movies. He would be laughing hysterically, no sounds at first, but full-body quaking at their zaniness. With a bleak outcome, he defied the odds and lived another robust forty years, always reminding me, "Think positively; it is the best medicine."

Frontier thinking in medicine emphasizes the power of belief, of positive imagery, and the effects that sound, light, color, and vision have on our healing. The thrivers in any disaster situation always see themselves in a better place; they believe in a brighter future. I am a strong supporter of using photographs and beautiful images (a bouquet of flowers at your bedside, a tropical beach poster, a view out your window) to invoke good feelings. Playing soothing music or toning chords are proven to rehabilitate brain injuries, foster wound healing, and calm hysteria and panic. Useful CDs or online access is available. Try Stillpoint.org, or TheUnexplainableStore.com.

We need to use the right stimuli for all of our senses when we are ill to help quell the runaway sympathetic nervous system branch and support the generous parasympathetic portion. Affirmations, meditation, and visualizations are enormously helpful. Accepting love and assistance from friends, neighbors, or even a support group helps us tip the scales from depression and anguish toward hope and healing. Though asking for help is so difficult for many of us, making this bridge really could be the critical turning point you require for healing. Going at it alone is only a stopgap, usually. Care from another is one of life's great balms.

The human being is enormously resourceful. We can, however, get stuck in bad ruts. When ill, we easily forget how to pull out of a pattern, and often dig in even deeper! The reflection of a friend's counsel or the love of a family member helps ground and nurture us. When we get fed emotionally and spiritually, many great body chemicals and hormones are produced. Turning on the positives of love, laughter, beauty, and hope always is helpful and healthful.

The body and mind are not disassociated as some professionals declared for certain generations. In fact, the antithesis is true. We have a massive conduit, the body-mind-spirit pathway, and once you learn how to tap into this roaring river, anything is possible! Turn to Mind-Spirit (page 327) for more information and exercises to facilitate this process. You can heal, grow, thrive, achieve, and do wonders for yourself and the world.

RESILIENCY

The trials of life can leave many of us battered and often scarred with physical or emotional woes. Some seethe with bitterness or anger after a divorce. Others may be plagued with allergies after a year spent nursing an ill parent. Yet someone else may be livelier and more confident than ever after two surgeries and a house fire. What makes some of us curl up and withdraw from the world and others keep on forging ahead, sometimes even with increased drive and passion?

Resiliency is the distinguishing quality that helps many people rebound and often grow with wisdom as they recoup from the hard knocks of life. In the world of natural medicine, we recognize resilient individuals have a lot of vitality, or a strong "vital force." We see children battling high fevers and many acute illnesses successfully, remarking on their innate vitality. When we see an adult bouncing back from severe illness or heavy emotional traumas, we recognize this resiliency as part of their strong "vital force." Some people seem to have an innate resiliency, but it can also be cultivated. How?

First off, let us look at the noted emotional stages of recovery we all experience when healing from a significant blow, whether it be a serious diagnosis or a dying parent. Shock and denial are first felt. "This can't be happening to me" or "This is a mistake" are common thoughts when facing any sort of tragedy or unexpected roadblock. In stage two, we begin to acknowledge the circumstances, but there is often still a sense of numbness accompanying it. Pain surmounts next, as we start to live the reality of this challenge, i.e., facing the months ahead in a body cast or the barrenness after a parent's death. Strong feelings of anger, fear, and sadness are commonly felt. Then comes adjustment, whereby plans and steps are incorporated into one's life. Relying on family for chores, learning to use a walker, or seeking out grief counseling show one is adjusting to the change. Finally, we come to a place of moving beyond, where resolution has been established. At this point in the journey, the resilient often note they feel even better than before the challenge surfaced. While tackling the illness you may find yourself developing a stronger self-confidence or a personal commitment to helping others with similar conditions. Or perhaps in reflecting on your deceased parent's life, you may find yourself more clearly and passionately identifying your own life's purpose.

These stages may flow smoothly in such succession or a few may be experienced simultaneously, or even in a different order. Some may be revisited a few times. We need to make it through them all, however, to recover fully. When we get stuck at a particular stage and cannot progress beyond it is when the complications arise. The bitterness and anger bubbles inside us, tending to cause easy conflict with others. Or the suppressed grief weighs down our immune system, breeding allergies or autoimmune disorders. Some of us do not know how to show or even inwardly connect with our feelings. When this happens we tend to try to use our mind to push the feelings away, or keep ourselves so busy that we can avoid confronting the lonely moments or the searing rage. We try to stop ourselves from entering these not-so-comfortable spaces.

Resiliency involves experiencing the feelings attached to each of these recovery phases. There are a myriad of ways to do this, and none is more right or wrong. Some people must emote dramatically: cry, yell, slam doors. Others will privately write in a journal. Another may talk to a friend, priest, or counselor. A fourth yet may find himself/herself taking long walks speaking to his/her departed beloved or spending many hours communing with nature or a special animal friend. Some need to run, paint, dance to experience their feelings. All methods are okay, as long as they help you make it through these phases. If you find yourself spending months locked in fury at your ex-spouse or feeling too insecure to drive again after an auto accident, it is time to seek help from a professional or a loving friend who can assist you in moving out of your locked place of recovery. Healing does take time, though—often many months after a significant blow. But we can heal, grow, and change for the better during this process.

Our bodies and minds hold the wisdom to heal. Our systems are designed to try and return to balance or homeostasis. Tears, tremors, or nightmares are emotional pathways our psyche will use to express and discharge feelings that threaten to wound or hamper us. Aside from accepting some of these processes as normal to the healing process, we can encourage the resiliency factor, too. The good news is that even though some of us may not consider ourselves that resilient, we can foster a greater allowance of it.

Psychologists have found certain attitudes and actions to be effective in encouraging greater emotional resiliency.

1. Accept responsibility for your life and actions. Some events are out of your control, but you can influence the emotional outcome.
2. Think positively. If you are struggling with this, just saying the words over and over, "everything will work out fine," is a good place to start.
3. Teach yourself to accept change. Rearrange your furniture or buy some clothing of different colors than your usual wardrobe. In accepting change during a low-stress time, you can better adjust when an unexpected change does occur.
4. Develop your self-confidence. Learning a new skill is the simplest avenue. Take sketching classes, learn yoga, train for

a 10k race. Outdoor education courses such as "Outward Bound" can be tremendous confidence boosters and make a significant difference in a short amount of time.

5. Be true to yourself by practicing authenticity. Façades end up limiting you severely in the end. Many people experience anxiety during this sort of self-discovery process. You may want to see a therapist or counselor for emotional support and confirmation of your self-identity during this blossoming journey.
6. Connect with your inner faith. Prayer, meditation, walks in the woods, and community service are all ways to tune in to your personal power and inner beliefs. Teach these things to your children. It will serve them well in life.

In the physical realm, some of us could use some boosting in terms of swift and effective recoveries. Good nutrition is, of course, important; fresh, non-processed, preferably organic food should be consumed. During times of stress the B vitamins, vitamin C, trace minerals, and immune supports such as echinacea and quercetin can be great aids. An adrenal supplement is wise, to keep too much cortisol from racing in your bloodstream and triggering the inflammatory cascade. Fresh air and circulation facilitate strengthened bodily function as well as mental balance. As a homeopath I must say that the use of homeopathic remedies during times of any difficult challenge in life, whether it be physical or emotional, is one of the most dynamic components in positive recoveries that I have seen. Time and time again over the years I have witnessed very difficult situations eased and softened by the wondrous influence of these gentle substances from nature. "Rescue Remedy" is a favorite standard.

The emotional tableau accompanying major life transitions is almost instantly modified for those turning to homeopathy. It seems that the psyche is touched in such a way that inner understanding and acceptance emerges amidst the overwhelming cascade of dominating difficult feelings, finally emerging from the shackles into a lighter and more knowing place.

Resiliency runs in families. Some of the strongest characters I know in my life are the individuals who have faced life's truest perils and have not caved in, but with optimism, fortitude, faith, and asking for help when needed have recovered from serious diseases, intense injuries, ugly divorces, or death of a beloved. Your spirit is mighty, and giving yourself time to move through the phases of trauma and recovery, without getting caught in fear or self-pity or self-neglect can make for a resilient swingback.

We learn by example. Children are imprinted by their primary caregivers by the time they are seven or eight years old on how to manage situations, people, and their feelings. If your family ancestors were survivors of resilient attitude, chances are you are instilled with that power set of will and fortitude and optimal visions of a better future. If not, do not pale, but use these pages to help ignite the phenomenal mind-body healing pathway in the chakra lesson chapters to come, and believe in your greatest potentials!

"Out of suffering have emerged the strongest souls; the most massive characters are seared with scars."

—Khalil Gibran

THE POWER TO HEAL

No one likes to be ill or injured. Unfortunately, it is a rare person who does not experience the occasional incapacitating illness or accident that sidelines us. Whether we suffer a broken bone, pneumonia, or a more serious situation such as lupus or cancer, healing is the objective we are striving for.

Our intricately designed body has a deep-seated, primitive desire to heal. That healing force encompasses many seemingly miraculous abilities we conjure up during the recovery process. With the advent of so many modern medical therapeutic tools, many of us are not aware that merely a few generations back we were still losing our loved ones to systemic infections, childhood epidemics, and childbirth complications. We are not completely out of the woods in terms of overcoming all the ravages disease and injury can threaten us with. Many chronic illnesses and serious injuries still can take our lives. However, many of us do heal, in spite of seemingly insurmountable odds in some very dire situations. Just what are these powers within that can summon up such healing energies? Can any of us do this?

The internal healing force within us has not yet been completely harnessed, even in recent decades of astounding scientific discoveries. We can fly a spaceship to Mars, but we have yet to clearly pinpoint what our healing force is. We reason that it is a combination of various systems working together. The immune system includes white blood cells, lymphocytes, T-cells, and the endocrine glands such as the pituitary and thymus, which align somehow with the brain and its myriad of natural sedatives, endorphins, and other chemicals. We also create natural corticosteroids that keep inflammation down, fevers to burn out microbes, and bone marrow to create new blood cells. With all these symphonic workings, somehow we "right" ourselves. Such amazing interplay of actions happens at often split-second speed and many times without our conscious instructions to orchestrate the recovery.

Sometimes we feel as if it will be months or years until we feel well. In certain instances this is very true. We may recover in days from a minor muscle sprain or bladder infection, but it may take three years to battle back from a stroke or Lyme disease. Some of us stall and remain burdened with a chronic illness, yet others gather their internal forces and make a complete recovery. Tapping into such deep healing abilities seems to be more difficult as we age, yet we all know the remarkable senior who heals as quickly as his or her grandson.

Having participated, both as an ally and personally, in many healing journeys over my thirty years in the natural medicine field, I have witnessed some stunning recoveries. A combination of factors enable those of us with the drive to recover. My observations, coupled with the knowledge of critical thinkers, highlight a few key ingredients. Though not yet a well-posited formula, these pieces are relatively consistent and not to be overlooked.

EPIGENETICS

A frontier edge of current medical thinking coins a term called epigenetics. This refers to the relationship between inner healing qualities and how we "turn on" cells and actual DNA to prompt recovery, even when the odds are stacked against us. Bruce Lipton's famous book, *The Bridge of Belief*, breaks the physiological processes down thoroughly, showing how an actual gene set can be ignited, via prayer and belief, to stimulate the physical body into generating healthier new cells and optimal function.

We all know and admire survivors—those brave souls who made it out of some plane wreck, a war, or invasive cancer. They are tough to the core. There is a smaller group of survivors who are termed "thrivers", Dawson Church's book, *The Genie in Your Genes*, gives great evidence to this level of soul medicine. Thrivers are individuals who survive the hellacious house fire or shipwreck and go on to do extraordinary humanitarian things with their lives. They live beyond their ego, the disease they battled, or the decimation, and touch mankind.

All thrivers, according to Church, have ignited a specific gene pair, numbered on the DNA helix. Studies show that survivors and thrivers run in a family. Their gene pair is already fired up. These fearless, willful, creative people are not common, but we all know someone like this. The more remarkable notation is that every human being has the capability of igniting that thriver gene pair. That means all of us can overcome abysmal situations, heal, survive, restore, and be happy and whole, contributing to the world again, versus being dependent on meds or sidelined on a cane.

But, just how do we do this? It sounds like magic right now.

WILL

The first and most potent tool is will. I have seen and felt the brilliant "light" of will within ambitious patients. It is a palpable sensation to those in the room. There is a strong, clear, unvacillating desire to "beat this thing," evidenced by a focus and a commitment to adhere to outlined protocols (getting out of bed for an often painful post-surgery walk, adhering to exercises, following a specific diet, defying a physician diagnosis), coupled with a no-nonsense attitude about refusing to "baby" themselves. These people are going to do "it" (whatever it is) and no one can change their mind! Like mountain goats, they must summit.

REST

The drive to recover must also be coupled with a commitment to rest. Sleep and rest are some of the greatest healing tools. You may push yourself to cook your own healthy meal, but you will also lie down and nap, finding someone to watch the kids or run a load of laundry.

SUPPORT SYSTEMS

This is a very key ingredient. People who have others showing their love and support seem to do the best. Daily doses of companionship, physical caress, and warmth of expression are the biggest salve I have seen. When we are ill and down, we need the love of others—not a precursory visit or card (those are nice too), but true compassion and emotional support. The occasional blue mood may disappear with a pep talk or gentle shoulder massage. Knowing others are there to help puts us at ease. When we relax, our adrenals produce less cortisol and our parasympathetic side of the nervous system grows stronger, allowing happy brain chemicals to flow.

SELF-LOVE

Being kind to ourselves, amidst the frustration, sadness, and anger of a condition, is another key mental attitude. Self-love is hard-earned. Most of us find it easier to love another human being, a dog, or a job even, than ourselves! Take a moment, close your eyes. Say your name out loud. Then say, "I love you, [your name]." What do you sense internally, in your heartspace?

Was that comfortable, or awkward and strangely foreign? I felt rather shocked when I first tried this. "Katina" felt rather filmy and like a young girl to me, instead of the hardworking adult, mother, and friend I know myself as. When I was tragically ill, seeing the inner Katina and telling her I loved her brought tears to my eyes, because I saw in my mind's eye how little self-care I gave myself, but generously doled out in armfuls to others. An epiphany! This was a true turning point in my healing journey, and is for thousands. When you really, deeply accept the necessity for—and practice of—self-love, something beautiful opens up inside of you; a small glow, a piece of pride, or, initially, embarrassment. But, just noticing the feeling of loving yourself is a powerful step.

For the core truth is this: we live and die from our heart. When it stops beating, we die. Our heart houses our love. Love keeps us alive. The hermit or shut-in loves their plants or menagerie of cats. The stout, robust grandmother with children on her lap lives in a swarm of love. The survivors and thrivers share a sentence in common: "I kept thinking of my son (wife, daughter, husband) and knew I had to live to see them again." Love propelled them. Self-love turns on the gene pair; this ties into the last and perhaps slightly mysterious element.

FAITH AND POSITIVE THINKING

Some look to their religious beliefs, or a broader spiritual base, or merely the act of positive thinking. Whatever the label, this place of belief creates a trust or inner peace. Such an emotional state appears to be a catalyst for the production of an array of brain chemicals prompting our healing response. Such faith and belief in our ability to heal breeds a certain form of internal medicine. This internal spectrum of medicine can be more potent than any externally directed pill, or prop, or procedure.

What is crucial to understand is that you bear the power to heal! Let no one tell you anything otherwise. Bleak diagnoses, forecasted terminal language, and projected cure dates trap your mind and heart. Maintaining a conversation with your inner healer is your treasure chest. Honor this. Work with yourself. Our future chapters will deliver skills for you to develop.

WHAT IS MY ROLE IN MY ILLNESS?

Understanding our role in the illness and our emotional undertones as relates to physical symptoms is important. Discomfort is an opportunity for awakening. It shows us the dyad of illness and pain as flashlights illuminating trigger points within that we can embrace as vehicles rather than obstacles for growth. "Emotions" contain the word "motion." They involve feelings. Feelings have energy attached to them. Exploring the energy of a feeling is a starting point. Sense the energy of these moments. What does the energy you experience feel like? Is it hyper, erratic, dragging, heavy?

We can take notice of the anxiety roaring in our gut or head, or recognize those angry outbursts or irritability episodes when we snap at children or a mate. From here we can get in touch with what this emotional energy is doing to our being, to our body. Do you notice a tightness somewhere in your body during these moods? Or an emptiness? Or does a boulder or noose or vise grip sit elsewhere? Be aware. Write it down if that helps you. This now is an awareness point for you, and a realization that this organ or body part is under siege. Your emotional state has energetically started to lay an imprint on a physical system. Holding such an energy for long periods of time will affect us physically and ultimately create symptoms, then cellular changes, and in turn our glandular and organ function may be damaged.

Imagine holding a forty-pound rock for weeks on end—it would become tiring and drain you. Pain, exhaustion, collapse would ensue. Imagine holding a fidgety, frustrated puppy in your arms for hours. You would be scratched up, overwrought, and frazzled. Our emotions and feelings are similar forces.

Of course, we just want to drop the rock or the puppy and run away. It is the same with our discomforts. We want them to disappear. Some of us try distractions or escapes—drugs, shopping, food, drama—to make them disappear. Such "fixes" do not really dissolve the discomfort; they just temporarily palliate. Underneath, the unresolved discomfort lingers until we actually explore it, process it, and intentionally work to resolve the issue. Or do we just keep holding onto the forty-pound rock or fidgety puppy?

Our culture has evolved into a situation with an endless array of externalized props, exits, and consumptions. There is scant "training" support anymore in childhood to teach us how to reach within ourselves to the place of stillness, contemplation, and self-awareness. If we can cultivate turning within, being aware of our feelings (even at a young age), then not as many levels of discomfort will get built up or plaqued onto our psyche. Being emotionally aware helps us live in greater clarity. We are more alive and free, able to share, to laugh, to move with grace in relationships.

Your role in your illness most likely has been a disconnect, whether minor or major, at two prime levels. One is the misunderstanding of how emotions have energy forms. If held too long the energy of fear, anger, betrayal, animosity, loss, or anything else will affect body parts and induce biochemical, and then cellular, change, ultimately resulting in dysfunction in an organ, gland, or system, resulting in symptoms and eventually what we call illness or disease.

The second disconnect is not fully realizing you have the ability to change your symptom state by working with your emotions and using inner mindfulness tools. When we see the symptoms of discomfort and illness as vehicles for change and growth, then healing becomes something far more multidimensional than just externally directed "doctoring." We actually are gaining some control and personal empowerment by embracing illness as a wake-up call for transformation.

Place your hand flat on your stomach. Close your eyes and sense what you feel. Does a feeling or image come to you? Let yourself absorb this feeling, image, or message. Take note of any sensations you feel in your body. What adjectives come to mind? Restless, hollow, heavy, exploding, erratic? Write these sensations down, or the image you see, including the colors, the scene, the people, or just you. What you are gleaning is a sense of your present self and the state you are in as relates to your personal presence and power. For aside from all the organs and muscles that physically sit in this region, the metaphysical companion as relates to your hara is known as your "presence": the image our Self portrays in the world. From our core, this third chakra, our creative energy and physical prowess, is showcased.

I often refer to professional athletes as prime examples of individuals with strong third chakra energy. Think about a professional athlete you know or see on TV. They have well-developed muscles and stand tall and proud. We sense their personal power just by looking at them. They radiate those undertones I mention of strength, will, determination, and presence. No wonder major corporate sponsors tap into these individuals; they radiate willpower and accomplishment. Others desire this powerful essence and want to use or "claim" it.

Even though you may not be a professional athlete or heroic firefighter, talented public speaker, or creative teacher (other examples of strong third chakra individuals), you can easily learn how to kindle the absolutely life-changing energy of willpower and ignite the brilliant conduit of the mind-body healing pathway. You can overcome the "disconnected" position you have maintained, probably for years, and now connect with your inner willpower and intention to promote your own healing and accomplishment. Part V teaches these methods. Taking action in your recovery allows for the transformation to occur.

For now, be kind with yourself. The understanding about how our feelings and body interweave has not been instilled in many of us within recent generations of upbringing. We have consciousness around being publicly correct and treating others with greater respect and equality. That interpersonal transformation was a necessary and beautiful outpouring of societal growth in the later 1900s. Now the time has come for each of us to learn how to attune to our own body, mind, and spiritual needs, and the fascinating interplay. Once we can gain some skills in this arena your illness will not feel like it has "become" you, nor the dominating influence of your life. You will no longer frame matters as, "My MS prevents me from joining you at the theater tonight," and instead move toward, "I want to join you at the theater tonight. I hope you understand my energy is a bit low, but the show will lift my spirits."

Perspective; how we use our language, attitude, and effort go a long way in life. They shape us significantly. Start paying attention to your emotions and the sensations they induce.

PART II

Overview of Autoimmune Illnesses and Lyme Disease

OVERVIEW OF AUTOIMMUNE ILLNESSES AND LYME DISEASE

The incidence of autoimmune illnesses has spiked in recent decades, alongside the explosion of the Lyme disease crisis. From the natural medicine and integrative medicine models, as well as what the Lyme disease experts of the world understand, we deduce that there is more than one reason why people are tumbling from active, vital, even youthful status into compromised sickness. We are finding limited success from the "old" lens of medicine that says, "Your immune system has turned on itself and gone into overdrive, so we must suppress that mechanism."

Our newer vantage point, which digs deeper than the "flipped autoimmune switch," is that assorted reasons have compiled to make your body overburdened and unable to function comfortably or happily. We will delve into these pieces and offer restoration and mending advice in Part III, but now let us take a look at the most common autoimmune illnesses and their often intrinsic interplay to the infectious microbes of Lyme disease and other tick-borne diseases. The role of systemic-inflammation-producing microbes is not to be overlooked. Microbial systemic testing needs to be more highly refined and accurate. The many essential deficiencies and toxicities many folks are labored by must be accurately ascertained, too.

What is worth noting, too, is that some people do not actually have enough cellular pathological change to warrant a disease state manifested in a specific gland or organ, but have a constellation of uncomfortable symptoms that confound a "frank" scientific diagnosis and are termed a "syndrome." We are familiar with premenstrual syndrome or irritable bowel syndrome and now chronic fatigue syndrome and fibromyalgia (actually a syndrome). Diseases typically are pinpointed via laboratory results and scans or scopes that find "clinical" pathological cellular changes and irregularities severe enough to claim diabetes with extremely high blood sugar levels or coronary heart disease with soaring cholesterol levels. The good news about syndromes is that complementary natural healthcare practitioners consider them to be *pre*-disease states and fixable via restorative supplements, dietary changes, homeopathics, herbals, and more. Hope for help and remission and a better quality of life even is possible for many disease states with these approaches.

Now, let us take a look at the core autoimmune illnesses over 50,000,000 American and 250,000,000 people are plagued with worldwide!

CHRONIC FATIGUE SYNDROME (CFS)

Chronic fatigue syndrome (CFS) is the common name for a group of significantly debilitating medical conditions characterized by persistent fatigue and other specific symptoms that last for a minimum of six months in adults and three months in children or adolescents. The fatigue is not due to exertion, yet can be aggravated by typical exertion. It is not significantly relieved by rest. In fact, the CFS patient wakes up feeling exhausted even after ten hours of sleep or bed rest. CFS may also be referred to as myalgic encephalomyelitis (ME), post-viral fatigue syndrome (PVFS), chronic fatigue immune dysfunction syndrome (CFIDS), or by several other names. Biological, genetic, infectious, and psychological mechanisms have been suggested as causes, but the exact etiology of CFS is not fully understood. CFS is considered to fall in the realm of autoimmune illness and has been increasing in huge proportions in the last couple of decades.

In the early 1900s, this state was called "neurasthenia" and colloquially labeled as "rich woman's disease," evoking the image of a Victorian-era female in lacy white collapsed on her divan. The suspected causes back then were the advent of electricity in wealthier citizens' homes, perhaps upsetting the nervous system of a female who largely stayed at home with her roosting family. Now, we understand more about CFS and note definite endocrine, immune, cardiovascular, and nervous system interplay. Underlying this condition in many cases is the presence of Lyme disease bacteria and other tick-borne organisms.

Symptoms of CFS include malaise after exertion, unrefreshed sleep, widespread muscle and joint pain, sore throat, constant or frequent headache, cognitive difficulties, chronic and severe mental and physical exhaustion, and other characteristic symptoms, such as leg tingling, blurred vision, and breathlessness in a previously healthy and active person. Additional symptoms may be reported, including muscle weakness, increased sensitivity to light, sounds, and smells, labile or low blood pressure, digestive disturbances, depression, painful and often slightly swollen lymph nodes, and cardiac and respiratory problems. CFS symptoms vary in number, type, and severity from person to person.

Having lived through seven arduous years of this condition myself, I can attest that the fatigue is so extreme that simple tasks like brushing your teeth, showering, making a sandwich, or even getting across the room from the sofa to use the bathroom feel like you are climbing Mt. Everest. Lifting your arms feels like thirty-pound weights are attached. I used to say, "Breathing is tiring," and "This feels like the worst jet lag of my life." The world spins by outside your window as you watch from inside, forlorn and deeply confused as to why you feel so weak and why nothing is helping. Your body feels like it is filled with lead, your mind layered in cottony gauze, and too many parts hurt including your plummeting spirits. Patients often end up "doctor-hopping," getting propped up on antidepressant or anti-inflammatory drugs with no real help, merely mild palliation.

The quality of life for persons with CFS can be extremely compromised. Fatigue is a common symptom in many illnesses, but in CFS it is extreme. Assorted national health organizations have estimated more than one million Americans and approximately a quarter of a million people in the UK have CFS. These estimates could be vastly below the actual count, as many people never get an actual CFS diagnosis, but instead wade through life with severe exhaustion and no clinical diagnosis. CFS occurs more often in women than men and is less prevalent among children, yet is growing among adolescents.

Although there is agreement that CFS poses genuine threats to one's health, happiness, and productivity, various physicians' groups, researchers, and patient advocates suggest differing diagnostic criteria, etiologic hypotheses, and treatments, resulting in controversy about many aspects of the disorder. The name "chronic fatigue syndrome" is controversial; many patients and advocacy groups, as well as some experts, believe the name trivializes the medical condition and they promote a name change. In fact, one study discovered the fatigue a CFS patient experiences is four times more severe than that of a person afflicted with cardiac failure!

All CFS cases should be tested at IGeneX, Clongen, or NeuroScience Labs for Lyme disease and/or coinfections. If this underlying issue is at play, there is strong hope for recovery. Additionally, integrative medicine and natural medicine modalities can restore quality of life. Mitochondria dysfunction, adrenal deficiency, thyroid imbalance, trace mineral loss, amino acid imbalance, hormone imbalances, and many more depletions can be corrected.

Also to be considered are heavy metal toxins, such as mercury and lead, which can create paralysis, MS-style conditions, and many neurocognitive problems besides deadening fatigue. Chelation therapy can remove these heavy burdens from your body. Yeast/candida overgrowth is to be evaluated, as this overgrowth of normally present, yet excessive, fungi creates massive brain fog, weakness, lethargy, and all sorts of gut issues and even learning disabilities. Mold toxins from your current environment or damage from past exposure is a very strong cornerstone for many CFS cases. Clearing up the internal toxic swamp and remediating your environment are essential. Mold issues are often a "kingpin" issue to many autoimmune and Lyme problems. Read Dr. Ritchie Shoemaker's book.

Our health begins in our gut, as the proper balance of good to bad bacteria and other flora is critical to proper immune function, digestion, energy production, and assimilation. Our omega-6 top-heavy diet, layered with sugars and additives, creates an overly acidic environment, within which there is ample room for all sorts of organisms to proliferate. Even cancers have room to grow with a below 6.0 internal pH. Balancing the "bugs" is essential with CFS/ME.

CFS has a strong overlap with retroviruses such as Epstein-Barr, cytomegalia, coxsackie, and the Chlamydia pneumonia. Retroviruses are in the same family as herpes and shingles, meaning they never actually leave your system but instead move in and out of phases of dormancy and activity. Typically they cycle in four- to six-week flares, yet can become perpetual if the immune function goes haywire, as in autoimmune conditions, and the body attacks all organisms, good and bad alike. These viruses need to be addressed in most CFS/ME cases. Likely they have moved out of latency to active phases. Have your practitioner run more detailed panels of these than the standard testing. Lauric acid, derived from coconut oil, can be very helpful in putting retroviruses into dormancy. I favor Monolaurin from Ecological Formulas for helping me regain my health.

Homeopathy is a big player in helping CFS/ME. So many remedies exist to address the trembling weakness and insomnia or the deep muscle pains or breathlessness. Remedies for acute symptomology can be used clinically or even more powerful is the able assistance of a certified classical homeopath who can seek out your born constitutional type, which denotes what type illnesses or syndromes you are prone to. Certain constitutions are prone to lupus, others to RA, no matter what the infectious agent is or what heavy metals you are burdened by. See the appendix for some easy remedy suggestions. A certified classical homeopath (CCH) is strongly encouraged to hone in on the specifics of your constitutional type and symptom state.

Metaphysics: Chakra imbalances to be focused on in your self-care revolve around 1, 3, 4, and 5. Chakras 1 and 3 are central to all cases involving muscular pain and weakness. Chakra 1 issues zero in on the balance of *doing* vs. *being* in your life. Most with CFS have been over-extending and caring for others dominantly and not being still, quiet, or tending to their own self. Ask yourself the questions, "What is too heavy for me to carry?" and "What is my calling that I am ignoring?" Please see Part V for energetic healing exercises.

CROHN'S DISEASE/IRRITABLE BOWEL SYNDROME/COLITIS

Crohn's disease was first isolated in 1932 by two doctors at Mount Sinai Hospital in New York City, who described a series of patients with inflammation of the terminal ileum of the small intestine. The illness is named after Dr. Burrell Bernard Crohn.

This illness is very painful and causes inflammation of the lining of the small intestine and bowel. It is labeled as an autoimmune disease but acts a little bit differently than most autoimmune illnesses in that most of the symptomology remains primarily in the digestive tract rather than spreading throughout the body.

Crohn's disease exists much more commonly in developed countries of the world. It is more present in Europe and North America and less in Asia and Africa or amongst communities with unprocessed and unrefined foods. Men and women are equally affected and it tends to surface in the teens and twenties, though symptoms can emerge at any age. There is a strong genetic component with over seventy genes involved and often a prior relative being afflicted. Smokers are 50 percent more prone than nonsmokers!

Gastroenteritis is often an initiating factor. Much confusion exists about Crohn's—currently there is no cure recognized by the mainstream medical community, merely pain management and surgical procedures. Corticosteroids are often used in early diagnosis and then very strong drugs like Methotrexate or Thiopurine. One in five people with the illness are admitted to the hospital each year and half of those will receive surgery for the disease at some point in a ten-year span. Abscesses, bowel obstructions, and even cancers can be part of Crohn's disease. Scar tissue after surgery leads to even more difficulties and maybe more surgery!

Symptoms include lots of severe belly pain and irregular bowel patterns, often painful cramping diarrhea, with episodes of constipation. Quality of life can become difficult for many as you feel "trapped" at home, afraid to go out to the movies, to travel, or to go to a restaurant because you have to stay near a bathroom. Being doubled over with pain is not uncommon.

When we remember that medical doctors are not trained to integrate several bodily systems together, but instead focus just on the malfunctioning part, we can see the limitations a gastroenterologist may have with Crohn's and the sister conditions of irritable bowel syndrome (IBS) and colitis.

From the lens of natural medicine we look to many factors contributing to these inflammatory digestive lining conditions. We realize that like other autoimmune disorders, the inflammation cascade has become like a runaway train and the body is apparently "turning on itself," sending signals to produce more cytokines and inflammatory agents, further destroying your natural tissues.

Crohn's, IBS, and colitis are each often triggered by chronic stress or an inciting strong stressor that caused the adrenal glands to go into overdrive, then fail into depletion. It's also essential to consider grains (wheat, barley, oats, and rye) as inflammatory antagonists. Dr. Joel Wallach, renowned for his work with diet and chronic diseases, frames "gluten intolerance" in a very clear metaphor. He says "modern" gluten is an antagonist to the average individual, and it is like the contact dermatitis reaction poison ivy has on the skin. Gluten creates a contact enteritis in the digestive tract, inflaming the lining so as to prevent it from absorbing the ingested "wayward" GMO protein molecule into the bloodstream. Most of us are of a body that does not like these "newer" GMO grains, with higher starch and gluten contents. Dairy and lactose issues must be examined, too. Other food sensitivities and the probable link to an infectious agent such as parasite or bacteria should also be questioned (we know how much inflammation borrelia, bartonella, candida, and mycoplasma can induce!). Imbalanced gut "biome"—bacteria in the wrong proportion to the body's natural levels—is a key factor. Lots of tension or bottled-up feelings are common among those diagnosed with inflammatory digestive conditions, so the emotional component must not be overlooked.

The best first step is getting to an integrative medical practitioner and/or certified clinical nutritionist. Your gut is 75 percent of your immune function and with Crohn's, IBS, or colitis, multiple imbalances have been triggered. Removing the inflammatory foods is essential for two to three months, as well as ingesting inflammation-soothing aids like aloe vera juice, papaya fruit, digestive enzymes, and/or turmeric spice in a product called curcumin should be had between meals at least twice per day. Additionally, taking a digestive enzyme formula WITH meals helps you break down and absorb the nutrients fully instead of relying solely on your malfunctioning gut. By bringing in better nourishment, in turn the body can have more source to mend.

Adding to the healthy good flora biome, from a probiotic formula, is critical to help reestablish good populations of our naturally existing bacteria in the gut, which will help clamp down other bacteria that have caused inflammation. You want a product that has multiple different strains of bacteria including bifidus and lactobacillus. You want to see the number count in the billions for each of the strains. The best probiotic formulas are those that need to be refrigerated so that the cultures remain active. It is wise to take them between meals or first thing in the morning, so they have a good chance to enter the gut before food interferes. Foods like kimchi, miso, and lacto-fermented sauerkraut also provide your gut with healthy bacteria. All the ancient diets of the world include a fermented food in their menu. Anyone who has had several courses of antibiotics, has been on birth control pills, or taken steroid drugs or acid reducers and NSAIDs has likely tipped the balance of his/her good flora so that not enough exist in the digestive tract and other antagonistic microbes have had a chance to multiply in excess.

Reducing the bad bugs is also very important—when they have crept up into the small intestine, which is supposed to be a sterile environment, that is often when we get the crippling pains and abscesses of Crohn's disease. Sometimes the problem simply may have been induced by a parasite from a trip abroad or a bout of gastroenteritis from something you picked up from one of your kids, or tainted food anywhere. There are many wonderful herbal antimicrobials that reduce the presence of parasites and bacteria. See the entire Nutramedix line, as well as the immune regulators and antimicrobials from Dr. Joel Wallach at Lyme Light Minerals. Most importantly, Crohn's is not an illness to treat on your own. You need a really top-notch integrative medicine doctor or naturopath and clinical nutritionist.

However, the good news is that with really strict dietary adjustments and using natural methods to bring down inflammation and reestablish proper functioning of the adrenal gland, which has gone haywire, as well as balancing out the healthy balance of your gut's microbiome, much mending can take place.

It is important to arrest the autoimmune switch that has been "thrown" and a classical homeopathic practitioner is often a wonderful asset in helping recalibrate the body after this state has been induced. Please read the chapter on homeopathic medicine.

Metaphysics: Metaphysically, Crohn's disease and gut issues obviously focus around chakra number three. There is a crossover link to chakra number four, though, as the immune system has become involved. Most people should look into exercises at chakra number six as well, involving the endocrine system, as the inflammation from a poorly functioning adrenal gland is linked.

Ask yourself, "What is eating at me?" or "What is eating me up inside?" If those questions do not resonate with you, consider, "What can I not assimilate in my life?" Is there someone, something, or a difficult situation that is too much for you to process and absorb emotionally and spiritually, reeking tensions and worry and angst that lodges in your "gut"? Chakras 3 and 4 are important.

Let your thoughts evaporate and take the time to be with yourself and sense the feelings that arise when you ask yourself these questions. Somewhere along the way either a very dramatic incident, or a slow accumulation of incidents, or maybe a certain relationship has brought you into an emotional state where something is perseverating inside of you that you seem to be quietly internalizing. Energetically, this has lingered too long and has become too intense to hold onto. Listen to the messages you receive and begin working with the exercises in Part VI.

FIBROMYALGIA

I recall the exact moment when I realized fibromyalgia was not just a rogue condition but something of growing concern. It was late summer 1992, and I was checking out at our local organic food store. The woman at the cashier was someone I was friendly with from step aerobic class. She was in her late twenties, pretty, athletic, and outdoorsy. Stephanie said to me, "I finally found out why I feel crummy all the time and my muscles hurt and will not recover after step class." I looked at her quizzically; I had no idea she was possibly sick, as she looked robust and rosy cheeked, with lovely honey brown hair. "Fibromyalgia."

"No way?!" I replied. "You're so young and fit—that doesn't seem right. Are you very stressed?" I knew that it was typically those burdened with lots of stress in their life that fumbled through this debilitating illness.

"Well, you could say kind of, as I'm trying to finish up grad school and am working part time, too. They're starting me on an antidepressant that is supposed to help. But I was wondering if I could come see you at the office of homeopathy?"

"Definitely, come in for an appointment. Let's get on top of this—you don't need to suffer forever."

Only two weeks prior I had given an evening talk at a fibromyalgia support group half an hour away. That group fit the typical picture of forty- and fifty-year-old women lumbering along with full body pains, on-and-off headaches, digestive issues, and general low-grade depression. Most of them were a little bit overweight and seemed just draggy and saggy, which fit into the category of my knowledge about adrenal depletion, hormonal imbalance, and food sensitivities. They also fit into a general type of constitutions that we know in classical homeopathy are prone to fibromyalgia and chronic fatigue syndrome. Stephanie was too young and vital and "out of the box" for me to fathom this diagnosis.

She responded quite well to homeopathic remedies and good adrenal support and we cut out all the starch and dairy from her diet. Within several months she was mired in her last year of grad school and I actually lost touch with her when she graduated. Her case piqued my interest, though; why should a young, healthy woman like her develop this disorder?

The decades tumble by and here we are now almost twenty-five years later, and fibromyalgia rates have exploded! Amy Myers, host of The Autoimmune Summit, says statistics show that one in fifty people in the United States are afflicted with fibromyalgia. That tallies up to 6,000,000! Conventional medicine has not been able to pinpoint the cause of this condition and manages cases basically with pain medications and antidepressant drugs. The world of natural medicine believes there's a lot more to the equation.

Dr. Kenny de Meirleir, whom I interviewed from Belgium on my program Lyme Light Radio, says that their studies prove that 97 percent of fibromyalgia and chronic fatigue cases can be definitely discerned as long-term Lyme disease and tick-borne-organisms conditions, with proper lab work, unlike the faulty lab testing we rely on.

The symptoms of fibromyalgia include persistent muscle pain, fatigue, sleep irregularities, brain fog, cognitive difficulties, depression, and a general lethargy. There are painful and tender points throughout the body that flare up in exacerbation for a week or more at a time. The condition is sometimes preceded by a flu-like episode or seems to creep up over a matter of several weeks and months, to never really let up. Other vague symptoms may circulate like digestive disturbances or dizzy spells or intolerance of certain aromatics like perfumes or gasoline fumes.

People often end up doctor-hopping with this vague constellation of complaints until someone finally diagnoses the situation as fibromyalgia. For many years, this disorder was disregarded and women who had it were labeled as hypochondriacs or were told they were imagining their problems. Then a certain class of SSRI drugs seemed to address a lot of the depression, pain, and fatigue, and when used in a low-dose manner many people feel better, but are dependent on the medication. Why has this illness soared so significantly, or is it just that it is being diagnosed more regularly?

Both sides of the coin probably come into play—denial from the medical world for decades and a plummeting status of diet and health and hormonal and other sensitive brain transmitter imbalances, in recent generations. However, through the lens of natural medicine, we can see very significant factors that come together to allow fibromyalgia to occur. The good news is that much can be done to overcome this disorder so that those suffering from it do not have to be dependent on pharmaceuticals forever. Finding a naturopath or integrative medicine doctor and acupuncturist is key. Acupuncture and Chinese herbals are very effective with fibromyalgia. So are homeopathic medicine and really solid nutritional work. Here are a few key points to address with your practitioner.

THE ADRENAL GLANDS

Known for our fight-or-flight response, the adrenal glands also make natural corticosteroids to keep inflammation down, as well as hormones and antiallergy histamines. Please read the chapter that focuses on the adrenal glands. Adrenal dysfunction is the condition that underlies fibromyalgia, as the body is not able to make enough corticosteroids to keep the muscle fascia layer inflammation at bay. When the adrenal glands are severely taxed and are prompted to secrete a large amount of corticosteroids for a primary purpose, such as an accident or an injury or an infection, they can get depleted and then cannot catch up to speed. So, chronic inflammation persists and your body cannot make the right hormones to address it. You get caught in a vicious catch-22 cycle.

THYROID

The thyroid is another endocrine gland that is known to regulate metabolism and reactions to temperature. Many of us have slightly imbalanced function of this important gland, with fatigue, depression, sleep irregularities, and muscle pain being prominent indicators. The testing that traditional doctors use looks for clinical abnormalities of the thyroid, and many people who have an underactive thyroid that is marginally noted on lab tests are flying under the radar. Iodine and the trace mineral selenium are essential to make the thyroid gland work properly. Have your doctor make sure they run the free T3 and free T4 tests as well as their standard ones and do a basal temperature reading before you get out of bed every morning for a week. Good labs like Genova are real assets to specific testing.

GLUTEN

Gluten is a huge source of inflammation for the majority of us. The type of wheat we have been eating for the past forty years is a hybrid that has been modified to have two growth and harvest cycles per season, versus the old heirloom strains our relatives ate a hundred years ago that were a taller plant with only one harvest cycle. This hybrid we are eating has much more starch and a higher gluten content. The majority of us are gluten sensitive, not intolerant (the latter provokes celiac disease). Spelt or millet or organic corn products are safer choices for most of us.

MOLDS

Exposure to mold can damage the thyroid and create a toxic brew internally in your system. Some of us are very susceptible to mold toxicities and spore counts. A good testing company from RealTime Labs runs a urine mycotoxin test to evaluate if you have been exposed to toxic mold. I had to move out of a house that had toxic mold, because it was causing migraines and fibromyalgia symptoms, which then contributed to setting me up for a very severe case of neurological Lyme disease. Many people have found that toxic mold is causing or contributing to their fibromyalgia.

YEAST OVERGROWTH

The most common yeast-related condition is candida, which many of us remember from vaginal yeast infections. When yeast, a naturally occurring microorganism, becomes overproduced, the candida create toxic by-products that then give you a fuzzy-headed feeling of brain fog plus fatigue and lots of digestive issues, often along with body pain. Sugar, carbs, and birth control pills or repeated antibiotic use can all contribute to yeast overgrowth. An anti-candida diet (low sugar, low starch, and no caffeine) will help, along with candida-reducing products such as Candibactin from Metagenics.

MAGNESIUM

Magnesium helps muscles and our nervous system. Many of us have depleted magnesium levels because our soils are lacking in nutrient content. In addition, our diets often make our bodies too acidic, which causes us to lose many of our minerals. Magnesium is one of the master minerals our body needs to function properly. Taking magnesium citrate will often eliminate muscle pain and fatigue surprisingly quickly! Start with 800 or 1,000 mg per day and up the dose until you get loose stools; that is the signal that you were taking a little bit too much and should back down until stools are proper consistency. Shockingly, I needed 1,600 mg per day of magnesium for over two years when I was overcoming CFS, Lyme disease, and fibromyalgia.

VITAMIN D

We have discovered the hard way in recent generations that we are severely lacking in vitamin D, particularly in the Northern Hemisphere at the higher latitudes. Long gone are the days of fresh cream, herring, kippers, sardines, and cod liver oil, all loaded with vitamin D. We also wear sunblock that prevents vitamin D from being produced by the skin. Anything over screen level #8 blocks out vitamin D absorption, so take twenty minutes of sunscreen-free sunshine daily, then apply your lotion. Vitamin D is one of the primary supports for a healthy immune system as well as for nourishing the brain and producing healthy neurotransmitters. Low vitamin D brings upon depression, alcoholism, skin issues, and seasonal affective disorder very quickly.

LIVER STAGNATION

My fourth-generation Chinese physician used to take my pulses when I was very ill and say, "Stagnant liver." At first, I had no idea what she was talking about. Later I learned it meant my liver was not cleansing the bloodstream effectively and a lot of toxic debris was being accumulated in this giant filter. Many people who do not have enough of a critical molecule called glutathione, and do not properly produce the enzymes to help detoxify and purge, will experience this condition. Liver "stagnation" includes body pains, especially around the upper back, shoulders, and neck, headaches and lethargy, dullness of mind, and loping depression. You don't feel like doing anything, have no ambition, and nothing feels quite right. Getting the liver going is a big turnaround for fibromyalgia patients. Milk thistle in synergistic blend with other herbs like dandelion, plus alpha lipoic acid or glutathione supplements help enormously. See Pure Encapsulations and Integrative Therapeutics formulas.

A classical homeopath will be a great asset to you, and may recommend liver drainage products available from BioResources Inc. or Mountain State Health Products. Many brilliant Chinese herbal formulas can cleanse "stagnant liver" and mobilize energy production again readily.

Metaphysics: Reflect on, "What is immobilizing me?" "Why is it too painful to make a move?" "What creative work have I been ignoring that feeds my heart?" Chakras 3 and 4 are in dire need of energetic assistance. Look into chakras 1 and 5 (the endocrine system), too.

INTERSTITIAL CYSTITIS

Until you have had a bladder infection you probably don't realize how sensitive this organ is. Located in the lower abdomen, the bladder is a fist-sized balloon organ that collects the intercellular waste products our body produces and all the liquids our kidney filters. Typically, we urinate approximately seven times in twenty-four hours. The bladder fills and releases the urine, exiting through a slim tube-like structure called the urethra, which is a mere three inches long in females and six or more inches long in males. A common urinary tract or bladder infection can cause searing pain, urging and frequency of urination, and enormous localized discomfort. Typically, E. coli bacteria, normally residing in the lower bowel and rectum, have migrated up the urethra into the bladder setting up the infection. Sexual intercourse, wiping the "wrong" direction after a bowel movement, or even hot, sweltering weather can induce an acute UTI.

Sometimes, chronic bladder and/or urethra pain occurs. Multiple tests later and many months of suffering often surmount with an interstitial cystitis diagnosis, now considered to be part of the autoimmune category of conditions. This problem has been growing significantly in the last twenty years and is more common in females.

Interstitial or chronic **bladder pain syndrome** (also **IC/BPS**) is a chronic inflammatory condition of the submucosal and muscular layers of the bladder. The cause of IC/BPS is currently unknown in conventional medicine and the condition is regarded as a diagnosis of exclusion. IC/BPS symptoms include urinary frequency, urinary pain, repeated waking at night to urinate, and sterile urine cultures. Those with interstitial cystitis may have symptoms that overlap with other urinary bladder disorders such as urinary tract infection (UTI), urethritis (inflammation of the urethra), overactive bladder, and prostatitis. Yeast and sexually transmitted disease infections can also induce IC-type symptoms.

IC can be extremely compromising for a person, interfering with daily abilities, and sexual relations. IC/BPS can escalate to a quality of life comparable to that of a patient with rheumatoid arthritis, chronic cancer pain, or a patient on kidney dialysis.

In our natural healthcare model, we return again to the antagonists of chronic inflammation. All these disorders circulate around the same central themes: allergens (often food sensitivities), microbes, toxins, depletions, stress (physical and emotional), and diet. IC has a very strong crossover to two issues—food intolerances (gluten, dairy, soy, corn) and Lyme bacteria and specific coinfection of the bartonella bacteria and/or mycoplasma organism. Urinary issues, specifically IC, are classic indicators of bartonella, mycoplasma, and Lyme infections residing in the mucosal lining of the bladder and urethra, which house abundant nerve receptor sites. Besides the fact that these organisms love to inhabit the mucous membranes of the body, bartonella and mycoplasma in particular settle into the bladder walls. The ILADS annual conference, San Diego, CA, 2013 highlighted this subject with doctor presentation/discussion. Dr. Stephen Harold Buhner's book, *Healing Lyme Disease Coinfections*, discusses these organisms' breadth and depth of damage in detail.

Specific testing from the state-of-the-art Lyme disease and co-infection labs can potentially turn your life around, with the help of a Lyme-literate practitioner. If this infection can be reduced, the inflammation cascade arrested, and antagonistic foods eliminated while anti-inflammatory ones are supplied, mending is fully possible.

The other strong offender in IC is yeast and fungi overgrowth. This can often be systemic after multiple earlier rounds of antibiotics for apparent UTIs for so-called "chronic" ones. Most urologists do not use testing to look for systemic fungal infections. At best, you will get a practitioner who looks for mold or candida spores in a urine culture. Many do not even do this. Consider RealTime Labs' urine mycotoxin test that will screen for a variety of strains. If yeast/fungi is a factor, this could explain much of your story and can be addressed with thorough cleanses and detoxification, and of course repopulating the digestive tract with healthy bacteria through ultra-rich probiotic formulas.

Metaphysics: Look to chakras 2 and 4. Reflect on, what is so "urgent" in your life or emotions that you are not prioritizing? Also, ask, "What am I holding onto that it makes me burn with pain?" Emotional toxins reside in chakra 2 as well as the fluid waste system. Relationship issues are up for examination in this chakra of intimacy and bonds. Some bonds we hold are very deep, but not always so "clean." Wounds, patterns, and history "hold" us in certain ways. IC is screaming to you loud and clear in this realm.

LUPUS

Systemic lupus erythematosus (SLE) is one of the most diagnosed autoimmune illnesses in the world. Like so many of these disorders, there is not one exact, specific test but a conglomerate of findings from which doctors deduce the diagnosis. Symptoms are, in some ways, very similar to CFS, fibromyalgia, and MS with a slight variation, the primary one being no sign of demyelination on the nerve sheaths.

If you complain of consistent fatigue, headaches, joint pain and swelling, hair loss, anemia, fever, a "classic" butterfly-shaped rash across the nose and cheeks, edema, photosensitivity, ulcers in the mouth and nose, or Raynaud's disease, physicians are likely to pinpoint lupus. Obviously, multiple systems of the body are involved here and symptoms can come and go in cyclical fashion. The heart, kidneys, joints, and skin can be affected from an overwrought immune system.

Doctors look for internal and external organs that are inflamed, including the skin, kidneys, and circulatory system. There are specific autoimmune inflammation tests they check, such as these cited from the Lupus Foundation of America:

ANTIBODY BLOOD TESTS

The body uses antibodies to attack and neutralize foreign substances, such as bacteria and viruses. The antibodies your body makes against its own normal cells and tissues play a large role in lupus, and other autoimmune diseases. Many of these antibodies are found in a panel or group of tests that are ordered together. The test you will hear about most is called the antinuclear antibodies test, referred to as the ANA test.

Antinuclear antibodies connect or bind to the nucleus or command center of the cell. This process damages cells and can destroy them. While the antinuclear antibody is not a specific test for lupus, it is sensitive and does detect the antibodies that are present in 97 percent of people with the disease.

The ANA can be positive in people with other illnesses or positive in people with no illness. Test results can also fluctuate in the same person. However, lupus is usually the diagnosis when these antinuclear antibodies are found in your blood.

In addition to the ANA, doctors trying to diagnose lupus often look for the following specific antibodies:

Antibodies to double-stranded DNA (anti-dsDNA): These antibodies attack the DNA, the genetic material inside the cell nucleus. Anti-dsDNA antibodies are found in half of the people with lupus, but lupus can still be present even if these antibodies are not detected.

Antibodies to histone: Histone is a protein that surrounds the DNA molecule. These antibodies are sometimes present in people with lupus, but are more often seen in people with drug-induced lupus. This form of lupus is caused by certain medications, and usually goes away after the medication is stopped.

Antibodies to phospholipids (aPLs): These antibodies can cause narrowing of blood vessels, leading to blood clots in the legs or lungs, which can cause stroke, heart attack, or miscarriage. The most commonly measured aPLs are lupus anticoagulant, anticardiolipin antibody, and anti-beta-2 glycoprotein I. Nearly 30 percent of people with lupus will test positive for antiphospholipid antibodies. Phospholipids found in lupus are also found in syphilis, a spirochete like Lyme, and the blood test cannot always tell the difference between the two diseases (or Lyme disease). A positive result to a syphilis test does not mean that you have or have ever had syphilis. Approximately 20 percent of those with lupus will have a false-positive syphilis test result (consider Lyme disease, too).

Antibodies to Ro/SS-A and La/SS-B (Ro and La are the names of proteins in the cell nucleus): These antibodies are often found in people with Sjögren's syndrome. Anti-Ro antibodies in particular will be found in people with a form of cutaneous (skin) lupus that causes a rash that is very sun-sensitive. It is especially important for your doctor to look for the Ro and La antibodies if you are pregnant, as both autoantibodies can cross the placenta and cause neonatal lupus in the infant. Neonatal lupus is rare and not usually dangerous, but it can be serious in some cases.

Antibodies to Sm: These antibodies target Sm proteins in the cell nucleus. Found in 30 to 40 percent of people with lupus, the presence of this antibody almost always means that you have lupus.

Antibodies to RNP: These antibodies target ribonucleoproteins, which help control chemical activities of the cells. Anti-RNPs are present in many autoimmune conditions and will be at very high levels in people whose symptoms combine features of several diseases, including lupus.

OTHER BLOOD TESTS

Some blood tests measure levels of proteins that are not antibodies. The levels of these proteins can alert your doctor that there is inflammation somewhere in your body.

COMPLEMENT

Complement proteins protect the body from infection by strengthening the body's immune reactions. Complement proteins are used up by the inflammation caused by lupus, which is why people with inflammation due to active lupus often have low complement levels. There are nine protein groups of complement, so complement is identified by the letter C and the numbers 1 through 9. The most common complement tests for lupus are CH50, C3, and C4. CH50 measures the overall function of complement in the blood. Low levels of C3 or C4 may indicate active lupus. A new combination blood test is using a subset of the C4, called C4d, to help physicians "rule in" lupus and "rule out" other diseases and conditions. C4a is often used to detect levels of inflammation in those with chronic illness. The higher the value, the higher the inflammation. (This is an important test to study when Lyme disease is a suspect in lupus.)

C-REACTIVE PROTEIN (CRP)

High levels of CRP, a protein produced by the liver, may mean you have inflammation due to lupus or any other chronic illness or infection. High CRP can lead to cardiovascular disease.

ERYTHROCYTE SEDIMENTATION RATE (ESR OR "SED" RATE)

The ESR test measures the amount of a protein that makes the red blood cells clump together. The sed rate is usually high in people with active lupus, but can also be high due to other reasons such as an infection or inflammation like Lyme disease or a coinfection.

BLOOD-CLOTTING-TIME TESTS

The rate at which your blood begins to clot is important. If it clots too easily, a blood clot (thrombus) could break free and travel through the body. Blood clots can cause damage such as a stroke or miscarriage. If your blood does not clot quickly enough, you could be at risk for excessive bleeding if you are injured (common with Lyme disease, especially if the mother is a Lyme carrier, leading to possible SID in babies and stillbirths. See research and findings of Dr. Joseph Burrascano).

Prothrombin Time (PT): This test measures blood clotting and can show whether you may be at risk for not clotting quickly enough at the site of a wound.

Partial Thromboplastin Time (PTT): This test also measures how long it takes your blood to begin to clot.

Modified Russell viper venom time (RVVT), platelet neutralization procedure (PNP), and kaolin clotting time (KCT) are more sensitive blood-clotting-time tests.

Fibrinogen: Measures the level of fibrin in the blood. If high the risk of blood clot increases. Fibrin is also a component of biofilm, which is formed by many bacteria and fungi to hide in and avoid detection by the immune system. This is the mechanism by which infection persists. Tick-borne organisms are known to populate biofilm. No conventional treatment can reach bugs that are hiding in biofilm (outside-the-box thinking includes energy frequency modalities).

URINE TESTS

Urine tests are very important because lupus can attack the kidneys, often without warning signs. The kidneys process your body's waste materials. Testing a sample of urine (called a "spot urine" test) can reveal problems with the way your kidneys are functioning.

The most common urine tests look for cell casts (bits of cells that normally would be removed when your blood is filtered through your kidneys) and proteinuria (protein being spilled into your body because your kidneys are not filtering the waste properly). A collection of your urine over a twenty-four-hour period can also give important information.

The common conventional medicine approach is, of course, to squelch unpleasant symptoms. Typically a diuretic or pain medicine will be started, along with an anti-inflammatory corticosteroid like

Prednisone or cortisone. If these measures do not work, then the more powerful pharmaceuticals that suppress the immune system are turned to such as Plaquenil and Enbril. If there is underlying infection, then use of steroids and immune system suppressants can make treating them more challenging. And, make the person feel worse.

All medications have potential side effects, including blood disorders, cancer development, susceptibility to infection, kidney stress and failure, and muscle atrophy. Generally speaking, it is a cat-and-mouse game of trying to stay ahead of the symptoms with rotating medications and a lifelong dependency.

Without a shadow of a doubt all lupus cases should be examined by a Lyme-literate physician! The crossover component to infectious microbes being an underlying factor with this illness is chronicled again and again in clinical settings by practitioners well versed in this topic. Once again I refer to the brilliant work detailed in Dr. Richard Horowitz's book, *Why Can't I Get Better? Solving the Mystery of Lyme & Chronic Disease.* His understanding of these autoimmune disorders and chronic illness as pertains to tick-borne diseases could shape the future of healthcare.

In addition, the Epstein-Barr Virus (EBV), a retrovirus that caused mononucleosis when we were younger, can start to have cyclical breakouts like the herpes virus. EBV in a chronic form is a player in fibromyalgia, chronic fatigue syndrome, lupus, and many states of Lyme disease. For several generations, doctors have believed that once you test positive for this virus, you will always test positive and there is no use trying to monitor the organism. However, more subtle testing can indicate when the virus is in remission or active or in what we call convalescent stage.

Typical six-week breakout cycles are common; however, when the immune system becomes very compromised and we have other issues complicating the picture, EBV can then become chronic. You may manifest with an autoimmune-style disorder. More research is needed in this arena of all viral infections. Good news comes in the form of lauric acid, which is derived from coconut oil, with a helpful product called Monolaurin by Ecological Formulas, and could be of great help for those afflicted with lupus. Please seek out those specialty labs for testing. Some doctors would prefer to put you on an antiviral pharmaceutical, which does help many people at least temporarily, but may not treat the underlying issues. There are several antivirals specifically for retrovirus that might be of benefit also. However, there are several herbals that are antiviral, and for the long haul, herbals have fewer long-term side effects, unlike antiviral medicines.

Besides an infectious microbial component, there are other underlying issues at hand to cause the autoimmune condition of lupus to surface. Mold exposure and the toxins they produce can be devastating and have the same symptoms as Lyme, CFS, fibromyalgia, some viral infections, and autoimmune disorders. Most doctors do not know to use the sensitive lab testing for mycotoxins and instead merely look for spores. See RealTime Labs for their state-of-the-art urine test for mold toxin.

The issue of gluten and other food intolerances is critical with lupus! As we have highlighted, gluten can create all sorts of inflammation and pain, cognitive issues, sleep disturbances, neurological symptoms, fatigue, and depression when we ingest it daily. All carbohydrates also turn to sugar in short order and then give us energy ups and downs and cravings for more sugar and carbohydrates. Our neurotransmitters become involved, as well as the adrenal glands and pancreas. A whole yo-yo of associated symptoms surface, in addition to the toxins, making us feel sick and creating many lupus symptoms. *10-Day Detox Diet* by Dr. Mark Hyman is a great book to explore this issue in full.

Heavy metals, specifically mercury and lead, create all kinds of symptoms in our body and are a significant factor with chronic fatigue syndrome, all the autoimmune illnesses, and many neurological conditions. Heavy metal exposure needs to be examined closely. Chelation therapy may be helpful for many lupus patients.

The ever-dominant issue of yeast and candida domination must also be addressed. Overgrowth of candida and other fungi can occur when your gut flora become unbalanced and your beneficial bacteria are overwhelmed or die off due to antibiotic use. Then any starch or sugar you eat becomes available food for these organisms and they multiply in excess creating bloating, gas, stool irregularities, and severe fatigue, headaches, rashes, and more typical lupus symptoms. Cleansing the system of candida can take months, even with dietary changes and the help of supplements like Candibactin, oregano oil, berberine, and caprylic acid. Systemic yeast is a big issue with lupus, especially when the butterfly rash is present. The diet can feel very limiting, and you may want to give up, but please do forge on, as once you get your flora rebalanced in your gut, your health can change in a dramatic way for the better!

Adrenal gland involvement, especially adrenal fatigue, is a component of autoimmune illnesses and other chronic problems. Stress in today's world, as the early portion of this book portrays, is a staple for most of us and we pump out adrenaline (cortisol) every day, all day and night. This wreaks havoc throughout the body and mind. Mindfulness and learning how to center ourselves and decompress are essential in the modern world. We must also learn how to find quiet time, reflection, and meditation to help heal these tender glands. There are great supplements to nourish and support the adrenals, like vitamin C and vitamin D3. Additionally, adrenal glandular products like Adrenaplex from EuroMedica are very helpful.

Integrative medicine practitioners, naturopaths, acupuncturists, and homeopaths are well versed in lupus. A bright future awaits you and hopefully you can rebuild the depletions and overcome damages that have been induced to regain a quality of life that is unlimited.

Metaphysics: Lupus involves every chakra! Do all the exercises in Part VI. Most important is chakra 4. Lupus, like Lyme, asks for a full life makeover. You are being asked to take a major "time out"—the old grid you are living upon is not working for you any more. Deep reflection, stillness, and evaluation are asked of you. "What is my heart calling for?" Are you really feeding the true essence of your purpose in this lifetime? What dreams and creative urgings have you ignored, shelved, or felt you could not find time to focus on? This is very real, lifesaving information for you to explore. Seek a spiritual healer, go on a weekend retreat, attend a workshop, or even find a life coach. There is ample room and space inside of your soul to explore ways to follow your passion and your heart. You are too precious to ignore. Lupus wants you to let go of old ways, thoughts, and beliefs and begin to dream and create your new tomorrow, your new path, and your healthier future.

MULTIPLE SCLEROSIS

Multiple sclerosis is a condition that affects the nerves and brain of a vastly growing population. It appears more frequently in the Northern Hemisphere of the world with a suspicious link to low vitamin D3 levels, Lyme disease, C. pneumonia, and other tick-borne organisms.

The diagnosis is made clinically, usually by a process of exclusion from other illnesses. There is no specific lab test to confirm MS. The leading characteristic symptoms are numbness and tingling in the extremities and vision problems—sometimes simply blurred vision and other times, complete blindness. Weakness in the legs and muscle tremors are common, as are balance issues. Any part of the body that receives innervation can be affected.

Some people deteriorate consistently over time while others plateau or even go in and out of cycles of remission and activity commonly called "flares." A mild fever sometimes accompanies these outbreaks and the state is reminiscent of malaria, with relapsing fevers and sweats. (A tick-borne organism called the babesia is often aligned with these states, along with Chlamydia pneumonia and borrelia relapsing fevers.)

Physicians look at MRI scans to evaluate demyelinization of the myelin sheath, the protective layer covering the nerves and brain, depicted as white spots on an MRI. True MS typically manifests with numerous white lesions in the brain and the spinal nerves, (not just a few random spots), specifically in the cervical and thoracic areas. These white spots are also found in bartonella infection. Many transient symptoms come and go with MS patients. One of the most notable is intolerance to heat and humidity, as well as a relationship to lunar cycles (suggesting parasites or worms?). Pain and headaches can also occur.

MS along with RA are among the most frequently misdiagnosed conditions in the autoimmune spectrum with a crossover to Lyme disease and tick-borne coinfections. In fact, the symptom of weakness in the extremities with tingling, along with fatigue and white spots on brain MRIs, are often the same for Lyme and bartonella as for MS. The problem is most neurologists are extremely under-educated about proper testing and diagnosis for Lyme disease and the coinfections. The Western blot test, done at IGeneX Lab, is the best for confirming the diagnosis of Lyme. The confirmation of a diagnosis for Lyme requires positive bands on the Western blot test that are specific for Lyme and include bands 18, 23 to 25, 28, 31,34, 39, and 83 to 93. The CDC requires that an Elisa Antibody test be done for Lyme before the Western blot, which is usually a false negative test about 65 to 75 percent of the time. In actuality, Lyme disease is easily missed with this type of test. If a patient comes up with only one of the positive bands specific for Lyme, the CDC does not qualify this as a positive Lyme case, as they require at least five-plus bands on the IgG and three-plus on the IgM test. Actually, confirmation of any one of these bands suggests Lyme (see lab testing chapter). Unfortunately, most doctors will skip the Lyme testing and diagnose the patient with MS, proceeding to prescribe strong pharmaceuticals that may produce many side effects without true healing. These medications can also impact the ability of someone to recover from Lyme if they have it as the underlying illness, by destroying the immune system further.

Known as the "great imitator," Lyme disease is capable of creating inflammation anywhere in the body, and MS symptoms are a vivid example of the potential of these organisms inducing central nervous system involvement. There are other culprit organisms that ticks (and vector insects like red ants, mosquitos, and fleas) inject into our bloodstream, which include mycoplasma, Chlamydia pneumonia, erhlichia, borrelia relapsing fevers, and bartonella. Mara Williams, author of *Nature's Dirty Needle*, cites, "C. pneumonia has been identified as an instigator of central nervous issues and a trigger for MS, but for some reason, few doctors seem to consider this." If you have an MS diagnosis and haven't fully ruled out Lyme, find a Lyme-literate physician, ideally someone trained by the famous International Lyme and Associated Diseases Society (ILADS).

There are a few other factors that underscore this chronic autoimmune-style disorder. As we know, all these conditions require multiple modalities for recovery. Contributing factors that need to be assessed include heavy metal toxicities in your system, particularly mercury and lead, which are known to damage the nerves and creep up to the spine with progression to the brain. Lead and copper piping lead to heavy metal toxicity. Also, some vaccines still contain mercury (thimerosal) and dental fillings are also responsible for mercury leaching in the system. The good news is, chelation therapy can help eliminate heavy metal toxins. Specialty lab blood testing and hair analysis can help identify your heavy-metal toxic load. Use of zeolite clay and cilantro help to pull heavy metals out of the tissues.

Another factor is B12 deficiency, which classically creates tingling and numbness in hands, feet, and extremities, as well as weakness and fatigue. This can be corrected with B12 injections. B12 is water-soluble and can be depleted readily with even minor levels of stress and a strictly vegetarian diet. B-complex vitamins are a must in our modern world. Remember, not all supplements are created equal. You want to find either methylcobalamin or hydroxycobalamin for B12 and folate, and P5P for B6, not folic acid.

An integrative physician or natural healthcare practitioner will have access to very subtle, accurate metabolic profile analysis tests and they know how to run mineral vitamin deficiency testing as well. Magnesium depletion is often a factor in MS, as the muscles and nerves of the body are nourished by this mineral and it is heavily leached out of our soils and food sources. Repetitive migraine headaches and epileptic seizures can also be indicative of a magnesium deficiency.

One woman I met from Norway had close to one hundred lesions on her brain and spine with so-called classical MS. Over a six-year period of treating with antimicrobial herbs and restorative work at the level of depletions, all of the lesions have disappeared and she has gone from bedridden to extremely active, working, and traveling again. Go Laila!

Metaphysics: Chakras 1, 3, 4, and 7 should be nurtured. Questions to reflect on are, "Why have I abandoned my inner authority or wisdom?" and "Do I bear a broken 'link' to spirituality?" "Why am I unable to move forward with my life's passion or creative work?" Think about this. Remove the BLOCK! Or start thinking about how to. Sometimes there is a shocking or upsetting incident that occurred before your symptoms surfaced. If you have ocular symptoms think about what you "saw" or witnessed that frightened, upset, or shocked you.

There is a great deal of work that can be done at the spiritual and metaphysical levels to help recalibrate an obviously disturbed seventh-crown chakra as well as the emotional underpinnings that develop after years of struggling with any chronic illness. There is too much good work available out there in the world for you to have to suffer endlessly—keep seeking!

RHEUMATOID ARTHRITIS

The majority of individuals with rheumatoid arthritis recall a "flu-like" illness state when their complaints first surfaced. My former sister-in-law, as well as many clients and friends, recount a fever with joint pains, fatigue, and headaches or swollen glands or a sore throat days for weeks before the more smoldering joint pain surfaced. Yet, most physicians do not connect the dots with the so-called suspicious flu-like condition and the persistent RA state. Pregnancy and menopause can also incite RA. The most current-minded physicians and practitioners recognize multiple issues coalesce with this illness.

As the years progress with RA, your joints can become so severely inflamed that even the simplest tasks, like brushing your teeth, opening a car door, or stepping out of bed in the morning onto the floor, are impossible. RA can make you wheelchair- and bed-bound. Once afflicted, traditional medicine has rare success in eradicating the illness, and palliative treatments involving chemicals as extreme as chemotherapy (metholtrexate) suspend a person in dependency and flare-ups for a lifetime.

Symptoms and severity of rheumatoid arthritis can vary from person to person, but common signs include joint pain, swelling, tenderness, stiffness and deformity in the joints or fingers, nodules or stiff bumps under the skin, fatigue, unintentional weight loss, and frequent urinary tract infections. Fever is common at onset.

Clinically, rheumatoid arthritis (RA) is defined as an autoimmune condition that occurs when the body begins attacking the joints, mistaking cells of the lining as foreign invaders. The body attacks the thin membrane surrounding joints, allowing fluid and immune complexes to build up in the joints and cause significant pain. Normally, these immune complexes filter out of your blood naturally, but when there is a buildup, they tend to settle into different joints and cause local inflammation and tissue damage. When these immune complexes build up in the joints, they can induce pain, stiffness, and swelling characteristic of RA. The inflammation prompts MORE fighter cells and then the situation cycles around again and again, triggering the autoimmune switch to flip!

Typically, RA appears first in the small joints of the hands, fingers, and toes. From there it progresses to larger joints like the wrists, ankles, knees, and hips. Shoulders, neck, and the spinal vertebrae can be afflicted, too. The pain and swelling are usually on both sides of the body or in bilateral joints. In some people, the joint pains migrate once the illness has become entrenched, meaning some days your knee and elbow can be inflamed and a few days later, the pains migrate to another location, like the hip or wrist. Weather, foods, stress, and menstrual cycles can induce symptom aggravation. Many women go into remission during pregnancy.

If someone in your family has RA or any autoimmune disease, then you are more likely to develop RA in your lifetime. Genetic constitutional predispositions create such tendencies. According to Dr. Amy Myers, if you have already been diagnosed with RA, then you are three times more likely to develop a second autoimmune condition. Additionally, she states, studies using identical twins found that genetics only account for 25 percent and environmental factors account for 75 percent of all autoimmune conditions (www.AutoImmuneSummit.com).

Making a traditional orthodox diagnosis for RA is based on a combination of symptoms, plus a physical exam and blood tests.

Typically, the doctor will order one or more of the following blood tests to look for signs of inflammation as well as autoimmunity issues: Anti-nuclear antibody (ANA), rheumatoid factor (RF), anti-citrullinated peptide/protein antibodies (anti-CCP), erythrocyte sedimentation rate (ESR), or high-sensitivity C-reactive protein (Cardio CRP). An x-ray of the affected joint or joints may also be ordered. Most physicians or rheumatologists do not ordinarily run the Lyme disease and coinfection tests. If they do, 99 percent will use a commercial lab that relies on the 70 percent inaccurate ELISA test and a very limiting CDC criterion Western blot Lyme test, concluding you do *not* have Lyme disease, even if you do. They also do not typically screen for the instigating tick- and other insect-borne microorganisms mycoplasma and bartonella.

Millions of cases of RA actually pertain to an underlying microbial infection rarely diagnosed accurately. Dr. Richard Horowitz and Dr. Joel Wallach both cite mycoplasma infections as a key initial inciting incidence of RA. They have demonstrated curative success by treating this underlying infectious microbe, which would account for that initial "flu-like" incident so many people recall. Way back in the 1930s, Dr. Thomas McPherson Brown isolated mycoplasma as the link to RA.

History: The Road Back Foundation, in Boston, MA, has focused on the infectious illness component as well as the research and methodologies of the late Dr. Thomas McPherson Brown. His groundbreaking work illuminated the mycoplasma organism to trigger the inflammatory joint and autoimmune condition of RA as well as connective tissue diseases like lupus and scleroderma. But, in the same era, the powerful drug cortizone was created, prompting physicians to jump on using this "wonder drug" with its quick-fix effects of squelching fiery inflammation versus following Dr. Brown's studies and theory.

His initial book *The Road Back* and then decades later *The New Arthritis Breakthrough* by Henry Scammell illuminated Dr. Brown's work and success with low-dose doxycycline (minocycline) to eradicate the mycoplasma infection. Cutting-edge practitioners in the Lyme disease/tick-borne disease arena understand the interplay of mycoplasma with RA and certain autoimmune conditions and treat the mycoplasma infection as well as address the associated issues of gluten and food sensitivities, adrenal compromise, possible heavy metal and environmental toxicities, and the other autoimmune triggers highlighted in earlier chapters. Without a shadow of a doubt, mycoplasma, the parasite bartonella, and Lyme disease infections *must* be examined with RA. Visit Dr. Joel Wallach's website www.LymeLightMinerals.com to learn more about the correlation between RA and microbial infections, plus the value of addressing trace mineral depletions, alongside immune system recalibration.

Metaphysics: RA patients will find chakras 1 and 3 to be key targets to work on at the inner personal energetic level. However, looking through The Map (see page 317) you will discover that other chakras are pertinent, too. Chakras 4 and 6 are secondary for RA patients. Think about and reflect on these questions: "What immobilizes me?" "What prevents me from making a move or hurts too much to make a move?"

THYROID: GRAVES' DISEASE AND HASHIMOTO'S THYROIDITIS

The thyroid is a prominent player in the masterful symphony of our endocrine system. Situated in the front of the neck close to the clavicle bones, this gland is responsible for running our metabolism and is linked in to how much energy we feel as well as sleep patterns, skin, hair, and sexual libido. The thyroid contains three lobes and also a smaller portion called the parathyroid.

Many of us have heard of the thyroid gland, but we do not realize how very sensitive it is and that sadly it is one of the most vulnerable glands in our entire body, easily becoming injured or malfunctioning. I often think of it as the canary in the coal mine, as this wondrous gland screens so much for us at the level of toxins, food intolerances, stress, and emotions. One simple mineral deficiency can throw the entire function off! Additionally, any inciting stressor from our tumultuous lifestyle, or even a shocking event, can trigger the thyroid to go awry.

The typical doctor or endocrinologist uses tests that look at clinical abnormalities only. This means they use a blood-testing reference range that looks for unbalanced results that are significant enough to indicate the thyroid has developed "pathological" cellular changes. If these tests indicate your thyroid is off-kilter, it means your thyroid has been malfunctioning to such a degree that it can't run properly at all, and often drugs such as Synthroid are used to help it perform its basic function. The problem with this method of testing is that the refinement is not there to pick up subtleties of thyroid imbalance at what we call the subclinical or pre-pathological state. In other words, your thyroid might not be running at 100 percent and because of this you are feeling some symptoms, but most tests are not finely tuned enough to show any problems. I suffered with this issue for decades!

In my early twenties I had terrible anxiety, could not sleep properly, was starving all the time, and my digestive tract was irritated. I became a nervous wreck and actually ended up vomiting on many occasions over a six-month period. The regular thyroid test suggested nothing wrong, but inside I sensed something was not right, including the fact that I had terrible neck pain. Coincidentally, when I had an injection of radioactive iodine for a CAT scan of my neck, my mother and I both noticed that within thirty minutes my anxiety, hunger, and digestive issues disappeared. The scan showed no irregularities, but the doctor confirmed that in some cases the dose of iodine is enough to reset someone's thyroid!

My mother's sister was a string-bean skinny woman like I was, and we all chalked it up to our thyroids tending to run a little bit on the fast side. Little did we know I had most likely been infected with Lyme disease a month or two prior when I had a wicked migraine and severe bout of neck inflammation that lasted for almost a year, and the bacteria was attacking my thyroid too! I had accidentally fallen on homeopathic medicine and within a matter of a few months all of my symptomology cleared up and I was on a healthy track of vitality for the next twenty years.

However, when I went crashing down in the summer of 2000, with a second infection of Lyme disease that did not get diagnosed for another five years, leaving me bedridden and maimed at all levels, I also developed symptoms of what we would now call hypothyroid—extreme lethargy and fatigue along with weight gain and water retention, irregular sleep patterns, shedding of my hair, anxiety alternating with depression, and sweats in the night. I kept harping on every doctor I saw that I felt like my thyroid was not running right. They would run tests and say, "No, Katina, your thyroid is just fine." However, my body temperature, when I tested it first thing in the morning on waking, was always very low—less than 98°—a spot-on indicator for low thyroid function.

The PhD clinical nutritionist, who finally discovered the hidden Lyme bacteria underlying the nightmare of chronic fatigue syndrome, fibromyalgia, irritable bowel syndrome, and constant migraines, had my regular GP run a reverse T3 test. This test is not commonly used by GPs or even many endocrinologists and is often the one, along with a free T4 test, that discovers peripheral thyroid malfunction. This means that certain hormones are not being probably converted into the thyroid T3 and T4 that need to make it run properly. So I was correct: I was limping along at half speed.

The good news is that the thyroid responded beautifully to many supportive modalities of natural medicine—selenium was a huge helpmate! But the sad truth is that millions of Americans are suffering with imbalanced thyroid function. If you stand in line at any grocery store or shopping mall or even at an athletic event you will notice that at least half of our population is overweight. Besides the imbalance in our diet of too many carbohydrates, sugars, and hydrogenated fats, the fact of the matter is that many of us have sluggish thyroids and do not even realize it.

Dr. Mark Hyman says that figures calculate one in five women and one in ten men have thyroid problems, translating to 30,000,000 women and 15,000,000 men in the United States! This gentle yet intrinsic endocrine gland could be a kingpin to why many of your symptoms exist, and is definitely a root cause issue of many of the autoimmune illnesses. There are two very frank thyroid conditions that fall in the autoimmune classifications that are specific to the thyroid: Graves' disease and Hashimoto's thyroiditis. Both involve inflammation states of the thyroid whereby proper hormones are not being produced in correct proportions and, like all the autoimmune illnesses, the body has become non-discriminating and has started to attack its own tissues.

Graves' indicates an overactive thyroid, running your metabolism too quickly and hyping you up, then burning you out. And, Hashimoto's is the opposite; a flagging thyroid often producing lemon-sized goiter swellings of the neck. Mainstream medicine uses drugs, while natural medicine looks to all our means of rebalancing this delicate gland, changing the diet, adding in minerals such as potassium iodine and selenium, reducing infections and inflammation, and very closely looking at emotional issues. Some people require an interim support of a natural thyroid support called Armour Thyroid or glandular extracts (the best ones are from New Zealand) while your practitioner is helping "clean up" your body and spirit.

Metaphysics: Thyroid issues focus on chakras 4, 5, and 6. Ask yourself, "What do I need or envision for more spiritual support?" and, "How can I pace myself? Am I running through life?" Or "What is making me labor so? How can I lighten my load or pick up the tempo?" Tempo and timing, pacesetting in the rat race we live in, are essential points to consider.

THE LYME DISEASE AUTOIMMUNE ILLNESS CROSSOVER

The crossover diagnosis between Lyme disease and autoimmune conditions is a critical factor to consider if you are ill. The bacterium of Lyme disease known as *Borrelia burgdorferi* causes a multitude of symptoms, many of which appear in the autoimmune classifications as well as neurology and cardiology literature. There are over one hundred strains of Lyme disease in the USA and 300 strains of borrelia worldwide. Commercial laboratories usually check for only one strain and therefore this organism is missed in thousands of clinicians' offices. Additionally, Lyme disease can mimic autoimmune illnesses or actually trigger them. The entire topic is in need of serious scrutiny and hundreds of millions of research dollars, because if this web can be unraveled, there could be deep restorative solutions to millions of people's suffering worldwide.

Dr. Alan MacDonald, a premier research pathologist and featured in the riveting Lyme disease documentary *Under Our Skin*, conveyed to me some incredibly pertinent data about Lyme's effect on the brain. His studies in 1989 at Southampton Hospital, on Long Island, New York, proved that seven out of ten Alzheimer cases showed Lyme disease spirochetes in their brain! Yet, he could not get the government assistance research money he needed to further the studies. However, since then Dr. MacDonald has been putting his attention on the crossover between Lyme disease and multiple sclerosis. I have had the good fortune to interview him on my radio program, Lyme Light Radio. Please visit the archived podcasts and listen to his groundbreaking details pertaining to MS, Alzheimer's, Lou Gehrig's disease, and Lyme disease at LymeLightRadio.com.

The nuts and bolts of it are that *Borrelia b.* thrives on fatty acids and fatty tissues. When the organism has augured its way from the bloodstream into the tissues of the body, it quickly gobbles up the fatty layers that are found on the nerve myelin sheaths and the muscle fascia. Organs such as the heart and brain also can be attacked this way. Another way that *Borrelia b.* can affect the nervous system in some individuals is by a process called "molecular mimicry." Our immune system tries to attack and kill the bacteria, but attacks our nerves instead, causing demyelination. The MRI scans then show lesions that are usually labeled as MS. These cases need to be evaluated for tick-borne diseases, according to Dr. MacDonald and other Lyme disease experts. These demyelinating lesions may be instead locations where the microorganism has chewed away the fatty layer and lining.

MS and Lyme disease share many common symptoms: weakness, difficulty walking, tingling and numbness in the extremities, visual disturbances, urinary difficulties, fatigue, sleep disturbance, and temperature dysregulation, as well as lesions on an MRI scan. They also can cause similar elevations of proteins in the spinal fluid, such as elevated levels of myelin basic protein (MBP) and oligoclonal bands, typically thought of as abnormalities only seen in MS. One way to differentiate between Lyme and MS, according to Dr. Richard Horowitz, a Lyme disease specialist, is that MS typically will exhibit more demyelinating lesions on a brain MRI than Lyme disease, have higher levels of MBP and oligoclonal bands on a spinal tap, and in

MS those lesions can also be found on the cervical and thoracic spine, which is not usually the case in Lyme disease. However, the boundaries between the two diseases can easily be blurred, and many cases of MS are actually *Borrelia b.* having found its way to the nerves and/or brain of the body.

Dr. MacDonald points out that MS is rampant in the most northern latitudes of the globe—across North America and Canada, Scandinavia, northern Europe, Russia, and Japan. This may be in part due to vitamin D deficiency, as well as where the Lyme disease epidemic is surging the most fiercely. The NorVect Conference held in Oslo, Norway, each autumn features speakers and authorities addressing the rampant surge of Lyme disease in Europe.

Norwegian doctors are cooperating with Dr. Alan MacDonald to continue his important studies on the crossover between Lyme disease infections and the occurrence of multiple sclerosis. Anyone can participate in Dr. MacDonald's MS study for free. Please visit the website www.Lyme-MS-Pathology.com to learn more.

These two illnesses are only the beginning of the story for autoimmune disease. Dr. Joel Wallach, famed naturopath and veterinarian of over fifty years and author of over fourteen books, proclaims that rheumatoid arthritis is addressed by going after the tick-borne organism mycoplasma and getting the patient off of all gluten products. Research from Dr. Brown from the 1930s backs up this very same conclusion about mycoplasma and RA. Lyme disease and the coinfections are also known to burrow their way into the synovial linings of our joints and create rheumatoid arthritis-type inflammation and pain, along with causing the classic "butterfly rash" seen in lupus.

Dr. Richard Horowitz, premier Lyme disease specialist, focuses on the crossover from Lyme disease to rheumatoid arthritis, MS, and other autoimmune disorders in clear detail in his *New York Times* bestselling book *Why Can't I Get Better? Solving the Mystery of Lyme and Chronic Disease*. He explains that Lyme disease and certain tick-borne bacteria can mimic and/or trigger autoimmune disorders, creating a confusing clinical picture for general practitioners as well as rheumatologists, neurologists, cardiologists, and endocrinologists. For example, it is not uncommon to find someone with Lyme disease develop a condition like Hashimoto's thyroiditis, an autoimmune thyroid disorder, or have Lyme disease affect other hormones of the body, subsequently leading to low testosterone, low female hormones, or low adrenal function. This is because Lyme can affect the pituitary gland, the master regulator of hormones in the body.

Lyme can also create specific auto-antibodies against the nerves, called antiganglioside antibodies, leading to low blood pressure and elevated heart rates, a condition called POTS (postural orthostatic tachycardia syndrome) or dysautonomia. In these patients, their resistant fatigue, dizziness, palpitations, and brain fog are not just due to an active infection with borrelia, but also an autoimmune process affecting the autonomic nervous system. This is the part of our nervous system that controls blood pressure, heart rate, and digestion. Some patients will require extra salt and fluids, adrenal hormones, and/or immunoglobulin therapy (IVIG) if the small nerve fibers have been affected by the autoimmune process in Lyme. It is also not unusual for patients with one autoimmune manifestation to develop another one, which suggests something deeper at play than just a faulty switch in your body being triggered to flip the immune system into overdrive.

Quoting Dr. Horowitz from his marvelous book: "Simultaneously treating the I's of Lyme disease—infection, inflammation, and immune dysfunction—may be the key to alleviating chronic pain. Blebs, secreted from the surface of *Borrelia burgdorferi*, can cause a nonspecific stimulation of the immune system (apart from the role of coinfections such as babesia, bartonella, and *Mycoplasma fermentans* previously discussed). Blebs are shed particles containing partial DNA from *Borrelia burgdorferi*. These blebs are highly stimulatory to the immune system, and intercellular blebs convert host cells into targets for the immune system. We also discussed the role of biochemical pathways, such as the nitric oxide (NO) pathway and its ability to increase oxidative stress and increase inflammatory cytokines in Lyme disease, fibromyalgia, environmental illness (EI), and chronic fatigue syndrome. Diverse stressors, whether viral, bacterial, physical, emotional, or exposure to volatile organic solvents or pesticides can all increase nitric oxide and its oxidative product peroxynitrite, leading to an increase in cytokines, causing fatigue and pain syndromes. This would be one of the common mechanisms linking these different diseases, which all have similar clinical presentations. Finally, inadequate phase I and phase II liver detoxification, with inadequate production or overutilization of glutathione, and the subsequent inability to remove neurotoxins and cytokines often seen with Lyme-MSIDS, will also result in pain."

This sums up the "mystifying" scenario quite succinctly. Dr. Horowitz often uses specialty lab IGeneX in California to identify the presence of the Lyme bacteria and suspicious coinfections. Most Lyme-literate physicians also do not limit themselves to the CDC definition for Lyme disease, which according to the CDC, is only meant to be used by the health department to epidemiologically screen large populations for the disease. Using the CDC definition in the clinical setting has the potential to miss hundreds of thousands of cases annually.

According to the renowned Lyme disease specialist Dr. Kenneth Liegner, there are maybe only fifty or sixty doctors in the entire United States who understand the crossover of Lyme disease infections to autoimmune illnesses. A pioneer in the field for over three decades, one of his strong pleas is, "We need practitioners who can cross disciplines and work together and not get stuck in dogma. It is incumbent on a physician to make allies with the other one treating a patient with a complexity of these autoimmune crossover conditions. It can be like the 'blind men and the elephant'—not grasping the "whole" picture with a lack of comprehension that something may be "driving" the autoimmune process. This can sometimes be an infectious agent and antimicrobial treatment can sometimes improve the situation, although immune-modulating therapies of various kinds may still be necessary at certain points."

Each one of us has certain genetic predispositions, determining whether we will be susceptible to flipping on the autoimmune switch when exposed to *Borrelia b.* An overstimulated immune system from a Lyme infection can cause the production of auto-antibodies seen in rheumatoid arthritis (rheumatoid factors, i.e., RF), or create auto-antibodies seen in lupus (antinuclear antibodies, i.e, ANAs). Some cases will test positive to both a Lyme antibody and a rheumatoid (RA) antibody test. Others will test RA negative and ANA positive and be crippled with deforming joint swelling and pain, and given an RA diagnosis plus a lupus diagnosis too. However, these autoimmune markers are not specific for rheumatoid arthritis and lupus, and all of these cases according to Dr. Liegner and Dr. Horowitz need to be examined for tick-borne infections, not just put on immunosuppressive drugs. According to Dr. Horowitz, there are antibodies that are more specific for lupus, such as the double-stranded DNA test (dsDNA), and specific markers for rheumatoid arthritis, such as the cyclic citrullinated peptide test (CCP), and these should be done to differentiate a true autoimmune disorder from one caused by Lyme and coinfections like mycoplasma. Getting to the root cause of the disease and finding underlying infections could lead to a cure and not just palliation of symptoms. Often, with successful treatment with antimicrobials—if the diagnosis of underlying tick-borne infection is correct—the autoimmune markers will diminish over time as treatment is applied. This can and often does occur with RF, CCP, and ANAs. Sometimes antimicrobial treatment, although needed, is not sufficient, and a combined application of antimicrobials and immune-modulating treatment is necessary and collaborations with open-minded immunologists and/or rheumatologists and/or neurologists are essential for the well-being of the patient.

Why are autoimmune symptoms so common in Lyme? The autoimmune system goes into overdrive when *Borrelia b.* goes inside cells and secretes pieces of DNA called blebs, which act like decoys for our immune system, setting up the immune system to go after them, as if it were a foreign agent! This is how our immune system attacks our own cells. It is as if the cells have been hijacked and seen as a foreign entity. Then there is the process of molecular mimicry, where the immune system tries to go after the tail (flagella) on a spirochete, but ends up attacking the myelin sheath of our own cells instead. These spirochetes are very "clever" and are likely to be a causative factor in many chronic inflammatory conditions, according to these brilliant doctors out in the field, with decades of clinical experience and knowledge under their belt.

To add more fuel to the fire, other culprits in autoimmune disease are certain strains of borrelia called *Borrelia miyamotoi*, which are a relapsing type of fever bacteria that have been around for a long time according to Durland Fish, PhD, Medical Entomologist, now at Yale, but only came on our radar screen five years ago, when Russian researchers published an article on it. That led Peter Krause, MD, to bring the information to the Imugen conference in Boston 2013, with a new lab test. Apparently, this strain is commonly found in deer ticks in the northern reaches of North America, and has mimicked autoimmune conditions for generations. Since the 1900s relapsing fevers of this sort, transmitted by ticks, were treated successfully with antibiotics in Africa. Some of this old information needs to be looked at with a new lens.

Other acclaimed physicians, such as Dr. David Perlmutter and the breakthrough functional medicine doctor Amy Myers, all suggest that infectious agents such as Lyme disease and mycoplasma be scouted out when looking at any autoimmune case. These agents cannot be dismissed any longer, as too much evidence is linking them to autoimmune manifestations. When combined with heavy metals, gluten, and other toxins in the bloodstream such as molds and plastic derivatives, our systems become severely compromised and when the infectious tick-borne microorganisms enter the equation, a perfect storm brews! In fact, it seems almost impossible not to have the autoimmune switch flipped when we understand the scenario at these levels. Cleaning up the inner terrain of the body, as well as isolating infectious microbes, is a much more functional approach to addressing the wide array of autoimmune illnesses than just taking an immunosuppressive drug.

The time has come for us to take a much broader view of autoimmune conditions, and look at our lifestyle, dietary habits, and environmental issues in concert with chronic infections, if we are to effectively deal with skyrocketing rates of Lyme disease and autoimmune conditions. As Dr. Liegner so wisely said, "No one physician can 'do it all' and it is often necessary and desirable for physicians trained in different disciplines to cooperate in the care of these patients with very complex illness. Physicians must cross the barriers and work together," just as personally we need to individually not just curl up inside ourselves and wait for help, but seek qualified alternative resources and work with our own inner healing powers.

LYME DISEASE BASICS

We have learned the hard way, after forty years of clinical findings, that Lyme disease is much more than an acute infectious illness limited to the North Eastern USA. It exists throughout the United States and over the globe in an exploding epidemic strata. In the USA, Lyme is spreading four times faster than HIV and is entrenched and misdiagnosed daily, due to lack of awareness, poor doctor education, and faulty lab testing. The common commercial ELISA lab test has a 70 percent false negative error rate, meaning hundreds of thousands of people are told they do *not* have a Lyme disease infection, though they feel awful or have odd symptoms, and get misdiagnosed typically for an autoimmune illness or are labeled as hypochondriacs or "emotionally imbalanced." This scientific neglect and huge vacuum of denial regarding this surging infectious illness needs immediate attention at the awareness, research, government involvement, and physician training levels. Millions are suffering worldwide needlessly!

Lyme disease is a bacterial infection caused by an organism known as *Borrelia burgdorferi*. There are also variant Lyme tick-borne co-infections caused by similar microbes, ehrlichia, babesia, bartonella, and mycoplasmas. These microorganisms and as many as 300 other strains related to Lyme disease all cause a similar set of symptoms with some minor yet detectable characteristics differentiating them. *Borrelia b.* is classified as spirochete, or corkscrew bacteria, which is in the same family as syphilis, yet Lyme is considered to be stronger and more virulent. Like syphilis, Lyme initially starts with seemingly mild acute symptomology, but over time, if untreated, it can cause devastating effects to the central nervous system, heart, kidneys, endocrine, skeletal, and immune systems, with sometimes permanent repercussions. This panoply of systemic symptoms mimics many autoimmune-style disorders.

The bacterium is spread by a blood transfer. It's most commonly transmitted by the bite of a very tiny insect, the deer tick. These ticks are the size of a pinhead or small freckle. It has been commonly assumed that the tiny deer tick (*Ixodes stapularis*) is the only variety infected with *Borrelia burgdorferi* bacteria. This is incorrect. All species in the USA, Europe, Canada, Australia, Africa, Asia, and South America *can* be infected with Lyme disease (bb) and an assortment of coinfections. The Lone Star tick, found throughout the southern tier of the USA, is particularly aggressive and quick to latch on to a host. It carries borrelia bacteria and other coinfections linked to many autoimmune-style disorders.

These coinfections are very tricky to diagnose properly via lab testing, still! A PCR test can sometimes confirm the organisms' presence. A clinical diagnosis is obtained via signs and symptoms collated by a Lyme disease specialist practitioner, most thoroughly trained beyond traditional medical, chiropractic, or naturopathic school, but also by the International Lyme and Associated Disease Society (ILADS) or Tick-Borne Disease Alliance (TBDA). If your practitioner claims you do not test positive for Lyme disease and they are not ILADS or TBDA trained, seeking a second opinion is prudent.

The common coinfections include bartonella, babesia, ehrlichia, mycoplasma. Also, Rocky Mountain spotted fever, heartland virus, and more are transmitted via ticks and vector insects (fire ants, fleas, mosquitos).

Note: Lyme disease is technically caused by the bacteria *Borrelia burgdorferi*. The similar coinfections are either bacterial, parasitic, or mycoplasma. For brevity's sake, the rest of this section will refer to Lyme disease, even though we include the coinfections.

Sexual relations may possibly transmit a form of Lyme disease, noted in a January 2014 study including Dr. Ralph Stricker and Dr. Eva Sapi. Pregnant mothers may transfer the bacteria to their baby, as Lyme bacteria are capable of passing to the fetus through the placenta, as well as in breast milk in approximately 33 percent of mothers. Interestingly, however, some infected mothers do not spread the actual bacteria to the fetus, but the baby can be affected by central nervous system issues; ADD/ADHD, food allergies, autism, Tourette's syndrome, OCD, or other syndromes. The miasmatic influence from the mother instead sets up a host of sensitivities, allergies, or imbalances in the offspring. This is referred to as PANS (peripheral autonomic nervous system).

Sharing food, drinks, eating utensils, or shaking someone's hand has not been proven to transmit Lyme disease. It's potentially contagious through mucous membranes and saliva, but this is not confirmed. Our blood banks are contaminated and need screening. You can't catch it from your pet through natural contact, such as by grooming or caring for them. You can, however, get bitten by a tick carrying Lyme that is on their body and moves to yours. Sleeping with pets is discouraged. Washing their bedding and dousing them with repellent such as Vectra is wise.

Lyme disease is a rampant epidemic in the twenty-first century. We have not understood the mammoth influence these organisms have inflicted upon our health for decades, creating a smoldering explosion of chronic disease in several generations by now. In August 2013 the Center for Disease Control announced over 300,000 people are infected yearly, yet 90 percent of these cases are not actually diagnosed or treated in acute onset form. Many authorities project that actually over 1,000,000 cases are contracted annually in the USA. Lyme is now the most rampant infectious disease in the United States. In my own county in New Hampshire, it's been increasing at a rate of over 100 percent per year over the last five years, with over 75 to 90 percent of deer ticks infected with Lyme bacteria in certain counties.

The Eastern Seaboard and West Coast are under particularly fierce assault and the southern states are undereducated on the matter. Cases are multiplying in large numbers in the Ohio River Valley, across the Midwest, and along the Great Lakes as a wide variety of ticks now carry the disease. Mild winters do not kill them off. Eighty-nine countries of the world now report Lyme disease. Ticks themselves carry an array of other infectious illnesses such as Rocky Mountain spotted fever, various relapsing fevers, and viruses. Ticks are miniature cesspools. Essentially, they transfer what they are carrying from a former host into you during their feeding cycle.

Low-lying woodland areas, beach grass, open meadows abutting forests, low shrubs, and ground covers like pachysandra are all favorable environments for ticks to inhabit. Ticks typically find a small animal, such as a rabbit, squirrel, raccoon, dog, or deer to live on as their host. They rest on leaves and grasses, about thigh-high, climbing aboard a warm-blooded animal (including humans) as they brush by. The tick crawls on the body, looking for soft delicate skin as its entry point. They often gravitate to the nape of the neck, the armpits, and groin. They will bite the host and attach, often lodging themselves for hours or days, as they engorge on blood. Many times the tick will never completely lodge itself in its host, but merely just crawl about. It must lodge itself in order to transfer the bacteria. Some suggest the tick must be embedded for over twenty-four hours for the blood transfer, but data does not support this well-intended reassuring conclusion. It all depends on where the tick is in its feeding cycle when it adheres to you.

Spring is a particularly elevated time for tick numbers, as this is when their eggs hatch, releasing almost translucent nymphs, which are particularly hard to see. After a rain, their population can be heavier, too. Autumn brings another round of infestation. The most telltale sign of a new Lyme infection is the "bull's-eye" rash or bite from the tick. A red dot in the center, with an outer red circle, is the classic early warning sign. This target-shaped rash may be as small as a dime or as large as a softball. Sometimes it's a pale pink color, other times it's a vermillion red, even inflamed to a swollen, sore, black-and-blue degree. Sometimes people show just a welt. This "erythema migrans" rash is a 100 percent confirmation that you have been infected by *Borrelia burgdorferi* when a tick accompanies it.

Many people never notice such a bite. Only approximately 50 percent show the target rash. A small bull's-eye could also be in a not-so-visible place, such as your back or scalp. If you think a red welt or bite could be a common spider bite—also sometimes a red dot encircled with a red ring—again, please get it examined. With Lyme disease escalating so rapidly and its consequences being so dire, it's not worth brushing off such a bite as insignificant. You are not being a wimp if you have an insect bite examined!

Aside from the initial bull's-eye rash, other early symptoms of a Lyme infection can include an aching, flu-like feeling, often noted in the limbs, back, and neck. Mild chills or nausea may accompany these pains (RA and CFS cases often start out like this!). Occasionally, individuals exhibit a frank swelling or pronounced pain in their joints (the knee being the most common). A slight fever, rarely over one hundred degrees, is not atypical. Headaches, often severe, are the second most common symptom alongside the flu-like feeling. Dizziness, sore throat, fatigue, and swollen glands may all manifest as well. Depression is not atypical. Symptoms often ebb and flow in four- to six-week "flare states," which is common of many autoimmune illnesses.

Any constellation of the mentioned symptomology tends to linger beyond a few days without blossoming into the customary respiratory or gastrointestinal pathway of influenza. The heavy mucus production, sinus drainage, and cough of the flu usually do not occur. This is a very significant feature to note. If you're feeling unwell and flu-ish, but not progressing into the natural route of sinus and cough, think Lyme. What later sets in is the heavy malaise and pronounced fatigue, often accompanied by a "cottony" head sensation and mental dullness. Some cases occasionally bloom into a pronounced influenza state, whereby one discounts the notion of Lyme at all. Individuals with very strong immune systems may get these flu-like symptoms for only a few days, to relapse again weeks or even months later. Some people conversely say, "I feel like I was slammed by a truck! I have never felt so sick in my life."

Please note that children may not get all the mentioned symptoms. Instead, they most commonly manifest achiness and headaches, and maybe the bull's-eye bite. Because children so frequently experience mild fevers, sore throats, and tiredness associated with a touch of some passing viral infection going through their school or daycare, we tend just to ride out their discomforts for a few days or a week, assuming it will all pass as their active immune systems capably arrest the microbe invasion. Most often this mindset is adequate and the child ably recovers from common viruses.

If your child complains of headaches, is unfocused in school, is showing anxiety or restlessness, has a knee or other joint that hurts, or just doesn't seem to have his or her usual energy a few weeks after a seemingly mild cold or flu-like episode, again I encourage you to have them tested for Lyme disease. Children, teens, and very healthy adults often are misdiagnosed regarding early Lyme and co-infections, especially if they didn't exhibit the bull's-eye rash or you didn't find a tick on their body. Their immune systems are very active and strong, working aggressively to tamp down the borrelia right away. Emotional woes, ADD, anger attacks, tiredness, and sleep disorders are common even in healthy youngsters and teens. Headaches, depression, OCD, anxiety, malaise, and GI issues are very common in kids, and so may not raise suspicion. The result is early, undiagnosed signs of Lyme, then a quieter waiting period, with malingering symptoms sometimes resurfacing weeks or months later, whereby no one, doctor or patient, makes the correlation to the initial infection. This scenario is where most chronic Lyme cases have gone awry. They were not diagnosed in the office or via accurate laboratory testing and clinical assessment up front, setting up the individual for repeated suspicious outbreaks, eventually morphing into the mysterious and vague status of chronic Lyme disease, sometimes with serious neurological or cardiac consequences and autoimmune syndromes. Dr. Richard Horowitz clearly explains how the tick-borne disease infections trigger autoimmune illnesses in many of us. A lifetime of suffering can ensue if these infectious microbes are not eradicated.

One of my most important messages is that early diagnosis and detection of Lyme disease is critical. The sooner this bacterium is arrested, the more hopeful the prognosis is for a complete recovery. Do not hesitate to seek professional testing if you are at all suspicious you may have been infected by the bacteria. I can't stress this enough!

Many physicians aren't willing to acknowledge the concept of chronic Lyme disease, as the IDSA has not gotten completely on board with this condition, still claiming Lyme disease is only an acute illness of a limited duration, and calling lingering symptoms "post-Lyme syndrome." Yet chronic Lyme disease is a very evasive condition, defying a clear black-and-white set of diagnostic keynotes. It may attack one or more primary systems of the body, consequently creating a broad variety of symptoms variant from case to case. The endocrine system gets particularly skewed.

I have met thousands whose neurological systems have been attacked, resulting in various types of palsy, MS, ALS, Parkinson's, neuropathy, as well as Crohn's disease, Hashimoto's thyroiditis, bipolar disorder, obsessive-compulsive disorder, dementia, and hallucinations. I've counseled individuals who have heart troubles, such as pericarditis or valve problems from the Lyme bacteria. A friend's child had ocular Lyme and was blind until treated. Many people are hospitalized from Lyme disease, especially when the immune system becomes so overburdened that secondary infections, like pneumonia, Epstein-Barr virus, or cytomegalia, hit. Water on the knee, rheumatoid arthritis, stiff necks, fibromyalgia, migraines, CFS, and lupus are common signs of a chronic case of Lyme and errant testing.

Being that the musculoskeletal system, immune/lymphatic system, gastrointestinal, heart/circulation, neurological system, and skin each can be attacked, again variant from case to case, a panoply of sometimes perplexing symptoms can evade a clear-cut diagnosis. A clinical diagnosis is made by a symptom picture, hopefully but not always backed up with new state-of-the-art laboratory testing that identifies DNA fragments of Lyme bacteria and specific proteins more closely. With limited funds, a few valiant research docs are diligently working to crack the code, with a newer antigen test hopefully bringing us confirmative diagnostic results in days rather than weeks.

One of my greatest concerns regarding the millions of people with progressed Lyme disease cases is the broken spirits that can result from this debilitating, ruinous illness. A being can handle only so much. Lyme takes the physical, mental, and emotional stuffing out of so many people and their caregivers. Tending to the broken spirit is just as critical as mending a broken body. This rampaging epidemic has shown us its very ugly face. Hundreds of thousands of people are suffering at so many levels because of it. My plea is that we find resources to tend to those afflicted. Reach out to organizations such as ILADS, TBDA, LRA, Lymedisease.org, and Lyme-MS-Pathology.net to find studies going on, and donate your blood or financial support.

Integrative medicine and natural medicine practitioners have a great toolbox of resources to mend from Lyme and the crossover status to autoimmune diseases. Naturopathic physicians are strongly suited to tackle this illness, as they have training in all the supportive modalities to rebuild depletions and detoxify a burdened body as well as go about arresting an infection with appropriate antibiotics or antimicrobial herbals. Dr. Richard Horowitz's groundbreaking book *Why Can't I Get Better? Solving the Mystery of Lyme and Chronic Disease* presents a very thorough model of treatment physicians can become trained in to address the complex nature of Lyme disease and co-infections and how they cross over to autoimmune illnesses.

My great hope is that as the next decade evolves, the long overdue government funding we need to properly research tick-borne organisms is finally allocated to the cutting-edge researchers, as we could be looking at a "lock and key" situation here, whereby TBD organisms could be the long-overlooked and misunderstood root link to the enormous surge in autoimmune illnesses and childhood afflictions like ADD/ADHD, autism, asthma, food allergies, and mood disorders.

In the field for fifteen years now, and having met thousands of people all over the USA and Europe, as well as having the fortunate role to interview the world's leading experts on my Lyme Light Radio program, the evidence is blatant that this "hidden" epidemic flew under the radar for too many decades, labeled as a short-term infectious illness and reeking generations of damage.

A very valuable Lyme disease/autoimmune disorder symptom correlation questionnaire is provided in the appendix, to use as a checklist to see how many of your own symptoms "cross over." Any and all suspect cases really should be evaluated by a Lyme-literate practitioner, not your GP or neurologist or rheumatologist, unless they have had ILADS training.

Lyme disease is a confusing illness. Some people carry the microbe with no symptoms and others become stricken and maimed. A sector of us succumb to chronic inflammation and the "autoimmune switch" is flipped, whereby many conditions and progressive damage occurs. The best hope is early detection of a Lyme infection and swift antibiotic protocols before it burrows into tissues, organs, and glands. When this secondary process occurs, recovery is longer and requires a multipronged approach of integrative medicine processes. As I have long stated, Lyme disease (and autoimmune illnesses) asks us to marry the two hands of healthcare—the diagnostics and pharmacology of traditional medicine with the restorative therapeutics of natural medicine, for we all know two hands working together are better than one.

Education, awareness, better early lab testing, and research are needed in enormous proportions to unravel the confusion and denial surrounding tick-borne diseases and to ultimately put the pieces of the puzzle together regarding the gigantic surge in autoimmune illnesses in recent decades. I believe it is not a coincidence that as the tick population has exploded and the transmission of the infection has bloomed since the 1970s, so have all the autoimmune illnesses and so many "mysterious" symptoms people struggle with. We potentially are on the verge of a tipping point, whereby the right research could change the nature of doctoring.

Metaphysics: Lyme disease chakra issues include all seven chakras, depending on where your most prominent symptoms lie. Use The Map on page 317 to help you find a starting point. Strong chances suggest chronic Lyme cases will benefit from you working on using all the seven chakra healing exercises. All Lyme cases will ultimately require chakra 4 work, involving immunity/defense postures and what your heart desires as well as chakra 3 to invoke willpower and intention about your true "place" in the world regarding your life work and creative offerings.

LYME DISEASE LABORATORY TESTING

Lyme disease and the associate coinfections are not easily identified in the bloodstream of an individual via standard commercial laboratory testing. The trick is using the correct test and lab to identify the *Borrelia burgdorferi* organism's presence. Even then, accuracy is not 100 percent. We do not yet have one definitive Lyme disease diagnostic test. Lyme disease can be elusive. A clinical diagnosis made from an experienced Lyme practitioner is ESSENTIAL. Do not accept a negative "result" from a test done in an emergency room, by a general physician, or even a specialist, including a rheumatologist, neurologist, immunologist, or infectious disease expert. They typically use the large commercial labs or the local hospital lab, which are notorious for false negative results.

The more reliable labs are specialty labs like IGeneX, Clongen, NeuroScience, or Frye Labs. Doctors will too often dismiss a tick-borne illness when more investigation is warranted based upon poor lab tests. I cannot tell you how many folks have told me they are sick and were tested for EVERYTHING, including Lyme disease, but the test was negative. I ask the worried individual, "Did the doctor use IGeneX Labs in California?" The eyes looking back at me are blank, as who would know to scrutinize a doctor's papers? Likely chance the infectious microbes were missed and immune suppressive drugs and pain meds are what I next hear are commonly prescribed. So, a thirty-five-year-old, prime-of-life individual stands before me, in the grocery store or post office in my own town, telling me this tale. My heart beats and I am sad for them. So FEW Lyme disease–literate practitioners exist even in New England—the heart of the epidemic! State-of-the-art lab testing is vital.

Lawyers Susan Green (MD) and Monte Skall (VA) got a key piece of legislation passed in Washington, DC, by National Capitol Lyme. This bill states that a negative result on an ELISA Lyme disease test can NOT rule out the individual may have Lyme disease. It is the first state to clarify Lyme testing can be faulty and further evaluation is encouraged. This bill is valid in Virginia and every state needs to follow suit

The ability of Lyme and the coinfections like bartonella and babesia, to hide from our immune systems makes proving illness with lab tests challenging. Often, a person knows they are sick, yet the practitioner, hospital, or laboratory will tell them time and again that "Your Lyme test is negative. You do not have Lyme disease. You are fine." Meanwhile, the bacteria is silently embedding itself further into the person's tissues and organs. Often a diagnosis of an autoimmune disease like lupus, MS, or rheumatoid arthritis is made, missing the true underlying infection with Lyme. Hundreds of thousands are lumped into either fibromyalgia or chronic fatigue syndrome without finding the root cause of infection.

An important "take home" message to readers who are suspicious that they have been bitten by a tick or "sense" they may have Lyme disease, is to insist that your provider use one of the more sensitive labs (IGeneX, Clongen, NeuroScience) and their specific tests in order to obtain a more accurate result. Even these labs have a high false negative rate. IGeneX Western blot for Lyme is one of the more accurate tests for Lyme. As mentioned previously, the vast majority of doctors who do not specialize in treating Lyme disease have relied on the common ELISA (enzyme-linked immuno-absorbant assay) Lyme test. If this is negative then testing stops. If this is positive, a rare 35 percent of the time, they move on to the commercial lab Western blot, which is not reliable. Even if one band on the test is positive they will call it a false positive, when, in reality, it is the reverse. These two-tiered tests are extremely inaccurate and faulty, with up to a 70 percent false negative error rate.

The CDC and IDSA currently do not recognize the persistence of chronic Lyme infection, making it difficult for physicians to diagnose or treat when all they have is a negative test result on a patient. The current guidelines for treatment set out by the IDSA are inadequate, as they treat for no longer than a month with usually only one antibiotic. This too often leads to the persistent infection that they deny.

At the International Conference on Lyme Borreliosis and TBD in Boston, 2013, the concept of "post-Lyme syndrome" was acknowledged by the IDSA. This syndrome is the IDSA's response to continuing and debilitating symptoms, which the IDSA claims are associated with the "normal" activities of aging and living. The IDSA states that the recommended fourteen to thirty days of antibiotic therapy for acute Lyme disease is sufficient, and something else must be at play when patients end up with chronic symptoms; i.e., autoimmune illness and inflammation for example.

There is much more to unearth surrounding *Borrelia b.* and the common coinfections, which cause horrific suffering. Dr. Richard Horowitz, past president of ILADEF, has treated over 12,000 Lyme disease patients. He states that the coinfections are a significant factor in persistent cases. Currently, Lyme-literate practitioners make a clinical diagnosis and feel reassured when more than one lab test gives them positive confirmation.

Dr. Ahmed Kilani of Clongen Labs has devoted much time and research to Lyme disease. He confirms that when testing for *Borrelia burgdorferi* we are looking for merely one strain of the organism, and there are many strains of the bacteria and the coinfections.

His statistics cite:

117 total organism strains

32 Borrelia (up to 380 known internationally)

29 Bartonella
6 Babesia
6 Anaplasma
12 Ehrlichia
23 Rickettsia

This does not include different viruses, numerous species of mycoplasma, Rocky Mountain spotted fever, or other organisms such as FL1953 protazoa (Fry Labs) that a tick may carry. As few as seven co-infections are found in a tick, often many more. Other studies suggest 380 worldwide borrelia strains and the northeast corridor of the USA and California are heavily infected with *Borrelia miyamotoi*, one of the borrelia relapsing fevers, of which no testing is available at this time. It is no wonder upward of 1,000,000 people are infected annually with tick-borne diseases and a mere fraction are properly diagnosed.

Every six months or so a clearer lens into the mechanisms of the shape-shifting borrelia spirochete is illuminated. Researchers and laboratories are earnestly attempting to find an infallible testing method to diagnose borrelia's presence, both immediately upon infection (in the example of a tick bite), and with more persistent cases. The newest, most specific, and sensitive tests are major assets in battling chronic Lyme by making a more accurate diagnosis feasible. However, these infections are best diagnosed clinically through the patient's history.

There are tests worth considering and addressing with your practitioner. Both IGeneX and Clongen Labs have much more sensitive Western blot antibody tests, PCR, immune modulator tests, and co-infection tests than commercial labs. Even these can be false negative. The bands that show up positive on the Western blot test that help a practitioner confirm a borrelia infection are numbers 18, 23 to 25, 28, 31, 34, 39, and 83 to 93. The CDC requires that an Elisa Antibody test be done for Lyme before the Western blot, which is usually a false negative test about 65 to 75 percent of the time. In actuality, Lyme disease is easily missed with this type of test. If a patient comes up with only one of the positive bands specific for Lyme, the CDC does not qualify this as a positive Lyme case, as they require at least five-plus bands on the IgG and three-plus on the IgM test. The CDC initially used these numbers for surveillance criteria for epidemiological reasons and then adopted them as diagnostic criteria. Actually, confirmation of any one of these bands suggests Lyme.

DNA fragments of borrelia found in the urine are another confirmation. IGeneX's urine etiope test is one version, and the Ceres Nanotrap test, currently being put through rigid clinical trials at George Mason University, may be a breakthrough moment in Lyme disease diagnostics. This test works on examining antigens in the urine. Antigens are the first reactors to a microbial infection, versus the later-forming antibodies. This nanotrap test is currently the most clearly promising indicative tool for an early, acute infection.

Another test with growing success is NeuroScience Labs' iSpot Lyme(TM) test. This test relies on the activation of the patient's effector T-cells (immune response). It utilizes four antigens instead of two and detects signature proteins called cytokines. The results are qualified as a function of the increase in the levels of interferon gamma. iSpot Lyme(TM)is a highly reliable and accurate test, with an 84 percent sensitivity rate and specificity of 94 percent. Many doctors are turning to this method now.

Additionally, NeuroScience offers an ELISPOT, another antigen test, which confirms borrelia presence in many seronegative Western blot or ELISA cases.

Still in question are the blood culture tests being performed. A patient's blood sample is allowed to culture on specific "agars" for two to sixteen weeks, noting if borrelia or certain coinfections grow, akin to a urinary tract infection culture test. At first the outlook was promising. But now, two years later, the process is questionable, as there is a preponderance of "positive" test results, suggesting that the test may produce a false positive too often. The Advance Labs borrelia culture is very promising and is being confirmed by a few independent labs at this time.

TICK-BORNE COINFECTIONS

Tick-borne "coinfections" often cause great suffering and are challenging to diagnose if a practitioner is not experienced with them. A brief summary follows:

Bartonella is a bacteria that acts like a parasite, is commonly called "cat scratch fever" and has long been associated as being transmitted by a cat scratch or bite. Now we know ticks and other vectors can be carriers. I recall my hilarious father referring to someone who was fidgety and full of erratic emotions and energy to "be so high strung, he must have cat scratch fever." Knowing that bartonella affects the nervous system in a very profound way, I had personal experience with the roaring, frightening anxiety it produces, as well as fidgety feelings and blinding severe nerve pain. With me, bartonella hit the tri-geminal nerve, creating days of searing migraines. Others find sciatic and cervico-brachial plexus nerve involvement, Bell's palsy, and various types of tremor and headache, torticollis, plantar fascitis, and wicked intense joint pain that can be migrating, intermittent, or continuous. Often patients will describe the joint pain as if "their bones are breaking." A classic bartonella symptom is pain on the soles of the feet, especially when first stepping out of the bed—often it feels like you are walking barefoot on pebbles. Additionally, long streak marks, like "stretch marks," are seen. Swollen glands and lymph nodes can be troublesome. Also, severe gastritis and nausea with or without vomiting can be caused by this bacteria. Bartonella has a strong crossover to RA, lupus, MS, GI issues, IC (urinary), and anything neurological. Severe mood swings, violent rage, and even PTSD-like states are not uncommon. Panic attacks and unrelenting anxiety can be experienced. There are articles in the literature noting bartonella outbreaks in Iraq and that it is possibly a player in "Gulf War Syndrome," which is similar to Lyme disease and CFS.

Babesia is a piroplasm parasite that "feels" and acts like malaria in some ways, though with more pain. The day I was stricken with Lyme disease I noticed a sudden vertigo as my first symptom when turning at the counter of a convenience store. Then, strong clammy chills and the feeling of a boulder bearing down on my head, accompanied by exhaustion, ensued. I recall telling the doctor, "This feels a lot like malaria to me. I had it in Africa when I was fifteen." He just nodded his head and finished the cursory exam (never even thinking Lyme disease or checking for it in 2000). Though we never found confirmation years later on lab work, my eventual Lyme-literate physician felt I had a babesia coinfection. Key signs are drenching sweats, night sweats, body heat in the head and chest, intolerance to heat, vertigo, headaches, fatigue, muscle aches, air hunger, dry cough, severe depression, suicide ideation, and nausea and vomiting. Liver damage and anemia can occur in long-standing infections, similar to bartonella. Some people get very mild cases; however, those who are immune compromised or have no spleen can get severely ill. Bartonella and babesia are frequently found together. The PCR (polymerase chain reaction) test can detect babesia DNA in the blood. The FISH (Fluorescent In-Situ Hybridization) assay can detect the ribosomal RNA of babesia in thin blood smears. The patient's blood can also be tested for antibodies to babesia.

Ehrlichia involves two tick-borne rickettsial parasites both called ehrlichia that infect different kinds of white blood cells. In HME (human monocytic ehrlichiosis), they infect monocytes. In HGE (human granulocytic ehrlichiosis), they infect granulocytes. HGE was renamed anaplasmosis in 2003. Ticks carry many parasites. It is likely that the Lone Star tick transmits HME and that the deer tick transmits HGE.

Ehrlichiosis (HME) was originally thought to be only an animal disease. It was described in humans in 1987 and is now found in thirty states, predominately in the southeast, south-central, and mid-Atlantic states, Europe, and Africa. Anaplasmosis (HGE) in humans was first identified in 1990 in a Wisconsin man. Before that it was known to infect horses, sheep, cattle, dogs, and cats. It occurs in the upper Midwest, northeast, the mid-Atlantic states, northern California, and many parts of Europe. Studies suggest that in endemic areas as much as 15 to 36 percent of the population has been infected, though often it is not recognized.

The clinical manifestations of ehrlichiosis and anaplasmosis are the same. Each is often characterized by sudden high fever, fatigue, muscle aches, and headache. Ehrlichia can cause severe joint pain, especially in the shoulders and hips. The disease can be mild or life-threatening. Severely ill patients can have low white blood cell count, low platelet count, anemia, elevated liver enzymes, kidney failure, and respiratory insufficiency. Older people or people with immune suppression are more likely to require hospitalization. Deaths have occurred (LymeDisease.org). Coinfections are best tested using PCR methods. Also, IgG and IgM antibodies of these bugs are checked. It may be necessary to run several different tests and negative results should not be used to rule out treatment.

Ehrlichia diagnosis is limited by our current ability to test for only two species. Ehrlichia parasites multiply inside host cells, forming large mulberry-shaped clusters called morulae, which doctors can sometimes see on blood smears. The infection still can easily be missed. The doctor may suspect ehrlichiosis/anaplasmosis in a patient who does not respond well to treatment for Lyme disease. The treatment of choice for ehrlichiosis/anaplasmosis is doxycycline, with rifampin recommended in case of treatment failure* (LymeDisease.org).

Courtesy of LymeDisease.org, we find this informative material on the coinfections:

"Besides the diseases described above, ticks in different geographic areas may be infected with one or more of the following: Colorado tick fever virus; mycoplasmas; Powassan encephalitis virus; Q fever; Rocky Mountain spotted fever (Rickettsia); tick-borne relapsing fever borrelia; Tularemia (bacteria).

It is certain that we have not yet identified all the diseases that ticks carry and transmit. Coinfections complicate diagnosis and treatment and make recovery even more difficult. Doctors may suspect coinfections in patients who do not respond satisfactorily to antibiotics prescribed for Lyme disease.

There are other possible explanations for treatment failures. People with chronic tick-borne infections often have a weakened immune response. This allows other opportunistic infections to flourish, such as HHV-6, CMV, and EBV. These diseases are not necessarily carried by ticks but are widespread in the environment. PCR rather than antibody tests should be used to diagnose these infections. Some people may also have exposure to toxic metals. Specialists should evaluate these cases.

Colorado tick fever is caused by a virus carried by Rocky Mountain wood ticks. Symptoms are acute high fever, severe headache, chills, fatigue, and muscle pain.

Mycoplasma species—approximately 400 different mycoplasma have been identified—are found in ticks and other vectors. Smaller than most bacteria with no cell wall, they invade human cells and steal the nutrients found there. They disrupt the immune system, causing fatigue, musculoskeletal symptoms, and cognitive problems. Each different mycoplasma has an affinity to specific areas in our body. Testing is poor for all except Mycoplasma pneumonia, which is a common respiratory infection that is easily transmitted. Mycoplasmas can be treated with antibiotics and herbals. Nutrients must be replaced to recover from the fatigue and other symptoms.

Powassan virus causes tick-borne encephalitis (TBE). Symptoms may include fever, convulsions, headache, disorientation, lethargy, partial coma, and paralysis. Ten percent of patients die and survivors may have permanent damage.

Q fever is caused by Coxiella burnetii, a kind of bacteria carried by cattle, sheep, and goats. Symptoms are similar to those of Lyme disease. Q fever is likely to start with a high fever. Pneumonia and abnormal liver function also suggest Q fever. Doxycycline is the treatment of choice.

Rocky Mountain spotted fever is caused by bacteria called Rickettsia rickettsii that are transmitted by the bite of a tick. Patients develop high fever, rash, headache, and bleeding problems. Thirty percent of untreated patients die. It is treatable with antibiotics, especially doxycycline.

Tick paralysis occurs when certain ticks secrete a toxin that causes a progressive paralysis, which is reversed when the tick is removed.

The agents of **tick-borne relapsing fever**, *Borrelia hermsii* and *Borellia miyamoti*, are carried by soft ticks of the western United States. It is characterized by cycles of high fever and is treated with antibiotics. Doxycycline is the preferred antibiotic. Testing for *B. hermsii* is available but not highly accurate. Testing for *B. miyamotoi* does not exist at this time.

Tularemia, or rabbit fever, occurs throughout the United States. It is caused by the bacterium *Francisella tularensis*. Symptoms may include skin ulcers, swollen and painful lymph glands, inflamed eyes, sore throat, mouth sores, pneumonia, diarrhea, and vomiting. The most effective treatment is with fluorinated quinolones, like Cipro, which now have a black box warning due to the damage to tendons that they can cause up to a year after taking them.

Working with a Lyme-literate practitioner is a wise choice, especially if an autoimmune illness diagnosis has been suggested to you. A symptom questionnaire is included in the appendix to help you correlate if your symptoms are numerous enough to test for Lyme disease and/or coinfection. Personally, I believe anyone with chronic illness should be "screened" for Lyme disease and other tick-borne diseases. These small microbes can be linked to hundreds of illness states. They are very intrinsic players in the root cause of many autoimmune illnesses, fibromyalgia, CFS, ALS (clue is true ALS has no pain involved, according to Dr. Alan MacDonald, while Lyme/ALS does), and Parkinson's.

The average provider is uneducated about these specific tests or the specialty labs that focus on Lyme/coinfections. It is important to insist that these facilities be used or find a Lyme-literate physician/practitioner who understands this important subject. More insurance companies, including Medicare, now reimburse for some of the tests. Please explore these labs. They are helping to diagnose these infectious diseases. Read their web pages for the specifics. Your practitioner can interface with these labs on technical questions. Once a diagnosis is achieved, proper treatment can begin. Diligence, patience, and persistence are all critical to your healing.

A final note on potential early infection and "what to do?": Gently remove the tick with tweezers held very closely at the site where it is embedded, making sure to gradually pull back, not YANK, and ease the tick out. Suffocating with oils, vaseline, or touching with a burnt-out match, scares the tick and makes it regurgitate its stomach—which includes all it has been feasting on in your bloodstream and prior hosts. So, these methods actually do harm and force more microbes into your bloodstream.

Wash the tick bite site, apply an antibiotic ointment, put the tick in a small baggie with a bit of grass and dab of water for moisture. Send it off for testing at MainelyTicks.com or IGeneX.com. They can hopefully ascertain what microbes it is carrying. Mainely Ticks offers three test kits to keep at home for such purposes. I suggest three doses of the homeopathic remedy Ledum Palustre, 200c or 1M strength, at the time of tick discovery and again twenty-four hours later. Dissolve the pellets under your tongue with no food for drink within twenty minutes prior or after the remedy. Get yourself to a Lyme doctor for an exam.

Mara Williams, LPN, renowned author of *Nature's Dirty Needle*, who has worked at Gordon Medical Association in California as a Lyme expert, suggests this prevention treatment protocol to arrest a Lyme disease infection before it takes hold.

"We can do so much with preventing chronic tick-borne illness with proper treatment of an acute infection, which includes at least two months of two antibiotics and herbal antibiotics, liver support, and probiotics. I usually give a month of Doxycycline and two days a week of Tindamax or Clarithromycin and Omnicef, and then check an IGeneX Western blot IgG and IgM. If positive, I treat longer than two months. If negative I stop at the month, but I have found that 90 percent of those I tested had a positive test even without symptoms. And that is in California, not the East Coast, where borrelia and 'company' are more likely to be present in the tick. A few people will have a mild herx reaction at the start of treatment and that would cue me to treat longer, also, as they are definitely infected. It is not unusual to treat a new infection for as long as four months! Now, I add the herbs and a biofilm buster along with liver and probiotic and immune support to prevent chronic infection from developing."

Lyme disease is a very real and valid contributor to many forms of chronic illness. Some cases later in the book illustrate this. The potential link between a Lyme infection masquerading as an autoimmune disease is probable as well as the relationship between Lyme disease wearing a system so far down that the autoimmune syndromes can then develop. This all weaves together and the great good hope is that over the next decade science is able to unravel the mysteries and some quicker diagnostics, more effective treatment protocols, and actual reversal of chronic autoimmune and Lyme disease struggles can be resolved. In the meanwhile, focus your mind on mending.

PART III

Healing Disciplines

WHAT IS NATUROPATHIC MEDICINE?

Naturopathic medicine is a branch of holistic medicine that has been around in various forms for centuries. Modern naturopathic medicine, or naturopathy, as it is more colloquially referred to in the United States, has been formalized through a standing medical association and practiced in our contemporary world since 1901. Prior to 1901, eclectic physicians, herbalists, and midwives practiced variant aspects of what we now call naturopathy.

Naturopathy has grown rapidly during the past thirty years. Sixteen states, plus Puerto Rico and the US Virgin Islands, currently license naturopaths as primary healthcare providers, meaning these physicians can give examinations, make diagnoses, perform minor surgeries like lancing a boil, and address primary healthcare issues. Numerous insurance carriers, depending on your locale, cover naturopathic medical procedures. Some hospitals grant naturopaths hospital privileges, enabling them to work with MDs in an integrated setting. Naturopathic physicians are considered to be some of the most solidly trained and diversified practitioners of holistic medicine in the United States.

Naturopaths go through four years of postgraduate schooling akin to allopathic medical schools. All the essential medical sciences are addressed, such as anatomy, physiology, pathology, microbiology, radiology, immunology, gynecology, diagnostics, and much more. Throughout, there is training in therapeutic nutrition, Chinese medicine, homeopathy, physical therapies, and counseling. Although naturopaths rely on pharmaceuticals only when they are highly indicated, comparable attention is given to pharmacology during professional training so that practitioners' expertise is current regarding Western medicine's drugs and their side effects. Then the final two years include extensive rounds in an outpatient clinic setting.

In the formalized naturopathic colleges many students elect to continue with a fifth year of studies, whereby a specialty focus is elected. This advanced training is available in obstetrics and natural childbirth, Chinese medicine and acupuncture, or classical homeopathy. The modalities of treatment a naturopath employs focus on diet and nutrition, botanical medicine, nutritional supplementation, bodywork, hydrotherapy, and perhaps other alternatives such as full-spectrum light therapy.

The philosophy of naturopathic medicine resonates with other holistic disciplines. Naturopaths treat the whole person, not necessarily just the illness, recognizing that the body's structure and chemistry are interconnected with the emotions and psyche. Emotional stress can have debilitating effects on the immune, neurological, and endocrine systems, triggering an array of unique responses. Instead of relying on drugs to affect the body chemistry and various ills, diet, botanicals, and lifestyle management are employed as restorative modalities.

The root goal of naturopathic treatment is to find and treat the underlying cause of the patient's condition. Instead of palliating symptoms via the aid of pharmaceuticals, a naturopath attempts to regain internal balance and wellness, termed "homeostasis," within the individual by utilizing therapies that do the least harm. Perhaps the most unfamiliar belief to some coming to naturopathy for the first time is the high regard naturopaths have for the body's innate healing wisdom.

Fevers, muscle pains, or digestive problems are often signs that the body is attempting to reject toxins that have accumulated as the result of an unhealthy lifestyle, infection, or consequential to destructive emotional interplay. Feeling ill can thus be a sign that your systems are attempting to heal you. Various naturopathic methodologies can help propel this process along, employing safe and noninvasive means to support the process instead of camouflaging or interrupting it. Neglecting symptomology, however, is not encouraged. If something hurts or disturbs you, it's important to tell your naturopath about this.

Prevention is also a key piece of naturopathic medicine. Much counseling is available regarding how to live a less toxic, more healthful lifestyle. It has long been recognized in various cultures of the world that our body is essentially a temple; that is why we need to know how to respect and care for it. Diet, exercise, and emotional fitness are all important. A premium is placed on avoiding potentially harmful substances such as alcohol, tobacco, caffeine, and highly processed foods, especially those with chemical additives, hydrogenated oils, or GMO ingredients. Fresh, whole foods are supremely valued; organic, local sources are preferable; and commercially prepared items are to be avoided.

Lots of fresh air and sunshine, coupled with regular physical activity, keep our systems running smoothly. Our body is comprised of big, broad, capable muscles that need to be used often and rigorously. In today's convenience-oriented lifestyle, some of these commonsense basics are overlooked. Naturopathic medicine reminds us to care for ourselves when we are well and to turn to nature's bountiful resources when we are ill.

The Council for Naturopathic Medical Education (CNME) regulates the various teaching institutions in its capacity as an accrediting body. There are currently five fully accredited schools in the United States and two in Canada, graduates of which are able to qualify for the Naturopathic Physicians Licensing Exams (NPLEX). Upon passing these exams NDs are able to apply for a license in states that license NDs. These states do not recognize naturopaths receiving their training from the many correspondence schools that abound. The ND initials appear after one's name upon school graduation. If you are concerned about NPLEX status, do inquire of your practitioner.

Naturopathic medicine can be of tremendous support while undergoing autoimmune or Lyme treatment and recovery. In fact, my opinion is that a Lyme-literate naturopath is perhaps the most qualified practitioner to deal with Lyme disease. They have an ample toolbox of skills, and great access to finely tuned specialty tests that common physicians do not know of. Even if you are under an antibiotic protocol regime, naturopathic medicine can provide many restorative supportive nutritional and herbal formulas, or bodywork modalities, such as lymphatic massage and hydrotherapy, as the body rebuilds depletions and cleanses itself from the Lyme bacteria and die-off. Detoxification is a critical step in Lyme disease recovery. The toxins that accumulate from the Lyme bacteria alone are enough to cause disturbing symptomology within one's system. The horrid brain fog and memory issues are typical of the neurotoxin brew.

As the Lyme bacteria are killed off, more uncomfortable feelings, energy loss, brain fog, and malaise can continue. Detoxification processes will help eliminate and reduce much of this symptomology and improve one's level of vitality and energy. Naturopathic medicine is a perfect avenue to resort to when undergoing detoxification processes. Detoxification can be difficult to try to manage on your own at home without proper guidance from a licensed practitioner. It's strongly encouraged to turn to naturopathic medicine for these purposes. Most medical doctors are not educated about the various support measures that can be employed for detoxification, such as herbs, colon treatments, skin scrubbing, sauna therapies, and sunlight therapy. Naturopaths are highly skilled in these modalities. Please read the detoxification chapter included. This is a naturopath's forte, however. All of the autoimmune disorders will benefit from the vast scope of care that naturopaths possess. With an emphasis on restoring and supporting the human body, mind, and spirit, naturopathy is strongly encouraged.

The digestive tract can be a real mess, the lining irritated and permeable, the flora way off-kilter, enzymes significantly depleted. This alone is worth seeking a naturopath's advice, as 80 percent of immune function resides in the gut. However, immune restoration, yeast proliferation, nervous system exhaustion, hormonal collapse, and thyroid and adrenal compromise are all specific areas common to chronic Lyme and autoimmune illnesses. Naturopaths have valuable methods to correct these disorders, plus state-of-the-art specialty labs that are better attuned to addressing metabolic disorders than the conventional larger hospital and commercial labs, helping pinpoint exact imbalances and enabling custom treatment unique to each individual.

WHAT IS HOMEOPATHIC MEDICINE?

Classical homeopathy is a comprehensive branch of alternative medicine that has been in existence since the late 1700s. The founder, a German physician named Samuel Hahnemann, brought to light two intrinsic principals, which are the cornerstones of this healing discipline. The first, known as "the Law of Similars," states that something that can cause a disease can also cure it. The second is the "magic of the minimum dose," which is the least amount of a substance to be used for curative purposes, but not to induce side effects.

Dr. Samuel Hahnemann was a research scientist working on understanding why quinine, or Peruvian bark, was effective in curing malaria. The suspicion was that its highly bitter quality was the essential reason. Hahnemann was not convinced of that explanation. During his studies he elected to self-experiment and began taking quinine himself. Curiously enough, a couple of weeks into this process Hahnemann developed the symptoms of malaria. This struck him as odd, as he wondered why a substance that was curing an illness could also cause it.

Hahnemann stopped taking the quinine, and the symptoms cleared up. He recommenced it and the malaria symptoms returned. This sparked the scientist's thinking. He turned to the converse thought process that if something can cause an illness to manifest, it could, in turn, be curative to that symptom state. Thus classical homeopathic theory was born.

Hahnemann devoted the rest of his long, illustrious life to exploring hundreds of common substances and their curative capabilities. He hired dozens of associate physicians and scientists to do tests on multitudes of substances, ranging from traditionally used herbals like chamomile and leopard's bane, to the more dangerous medical substances of arsenic and mercury. The cataloguing of these tests and studies done on hundreds of human beings is compiled in the *Homeopathic Materia Medica*. It's a vast, brilliant piece of scientific work. Homeopaths still rely on this "bible" over two hundred years later.

Hahnemann was concerned about the dangerous side effects of taking too much of a substance, specifically arsenic and mercury, then used liberally for treating syphilis. This spurred him into experimenting with diluting amounts for curative work. Something sparked Dr. Hahnemann's thinking to shake or "success" each progressive dilution as it was made. He would start by making a mother tincture of a substance, akin to an herbal tea, then dilute it one part to ten and shake that mixture. He then took one drop of that newly shaken potency, which he labeled as 1x, and mixed that with another ten parts water in a new vial, shook that and labeled it 2x. One drop of the 2x was taken and diluted with ten parts water, shaken and became 3x. He continued this process of "potentization," discovering that the more diluted, yet energetically "shaken" potencies were faster acting and longer holding than the former one. So a 20x potency procured better results, eradicating symptoms more effectively than a 2x. This is the "minimum dose" principle of homeopathy. After the thirtieth dilution, mixing one part matter with ten parts water or alcohol, no medicinal substance is found in the remedy, yet its effects are remarkably more effective than taking the original mother tincture—energy medicine at its finest.

Homeopathy spread like wildfire across Europe in the 1800s, becoming favored in the French and English courts. It made its way to America and across the Great Plains on wagon trains. Most households in the late 1800s relied on the homeopathic remedies arnica, lycopodium, and Rhus tox for an assortment of ills. The world's greatest homeopaths, James Tyler Kent and William Boericke, flourished along the East Coast at the turn of 1900. Dozens of homeopathic hospitals and colleges prospered in the era. In fact the first medical society in the United States, known as the American Homeopathic Association (AHA), was founded in 1843, four years before the American Medical Association (AMA). The wealthy and famous, including the Rockefellers and Mark Twain, as well as the common man, found homeopathy to be gentle, effective, and reliable.

During the massive typhoid and influenza epidemics of the early 1900s, those who relied on homeopathic treatment fared dramatically better than those who turned to allopathic medicine. Homeopathic pharmacies abounded in all the major US cities well into the 1920s. Then, unexpectedly, things shifted with the advent of the Food and Drug Administration (FDA) and a quest to eradicate the "snake oil" sideshow charlatans peddling nebulous elixirs at fairs and on sidewalks.

Laws were created regarding patenting, a wise step, and a man named Abraham Flexner was installed to investigate the numerous "quack doctors" and lay-physicians trained at the knee of their father-physican or in the wards of a Civil War hospital. Homeopathy, unfortunately, became decimated in Flexner's single-minded ambition to preserve only modern MDs. By the 1940s, homeopathy, natural medicine, had essentially vanished from America's life, pharmacies boarded up, the schools' and homeopathic hospitals' licenses revoked. Only the Hahnemann Hospital in Philadelphia remained. Fortunately, FDA laws were passed regulating the manufacture of homeopathic remedies as standard over-the-counter aids, leaving them legally available. Still, with the advent of antibiotics and cortisone, both so-called miracle drugs, the pharmaceutical industry had planted itself front and center in our society, shoving aside all other modalities, unlike in Europe, Asia, and South America, which integrated homeopathy alongside Western medicine, enabling a more complementary practice of medicine to thrive in those continents.

Homeopathy embraces many ideals. Respecting the wisdom of the healing force within is one of homeopathy's tenets. The body wants to heal, continually attempting to right itself when off-center, using primary methods of discharge to purge toxins and emotional impediments. The essence of homeopathy is to honor these attempts, by providing the person with a remedy that actually mimics the constellation of symptomology, not counteracting the process already under way. Suppressing or counteracting symptomology, as allopathic ("opposite suffering") medicine does (i.e., via decongestants or muscle relaxants), is oppositional to homeopathic doctrine. Instead the simillimum remedy works by supporting and actually speeding up the healing process.

The two primary avenues of homeopathic application are acute and chronic care. Acute ills, such as sunburn, influenza, or bee stings, are self-limiting conditions and readily addressed with a remedy, often in a self-help vein. Chronic ills, like colitis, fibromyalgia, or asthma, are treated by a certified practitioner at a constitutional level. The concept of a "constitutional type" is another essential facet of classical homeopathy.

Each of us is recognized as being born with a particular given constitutional blueprint or type. Classical homeopaths are trained to identify one's constitutional type by a set of qualities: body type, coloring, personality traits, and tendencies when ill. Genetic strengths and weaknesses in individual constitutional types are prone to manifestation of particular ills when run down or weakened. One's natural characteristics and specific symptoms are all valued as illustrative measures, guiding a practitioner to the wondrously compatible substance from nature that most closely energetically resonates with each person and their innate life force. A Cimicifuga (black snake root) constitution will readily develop depression, migraines, joint pains, and stiffness. Meanwhile, a Silicea (flint) constitution shows easy tendencies to colds, ear infections, chronic fatigue syndrome, cysts, bowel irregularities, and often lack of self-confidence and social anxieties.

It's critical for homeopaths to understand the person for who he or she is, as it's the person, not the disease, who is being treated. Discovering whom each individual is and what makes them tick, how they react to the world around them, what inspires them, what deflates them, is the agenda of the homeopath. Constitutional prescribing helps restore harmony and balance within the individual, whereby the body is then able to right itself, throwing off the symptoms and illness of its own accord.

Classical homeopathy is still practiced essentially the same as it has been for well over two hundred years. Homeopaths pay close attention to the details of symptoms and their fluctuations. Observation is essential, as well as the patient's communication of their sensations and symptoms. The homeopath then matches the person and the remedy, thus coining the expression one knows so well with classical homeopathy that "like treats like." Allergy shots and vaccination principles have been borrowed from the homeopathy model of "like treats like." A minute amount of a particular ingredient is introduced to stimulate the body's own reactionary processes. Thus allergy shots, vaccinations, and homeopathic remedies all work in a similar way, though homeopathic remedies are administered sublingually and are energy medicine rather than biochemical preparations.

Homeopathy requires two years of postgraduate training plus a premed background. Homeopaths are not considered primary healthcare providers unless they hold a license in another profession, such as MD, DO, DC, or LPN. Classical homeopaths can't give exams, prescribe pharmaceuticals, or make a diagnosis. They will, however, make sure you receive the medical evaluation and care needed when indicated. Most have working relationships with allied healthcare professionals, often in a shared office or clinic. The Council for Homeopathic Certification examines candidates for national certification annually. A good homeopath must be an excellent listener, open-minded, and a keen observer. A strong memory helps, too, as homeopaths need to be intimately familiar with hundreds of remedies to pass the national exam.

It's a very tall order for a homeopath to pinpoint the one essential remedy out of over four thousand choices at the time of your first visit. Sometimes a few visits may be required before the perfect match is identified, but then a whole new feeling of well-being is found. Symptom alleviation can be rapid with an acute condition, often even when the remedy pellets are still dissolving under the tongue, as with an allergy spell. With chronic illness, regained wellness comes during a span of weeks and months as the body recalibrates.

Classical homeopathy experienced a resurgence in the United States in the late 1970s, when Dr. Bill Gray introduced Dr. George Vithoulkas, master homeopath from Greece, to the pioneering collective of doctors, nurses, vets, and laypeople who had held the remnants of this healing art in a protective clutch. Soon other great masters from South America and Europe came to train these followers. By the late 1990s homeopathic schools were reborn and pharmacies on the rise. Today, commonly used potencies, such as 6c, 30c, and 200c (in which c dilutions indicate 1/100 parts), are available in most health food stores and even allopathic pharmacies, and large, high-tech machines make it possible to potentize remedies up to the 50,000 dilution.

Homeopathy has not been studied at the scientific level during the technological mastery of the 1900s. It has ambled along, mostly disregarded as old-fashioned and a bit fantastical. Because it does not fit the scientific standards of pharmacology and deductive reasoning, much of our American medical system has tried to dismiss homeopathy as unproven and unscientific. It must be evaluated on a different spectrum, since its language and values are so divergent from allopathic medicine, being a system of empirical findings and data. Generations, however, testify to homeopathy's capable workings. Animals and infants respond to it unequivocally. Germany's, France's, and India's physicians are schooled in homeopathy.

Classical homeopathy offers highly valuable support in the treatment of all autoimmune illnesses and Lyme disease. Individual remedies may be prescribed to treat the various acute symptoms that plague the individual, whether joint pain, stomach irregularities, headaches, depression, anxiety, or insomnia. All such states are greatly aided by the fine workings of homeopathic remedies.

I, myself, found homeopathy to be indispensable in the circuitous journey I have traveled in overcoming chronic illness. I truly believe that without the assistance of this wonderful healing discipline I would not have made the most obvious strides I have. Please do not overlook this effective modality. Internationally, it is a well-respected and utilized healing system.

Homeopathic remedies can be found in most health food stores, or ordered online from the world-renowned pharmacy Boiron. There are dozens of singular homeopathic remedies pertinent to clearing acute Lyme (and coinfection) symptoms. Personally, bryonia, Epatorium perf, pulsatilla, natrum mur saved my life! There are also wonderful "combination formulas" that contain four to eight low-dose remedies in synergy to use at a purely physiological, or what homeopaths call "clinical symptom," level to help in either detoxification measures, fibromyalgia pains, neurotransmitter balancing, insomnia, and more. The realm is enormous actually.

Nuances and subtleties make all the difference in finding remedies that are a "direct" match for your case. Seeing a professional classical homeopath (CCH) or naturopath (ND) who specializes in homeopathy is key! Many practitioners call themselves homeopaths. They are not properly certified. This is not a good situation. Homeopathy gets misused and misrepresented and is often ineffective in the hands of an only partially trained practitioner. You want a master, not a dabbler. This healing art requires vast training, a very astute mind, and someone with great perspective and finesse. Practitioners can be found via the National Center for Homeopathy and the Council for Homeopathic Certification.

All homeopathics are labeled by their Latin name, so they can be found in worldwide pharmacies, versus their common name (e.g., wind flower or pasque flower for pulsatilla), which may vary by region. All remedies are to be taken with a "clean mouth," meaning no food, drink, toothpaste, gum, etc. fifteen minutes before or after a dose. Dissolve two pellets under the tongue, absorbed by the sublingual glands and bypassing the digestive tract. Some people note symptom alleviation in mere seconds under the tongue, others could require several doses for a change. Do not handle the pellets with your fingers, etc., as they are sensitive to oils, fragrances, and can become "negated." Just pop them in your mouth, a child's, even a pet's lips, quickly. Some people dissolve the pellets in two inches of pure water and sip the solution over an hour or so. Thousands of books are available on this wondrous healing art. India, Germany, France, England have relied upon it for centuries.

The appendix includes some basic remedies for self-help assistance while you seek a certified classical homeopath. See HomeopathicEducationalServices.org for a vast array of self-help books, DVDs, textbooks, materia medicas, and more.

WHAT IS ACUPUNCTURE?

Acupuncture is a three-thousand-year-old healing discipline heralding from China. Anecdotal evidence claims that this practice may actually date back five thousand years. Very little in this intricate yet straightforward approach to healing has altered throughout its history, primarily because the philosophy and practices of acupuncture have required scant improvement.

In 1949, Chairman Mao tried to eradicate the religious and superstitious mystical aspects of Chinese medicine and acupuncture, but when taken ill, his life was saved by this "folk medicine." So he allowed acupuncture to continue, but only as a less spiritual practice. In recent decades acupuncture has moved beyond the walls of China into the Western world. Many people arrive at acupuncturists seeking pain alleviation, which is one of its fortes. The realm of this healing discipline extends much beyond such a scope, addressing hoards of complaints and illnesses. The Chinese have relied on acupuncture and Chinese herbal formulas for treatment of organic disorders and conditions such as MS, asthma, colitis, infertility, stroke, insomnia, and more. The American Medical Association (AMA) has published a list of thousands of conditions that can be treated by acupuncture.

Looking at acupuncture in practice requires us to understand some of its philosophy. All living matter, whether it be a cat, a tree, or a human being, contains a life force or energy. This miraculous dimension, intrinsic to our existence, is rather difficult to evaluate through science. We all recognize that life energy, or qi (chi), as the Chinese call it, is vital to life yet is of rather nebulous boundaries. Western science has been unable to determine accurately where life energy comes from and why it disappears at the time of death. But it certainly is real, even if unseen by the naked eye or sophisticated test equipment. Just as we know emotions are real, so is life energy. We certainly can't see the energy of anger or sadness, but when you walk into the room of one who is in the throes of such an emotion, you can feel it radiating from them. Qi is similar.

Methodologies from many Asian cultures, such as tai chi, macrobiotics, feng shui, shiatsu, qi gong, and acupuncture, focus on this qi force. Chinese medicine suggests that within the body there lie fourteen energy meridians, which network the qi. These meridians run essentially in a longitudinal direction head to toe. Each meridian encompasses a pathway between various body parts, organs, and glands. Charts depict these meridians quite specifically. Practitioners also relate them to one of the five elements of nature as a way of describing one's system and the imbalances. You will hear an acupuncturist using terms such as Earth, Fire, Water, Wood, and Metal.

At various points in the body, a meridian channel runs close to the skin's surface, referred to as acupuncture points. When an organ is in a state of imbalance, these points exhibit a telltale signal via sensitivity and tonicity. These points have been empirically agreed on for thousands of years. Anatomical landmarks for where they are and unique functions that each point has attributed to it are undisputed in the profession. There has been some scientific research to determine noticeable differences at these points. Some studies have found a greater degree of salinity in the precise area of the points, while others have noticed increased electromagnetic readings. This research, however, is still underway and has yet to be completely verified.

The signs of disturbance along the energy meridians are rather subtle to the average person, yet practitioners identify them quickly.

Chinese medicine relies on another facet of diagnosis: pulse points. Several pulse points are located on each wrist. These spots specifically correspond to the energy meridians. Through keen appraisal of the pulse points, a trained practitioner is able to access the status of the varied meridians and the corresponding body parts. By correlating the findings the practitioner is able to determine such bodily imbalances as anemia, heart disease, kidney weaknesses, and much more. Most of us marvel at the accuracy of these assessments when they are then verified by laboratory findings.

Acupuncture is actually a component of the comprehensive system of Chinese medicine, including herbal formulas and diet. Illness or states of discomfort are eliminated by unblocking, redirecting, and balancing the qi forces within.

Once the acupuncturist has identified your imbalances, fine hair-like needles are inserted into the corresponding acupuncture points. Unlike a hollow injection needle, these solid ones cause no pain other than sometimes a minute pricking sensation. They are inserted very delicately into the skin atop the muscles or joints. Joints are like rocks or boulders in the streams of energy flow. Various stresses, such as thermal, physical, emotional, nutritional, and mental can also upset the qi of particular meridians. When such a situation lingers too long or is quite forceful, illness can set in. By activating the acupuncture points, the disturbed qi along the meridian is restored. When all meridians are experiencing adequate flow of the qi, the body functions in a perfect state of health and harmony.

Length and number of acupuncture treatments will vary, depending on several factors: acute or chronic condition, multiple meridian involvement, an individual's particular life force, and age. Chronic conditions typically require a series of treatments, while an acute illness may be corrected in one or two visits. Lyme disease in both acute and chronic forms responds well to acupuncture. It's both supportive and restorative, helping build up one's energy, immunity, and wellness. Multiple treatments are necessary, though, as Lyme disease is an aggressive illness. Some people need months of devout treatment.

The Chinese medicine herbal formulas are numerous, some millennia old. These formulas will vary for each individual, depending on your manifestation of symptoms and the nature of the state of imbalance. Two people coming in with lower back pain may end up with different herbal formulas and have needles inserted in different locations, since one person may have blocked liver qi and the other may discover that his toxic colon is to blame. With Lyme, several formulas may be selected, as so many systems of the body are affected. Additionally, as the Lyme bacteria are killed off, the liver and kidneys respond well to strong support via acupuncture treatments and certain herbal formulas to help flush out these toxins. Acupuncture is a wonderful helpmate in this detoxification process, which is an essential component of Lyme recovery.

Some insurance carriers cover acupuncture treatment. This is an exciting step in the progress of our healthcare system. There are a couple dozen accredited acupuncture and Oriental medicine graduate programs offered in the United States. Practitioners then sit for a national certification exam followed by state exams. The National Certification Commission for Acupuncture and Oriental Medicine (NCCAOM) and Clean Needle certificate course must be passed. State licensure varies from state to state. Some, like California, require separate exams for licensing. Each state also requires additional CEU (continuing education units) in order to maintain licensure. Your acupuncturist should be nationally certified by the NCCAOM and hold a current state license in the state in which you receive treatment. The NCCAOM can help individuals locate licensed acupuncturists in your area.

This fascinating branch of Eastern medicine can provide great benefits to many. Please do not gloss over its very capable workings during your journey toward wellness in tackling Lyme disease; I find it still to be a terrific asset even in the wellness capacity.

WHAT IS CLINICAL NUTRITION?

Many individuals question why they would ever seek out the advice of a nutritionist other than to lose weight. The fact of the matter is that highly specialized certified clinical nutritionists are very capable of addressing all sorts of healthcare conditions, focusing on the biochemistry of the body and its function or improper function. The best of the best in this field have made some breakthrough discoveries in their studies and clinical research while others have crafted marvelous formulas for healing deeply compromising conditions such as neuropathy, colitis, and assorted autoimmune diseases.

It was a certified clinical nutritionist whom I credit for saving my life. Five years of my life spiraled away from me until I was bedridden, bankrupt, and emotionally broken from misdiagnosed Lyme disease. Three false negative ELISA Lyme tests led me doctor-hopping through some of the most famous hospitals and to the most highly revered doctors in New England, and none could "fix" me nor give a reason as to why my health was deteriorating more and more every year. They had ruled out Lyme disease and chalked it up to autoimmune disorders and a migraine-anxiety complex.

Bedridden and wheelchair bound with chronic fatigue syndrome collapse, palsy, MS-style foot drop, crippling migraines, early onset dementia, and fibromyalgia, on a tangential stretch I reached out to a colleague of mine, whom I had sent "difficult" cases to over a ten-year span. I figured perhaps he would know what to make of my horrific decline in health and offer me some sort of restoration, as I had seen this brilliant clinical nutritionist work wonders on some very confusing cases in the past.

I recall the day in vivid clarity that I sat in the teal green armchair across the desk from my seasoned friend relaying my horrifying story to him, quaking in weakness and shedding a trickle of tears. Twenty minutes into my story the doctor says to me, "Katina, this is Lyme disease. You have an advanced case of neurological Lyme disease that has gone untreated and is wreaking havoc on your immune function and likely numerous other systems from what you are describing."

I sat stunned and muttered, "No, no I have been tested three times for Lyme and they said I didn't have it." And, that is when I learned the wretched truth about the faulty lab testing, the lack of physician education, and the enormous damage chronic forms of Lyme disease create.

The good out of the bad is that this clinical nutritionist knew of a state-of-the-art specialty Lyme-testing lab in California to use and we validated his suspicion with positive test results. Having dealt with the illness numerous times in his twenty-five years in practice, the doctor had three wise recommendations for me: "First we will open up your detox pathways, then assess and address the worst of your nutritional imbalances and depletions, and finally kill off the "bugs" with high-quality herbal antimicrobials. It could take two or three years of devoted work, but I believe you can regain 80 percent of your health and vitality."

Shocked, relieved, and angry all at the same time, I was in good hands. The metabolic profile analysis tests he ran illustrated the damage to my neurotransmitters, the imbalance of flora and rampant inflammation in my gut, and the extreme collapse of my adrenal glands and other hormonal imbalances. He tailored a diet for me as well as supplements. I saw him every six weeks and in five years I was 100 percent recovered!

All the while this astute, caring, and well-schooled practitioner was constantly assessing and delving into supplements and dietary or lifestyle changes I needed to make for recovery. Though at times I was taking handfuls of supplements, I did not care, because I was improving. The anxiety rapidly vanished with an amino acid glycine, and my chronic fatigue was gone in three weeks of Monolaurin. We rebuilt me from the ground up.

Not all clinical nutritionists are the same. The profession has a certifying body and a national exam. However, some people call themselves a nutritionist with merely an online degree and no classroom or practice intern relations. See the websites AmericanNutritionAssociation.org, www.cncb.org, and www.IAACN.org for more information.

Registered dietitians are different than nutritionists. They tend to work in institutional settings and are not focused on health disorders and healing, but rather on food groups and sanitation. See the descriptions below to clarify. Nutritionists get into the field generally because they either love biochemistry or are drawn to the health and disease relationship via foods and physiology. Their selective pathways to nourishing the malfunctioning body parts are fundamental to life and renewal.

Certified Clinical Nutritionist, CCN: A CCN is a highly qualified nutritional professional with a four-year bachelor's degree and a 900-hour internship, a fifty-six-hour postgraduate intensive study in clinical nutrition, or a master's degree in human nutrition from the University of Bridgeport or Bastyr University, and must pass the national board exam issued by the CNCB. The CCN focuses on how foods are digested, absorbed, and assimilated, and ultimately how food affects the body biochemically. Among the many aspects of nutrition research considered within this context are by-products of digestion, gastrointestinal health, neurotransmitter response, immune function, metabolic shifts and balance, allergic or sensitivity reactions, and systems and pathways of detoxification. The CCN's approach to diet structure is developed according to what is best for the individual—

not necessarily what is a standard recommendation for the general public at large, or for all people experiencing a particular health concern. Rather than strictly advocating a pyramid or food-group-style diet, the CCN will determine the healthiest and most effective program for the individual according to the latest nutrition research and the unique biochemical makeup of the individual.

Registered Dietitian, RD: An RD is a food and dietary professional, usually with a four-year bachelor's degree and 900 to 1,200 hours in a dietetic internship through an accredited program and passing a dietetics registration exam. Dietitians focus on calories (energy), sanitation, and avoiding spoilage and contamination, meal planning, evaluation of standard measurements of foods, specific diets for certain conditions, and eating patterns based primarily on food groups, such as the food pyramid, and other guidelines based on daily food intake strictly outlined by health organizations. Dietitians often work in health institutions as clinical dietitians, management dietitians, but can also work as community or consultant dietitians.

When facing the perils of autoimmune illness and chronic tick-borne disease infections, I suggest the skills of an expert CCN may be very advantageous for mending. Delving into your particular weaknesses, food intolerances, and toxicities is in their domain.

WHAT IS INTEGRATIVE/ FUNCTIONAL MEDICINE?

A philosophy in medical care that has been gaining ground over the past decade, due to the tremendous insight and hard work of the prominent physician and author Dr. Andrew Weil, is that of integrative medicine. Essentially this form of doctoring involves a traditional Western allopathic physician who is trained in a known established medical school who then goes on to continue his or her education with complementary medicine modalities such as clinical nutrition, herbal medicine, acupuncture, or other special modalities. These practitioners do not give up allopathic medicine in favor for alternative medicine, but rather they blend the two. The unification is integrative medicine or sometimes called complementary alternative medicine with the acronym of CAM.

Sometimes we find integrative medicine healthcare clinics that will include a traditional allopathic physician with other alternative natural medicine doctors and practitioners under the same roof. So you will find an acupuncturist, a homeopath, a massage therapist, a chiropractor, and/or a spiritual healer all working in harmony to bring the best of assorted treatment modalities to their clientele. In my opinion these are the healthcare centers of the future. Every town should have an integrative healthcare center. I'm very proud of my alma mater Duke University for creating an outstanding example of an integrative healthcare facility.

Joining an integrative medicine practice is how I got to New Hampshire way back in 1989—I was a classical homeopath who became part of an integrative healthcare center with eight practitioners working and sharing clientele, bringing them the best supportive and diagnostic treatment protocols available.

Europe and Canada have these types of facilities, and countries around the globe like France and England and even South America and parts of Asia have had integrative medicine established for centuries in their healthcare industries. The USA is behind the times and the explosion of chronic diseases asks for immediate care and attention in this form of treatments. Pharmaceuticals and drug palliation do not cure autoimmune illnesses—they just mollify symptoms.

Dr Andrew Weil succinctly sums up integrative medicine as follows:

> "Using synthetic drugs and surgery to treat health conditions was known just a few decades ago as, simply, 'medicine.' Today, this system is increasingly being termed 'conventional medicine.' This is the kind of medicine most Americans still encounter in hospitals and clinics. Often both expensive and invasive, it is also very good at some things; for example, handling emergency conditions such as massive injury or a life-threatening stroke. Dr. Weil is unstinting in his appreciation for conventional medicine's strengths. 'If I were hit by a bus,' he says, 'I'd want to be taken immediately to a high-tech emergency room.' Some conventional medicine is scientifically validated, some is not.
>
> Integrative medicine is healing-oriented medicine that takes account of the whole person (body, mind, and spirit), including all aspects of lifestyle. It emphasizes the therapeutic relationship and makes use of all appropriate therapies, both conventional and alternative.

The principles of integrative medicine:

- A partnership between patient and practitioner in the healing process
- Appropriate use of conventional and alternative methods to facilitate the body's innate healing response
- Consideration of all factors that influence health, wellness, and disease, including mind, spirit, and community as well as body
- A philosophy that neither rejects conventional medicine nor accepts alternative therapies uncritically
- Recognition that good medicine should be based in good science, be inquiry driven, and be open to new paradigms
- Use of natural, effective, less-invasive interventions whenever possible
- Use of the broader concepts of promotion of health and the prevention of illness as well as the treatment of disease
- Training of practitioners to be models of health and healing, committed to the process of self-exploration and self-development[3]"

Also in the same vein as integrative medicine is a growing term we have heard in the past three or four years, "functional medicine." Functional medicine is similar in its philosophy to naturopathic medicine; however, it involves medical physicians who have taken on a new philosophy toward doctoring.

Please read this wonderful quote from the website of the Institute for Functional Medicine:

> "Functional medicine is a personalized, systems-oriented model that empowers patients and practitioners to achieve the highest

[3] Brad Lemley, DrWeil.com News

expression of health by working in collaboration to address the underlying causes of disease. It is an evolution in the practice of medicine that better addresses the healthcare needs of the twenty-first century. By shifting the traditional disease-centered focus of medical practice to a more patient-centered approach, functional medicine addresses the whole person, not just an isolated set of symptoms. Functional medicine practitioners spend time with their patients, listening to their histories and looking at the interactions among genetic, environmental, and lifestyle factors that can influence long-term health and complex, chronic disease. In this way, functional medicine supports the unique expression of health and vitality for each individual.

'Disease is neither the starting point nor the end point of illness. It is a pathological process that may not be discovered until decades after the identification of an illness.' This insight has been the impetus for many of the new approaches to disease prevention and treatment that have emerged over the last thirty to forty years. Most of us—scientists and physicians alike—would rather not wait until we have a diagnosable disease to address the underlying problems that, over time, cause the signs and symptoms that influence the development of illness and disease.

A major premise of functional medicine is that, using science, clinical wisdom, and innovative tools, we can identify many of the underlying causes of chronic disease and intervene to remediate the dysfunctions, both before and after frank disease is present. People may wonder (quite reasonably) why preventing and treating chronic disease effectively requires something different than is usually available in our very expensive healthcare system. Perhaps the most urgent reason is that a rapidly spreading epidemic of chronic disease has compromised the effectiveness of our healthcare system and threatens to bankrupt both national and global economies. Alarming projections suggest future generations may have shorter, less healthy lives if current trends continue unchecked.

Our current healthcare model fails to confront both the causes of and solutions for chronic disease and must be replaced with a model of comprehensive, personalized care geared to effectively treating and reversing this escalating crisis. Consider the facts. Over the last century, there has been a dramatic shift in prevalence from acute to chronic diseases. By 2020, worldwide deaths from chronic disease are projected to total more than twice the number of deaths from infectious disease (50,000,000 vs. 20,000,000). It is estimated that more than half of all Americans suffer from one or more chronic diseases, and that the 8,000,000 Medicare beneficiaries who have five or more chronic conditions accounted for over two-thirds of the program's $302 billion in spending in 2004.

Of total healthcare costs in the United States, more than 75 percent are due to chronic conditions. In 2008, the US spent 16.2 percent of its GDP ($2.3 trillion) on healthcare. This exceeded the combined federal expenditures for national defense, homeland security, education, and welfare. By 2023, if we don't change how we confront this challenge, annual healthcare costs in the US will rise to over $4 trillion, the equivalent—in a single year—of four Iraq wars, making the cost of care using the current model economically unsustainable. If our health outcomes were commensurate with such costs, we might decide they were worth it. Unfortunately, the US spends twice the median per-capita costs of other industrialized countries, as calculated by the Organization for Economic Cooperation and Development (OECD)."

These words certainly feed into my very own belief system of thirty-five years and why I have been a devoted natural healthcare practitioner. Keeping someone well, or helping their body right itself with less expensive herbal and naturally supportive dietary and other measures keeps us healthier in the long run. I sense the "tipping point" has come, where the rate of chronic illness in the USA is forcing us to examine how to get well, stay well, and prevent becoming unwell. The evolution of integrative medicine is overdue and likely to be a key tool for many of you seeking better health and less drug dependency.

WHAT IS METAPHYSICAL HEALING?

Our body is an astonishing complex of cells, organs, glands, fluids, systems, and emotions that all interplay with one another every nanosecond. Constantly regulating, adjusting, and completing basic functions to keep us alive and moving each and every moment of the day and night, our bodies constantly amaze me with their extraordinary capacity to endure hardships as well as excel when we "ask" them to perform. The cohesiveness of the many systems, as well as our emotional and mental entwinement, procure the experience we call living. It is nothing short of miraculous!

Life is what we are each manifesting. Your life is happening at this very moment that you are reading these very words, most likely sitting somewhere, as you absorb them. You are processing these sentences and taking in information and making evaluations mentally and emotionally to my commentary, as well as the fact that quietly, or maybe in a grumbling way, your body is engaged in this act, too. There is a strong likelihood that many of you reading this book right now are not in perfect health and your body and mind may feel unwell. I understand. As you know, I endured ten painful, trying, and actually decimating years trapped in the rip cords of autoimmune-style illnesses. My body, mind, and spirit were miserable. The suffering of these conditions is not imaginary and you have the right to feel outraged, confused, and even abandoned when the traditional medical methods have not been bringing you healing results.

My goal is to help you reclaim wellness or a significant improvement in your health status. We are much more resourceful as human beings than we give ourselves credit for. This miraculous body we inhabit is outstanding in so many ways, endlessly aiming to help you perform or, when needed, to rest deeply. The symptoms it conveys are signals to help direct us—at the simplest level, when you feel exhausted, it's your body telling you to lie down and sleep, even if you are scheduled to be somewhere. A slightly more complex example is anxiety attacks. An anxiety attack is your body telling you you're in trouble. Honor this. Tune inside and listen to what your heart is saying—"I feel alone and cannot pay my bills," or, "My mate is distant and will not talk to me when I feel so sick." The anxiety bears a message worth listening to even if you cannot immediately correct it. But, the pearl of insight is significant and a directive we often ignore. I know I dismissed my intuitions for decades, brushing them off as merely my imagination or a weird transient thought.

The body and mind are unified and have an internal dialogue concurring that we do not always consciously note in the milliseconds of the interchange. Sometimes days, months, or even years pass until we recognize the "reasons" we are feeling so unwell. I know it took me over five years to understand why I was maimed and bedridden with CFS, migraines, fibromyalgia pains, and depression. Even after the hidden Lyme disease bacteria was properly diagnosed and I was a full year into recovery treatments, I could not put all the pieces of my puzzle together and understand what held me back from full recovery. I did, however, sense my emotions and spirit were still in bad straits. The biggest confusion to me was how to mend my broken spirit. Who should I see for that kind of thing? I felt completely lost in that department. I knew of no doctor or psychologist or pastor who was versed in mending broken spirits. In fact, I Googled "mending a broken spirit" and found nothing of real use. Do you know how to mend a broken spirit?

Sadness prevailed. I kept on meditating, praying, adhering to my new "Lyme diet" and laser-tuned arsenal of nutritive supplements and herbs, while willing myself with visual affirmations toward a vibrant, healthy future. I imagined myself happy and whole, sunning and swimming at a gorgeous tropical beach.

I wanted desperately to be well again! How I longed to escape from the clutches of disease and be active and happy. Stuck at home, I was relegated to floor and bed yoga because I was still too weak to walk more than a few blocks. Very relieved to be actually working on killing off Lyme disease bacteria, Epstein-Barr virus, and babesia infections, instead of just floundering on the sofa for too many amoeba-like years propped up with supportive yet not fully curative care, I noted that I was perhaps 50 percent improved but needed something more to move along my healing. What could that be?

How could I overcome all this loss and the fact that my spirit lay so low without a true sense of hope? Could I really ever swim or dance or work again out in the world? I missed my lithe athleticism with deep pangs, as well as all that roaring, hilarious fun I used to thrive in. Isolation of chronic illness does a real number on so many psyches. How could I pull through this dark vortex, even with a kind boyfriend hugging me nightly and telling me I was beautiful? I lay shallow and inert weeks on end, medical bills towering like Mt. Everest. My sweet eight-year-old son was a busy boy and soaring as a star Little League pitcher, and I could only lie on a blanket at the sidelines during a game. I was improving, yet my impatience was palpable and I felt strongly that I needed something more.

Grace arrived in the mail one spring afternoon. I received a postcard about a spiritual healing weekend retreat north of me in the White Mountains, to be lead by a renowned healer and teacher, Dr. Meredith Young-Sowers, author of a book I loved back in the 1980s, *Agartha: A Journey to the Stars*. Was I strong enough to attend? This workshop felt to be exactly what I had been praying for! My boyfriend surprised me by agreeing to attend too, so I could go.

The weekend was a miracle for me. Forty of us gathered in a ccathedral-ceiling post-and-beam carriage house, with a stretching fieldstone fireplace in the back. Sai Baba, Jesus, and Buddha photos and figures perched on the mantel and candlelight anointed our evening of arrival. Meredith guided us into the core of our souls with absorbing wisdom and deep truths of spiritual insight as I came to unravel the profound understanding of what metaphysical healing is about. We learned about the Seven Energy Chakras our bodies hold and the relationships between our minds and bodies, with our emotions as matchstick igniters for all sorts of symptoms and conditions. By the time we departed for home, forty-eight hours later, I had flushed away a huge collective of sticky emotional debris clogging my immune system and weighing down my once playful spirit. Relieved and awakened, I also found an answer to my question, "How does one mend a broken spirit?"

Metaphysical healing work was the pathway. I had blessedly fallen into the hands of a gifted teacher and healer. On that magical Easter weekend, with the soft green leaves of maples and poplars unfurling around us, I knew in my heart that if I embraced this sort of inner healing work, I could fully recover from all these autoimmune conditions and mend my whole self; body, mind, and spirit! Meredith opened a window into a realm of healing that may seem mystical to some, but actually made a great deal of common sense to me. Finding out that there is a strong, hardy conduit of healing energy inside of each of us and how to tap into it was extremely empowering and literally life altering. There was no turning back!

I had been caring for my body over the past year with high-quality professional-grade supplements and natural plant antimicrobials; now I could tend to my quaking spirit and emotions. When I viscerally experienced the patent workings of the mind-body healing pathway under Meredith's guidance, an entirely new paradigm appeared for me. We are not compartmentalized beings, but whole and resonant. Alit with new understandings and experiential process boosting me, I had rounded a corner, believing fully in my successful future!

The long and short of it all is that I went on to do a year-long metaphysical training program at Meredith's Stillpoint School of Integrative Life Healing. I healed 100 percent and actually gave the commencement speech for our class! My life expanded in so many ways, leading me to become a successful spiritual healer too, helping so many others now, and author of an award-winning book on Lyme disease.

Metaphysical healing is an absolutely essential healing path for those mired in autoimmune and tick-borne diseases. These conditions so often stem from—or are worsened by—a person not living out their heart's desire. You may have been thwarted and burdened, and shoved your essential soul or spirit's purpose for being here in this lifetime aside. For a myriad of individual reasons you may be out of sync with your gut and heart and mind. The illnesses take root because energetically, and eventually biologically, your body has become the voice calling out to you for help. We sadly overlook this spiritual request for so many reasons, and when ignored for too many long months and years, our body creates symptoms and disease states as a dire pleading for meaningful attention.

Pharmacology is rarely the full answer for these long-term illnesses. But thankfully, metaphysical work can be done on your own time by you! The beautiful piece of this healing domain is that you bear the tools. My job in these pages is to help guide you as to what they are and how to implement them. Ultimately, this skill set is yours to develop.

Metaphysical healing has a long relationship with indigenous cultures. Shamans, medicine men/women, priests, and magi, even ancient physicians, all worked with the understanding that the energy of thought forms can affect a person physically and emotionally. Metaphysicians value the unseen world as prominently as the seen world. Science only focuses on the seen or empirically collated tangible world. Our current medical system is science-based and has dismissed the value of the unseen, except in the domain of psychiatry.

Metaphysical healing is based on the belief that negative mental patterns, left unchecked, can eventually result in physical disease or illness. By reversing specific negative mental patterns into positive patterns we can promote healing.

Though Western medicine dismisses the notion of metaphysical healing, there is little doubt about the connection between the mind and body. Doctors routinely tell patients to keep spirits high and encourage visits from family and friends, understanding that anything that makes a patient feel better mentally and emotionally aids healing. Depression, on the other hand, tends to slow healing.

Metaphysical healing takes this principle to a very fundamental level, in exact ways. According to metaphysical insights, certain common negative thinking habits affect particular areas of the body. For example, financial worries tend to manifest as lower back problems. The logic here is that the back represents support. In metaphysical healing terms, if you are experiencing lower back pain or soreness, you would examine your thought process to see if you have been overanxious about money issues. Once the negative thinking pattern is identified and replaced with a new habitual positive pattern, the backaches, if caused by the old negative pattern, should subside. The correlations between assorted conditions and thought patterns are quite remarkable.

The idea behind metaphysical thinking is that the individual is his or her own healer, able to affect both health and illness. When we fall ill, in metaphysical healing terms, we recognize this was not by chance, but by mental patterns that can be identified and replaced. The type and point of origin of the ailment gives a clue where to look for the emotional reactions and thinking patterns. The body and mind are actually united in a "map" of sorts that ties the major systems together with set energy grids and corresponding emotions. We are not haphazardly designed, but actually fine-tuned, sentient beings. Seeing the summation of it all is quite fascinating, and it is a shame that it has been dismissed for a few hundred years in the Western world.

According to metaphysical healing understanding, the most compromising emotions to health are long-standing guilt, resentment, grief, and anger. The biggest healers are self-love, self-acceptance, and self-worth.

In the late 1800s, the most popular metaphysical healer and eventual religious leader was Mary Baker Eddy, the founder of Christian Science, who healed herself from spinal paralysis after an accident had left her bed-bound for many years. Her public talks and appearances would garner audiences in the tens of thousands, as well as launch the prominent newspaper, *The Christian Science Monitor*, which shares news without the "pang" of emotional content. Her book *Science of Mind* is still a wellspring of metaphysical knowledge. Eddy espoused the power of the mind and prayer with enormous success in a pre-pharma culture when lifestyle pacing was more purist. Her famous expression "mind over matter" is still touted, even though the religious aspect of her doctrines have come under controversy on many occasions, as science-based medicine with many of its miraculous procedures or antibiotic rescue measures has been rejected by Christian Scientist followers.

Arguably the best-known modern proponent of metaphysical healing is Louise Hay. Her books have sold tens of millions of copies, translated into twenty-nine different languages over thirty-five countries. She began teaching techniques for it in the 1970s. Hay had an opportunity to put her techniques to the test when she was diagnosed with vaginal cancer, and subsequently claimed to heal herself. Still vibrant in her eighties today, her imprint Hay House Publishing has produced many well-loved books.

Most proponents of metaphysical healing do not believe in shunning Western medicine, but do believe that illness is a by-product of an unhealthy mental pattern, and if the by-product is simply removed by doctors but the causation remains, the illness will return. Taking responsibility for our own well-being as much as possible can create better outcomes and less medical dependency.

PART IV

Recovery Guide

CAUSES OF INFLAMMATION AND AUTOIMMUNE TOXINS

The common denominator with all autoimmune illnesses as well as Lyme disease is systemic inflammation. Inflammation can occur anywhere in the body. Any system, organ, or gland can become inflamed, as well as a site such as a joint or your spine. Most of us recognize inflammation when we get a bee sting or twist an ankle. The sharp, often hot pain is notable minutes after an accident or sting.

What has occurred internally at a physiological level is a cue to the adrenal glands and nervous system that either a foreign agent (bee venom) or damage (pulled ligament or tendon) has occurred. As a self-righting and self-protecting organism, our body aims to arrest any further damage. Immediately, the affected tissues emit chemicals that alert the brain to go into survival self-protection mode. In seconds, the adrenal glands are instructed to make corticosteroids, natural auto-inflammatory and anti-inflammatory agents, which attempt to corral the afflicted area from getting further damaged and bleeding internally. By surrounding the injected venom or ruptured tissues, the inflammation keeps the agent from voyaging through the bloodstream to the heart and other major organs. Simultaneously, histamines and adrenaline are released, also as self-protective measures.

Inflammation initially is a good response. The body is attempting to contain the injury or the invasive agent. Injured muscles actually stiffen up in what we call "splinting" to prevent the already strained or torn connective tissue or muscle from bulging or tearing further. The awful pains of back or knee swelling are examples of natural "splinting" measures. These physiological actions hurt! And we want to stop the pain and swelling and spasms as soon as we can. We often turn to medications immediately. The advent of steroid creams, anti-inflammatory pills, and painkillers have become staples in every household. For injuries and allergies, Benadryl and Advil have helped millions through a rough patch of a sudden minor accident.

Autoimmune illnesses such as MS, fibromyalgia, Crohn's disease, RA, and CPS/ME all are purported to be situations where your natural immune system, your first and secondary lines of defense, have somehow gone into overdrive and your body has turned on itself, making too many inflammatory cytokines, histamines, and fighter cells and not enough of the natural corticosteroids. Western medicine says you have a "flaw" and an apparent autoimmune disease. The efforts are to assist an individual by stopping the symptom and stymie the immune system from working in overdrive. Usually a drug is used to tamp down a symptom—diarrhea, razor-sharp migraines, or excruciating joints. But we want to do more than just alleviate the symptoms—we want to put a stop to the underlying causes.

To do this, we must address two major questions:

A. What is triggering inflammation inside of me?

B. Why can my adrenal glands not make the normal corticosteroids I need to help my immune system do its job?

Here is a comprehensive list of all the instigating factors that can make you more susceptible to an autoimmune illness or chronic tick-borne disease. Remember, your body is a small microcosm, like a terrarium. Your skin is the outermost layer and all the systems and bones lie inside. We must keep the proper balance and ratios running smoothly to maintain good health. When several of the following factors coincide, it can create a negative chain reaction. Your pH becomes too acidic, microbes then have a fertile breeding ground to thrive in, whereby the endocrine system and the immune system disregulate. The result is damage to a vulnerable organ and the switch is thrown, so to speak, to set your immune system to leap into an overactive, self-protective mode. Inflammation soars and you feel awful.

Look at this list. How many of these topics are issues for you? Get yourself to an integrative physician or see a naturopath or a clinical nutritionist to run the proper blood tests to determine if any of these factors are contributing to your illness.

<u>Inflammatory-Inducing Agents</u>

- Foods
  - sugar
  - dairy (for those who are sensitive or lactose intolerant)
  - gluten (found in wheat, oats, rye, barley)
  - hydrogenated oils
- Mold damage: current or past exposure
- Heavy metals
  - mercury (tuna, swordfish, dental fillings, vaccines)
  - lead (paint, pipes)
  - copper (pipes, artesian wells)
  - cadmium (galvanized pipes, cigarette smoke)
  - fluoride (in toothpastes, water systems, dental sealants—it is a toxic halogen that suppresses thyroid function)
- Chemical toxins
  - environmental
    - glyphosate (Roundup)
    - paints, solvents
    - dry-cleaning solvents

    - pesticides
    - cosmetics
    - food additives, preservatives, dyes
    - drugs, including antibiotics and corticosteroids
- Plastics (leaching into foods)
- Imbalanced gut flora (candida, yeasts)
- Birth control pills
- Parasites (foreign travel, foods)
- Tick-borne diseases
    - Lyme bacteria
    - bartonella
    - babesia
    - mycoplasma
- Viruses: Epstein-Barr, cytomegalia, etc.
- Antibiotic overuse
- Vitamin and mineral deficiencies
    - A, B, C, D, E
    - trace minerals
    - selenium
    - potassium
    - iodine
    - amino acids
- Food sensitivities
- Genetic predispositions:
    - MTHFR (Methylene tetrahydrofolate reductase)
    - mitochondria disregulation

The assistance of an integrative medical doctor, naturopath, or certified nutritionist can help you scout out these contributing factors. There are many finely-calibrated lab tests to get clear information on which of these areas are plaguing you. Chances are you have several categories involved if you have become ill with Lyme disease or autoimmune illness.

The wonderful news is that all these facets can be addressed. Though cleaning up toxic burdens can take time, and repairing damage from molds and bacterial infections requires dedication, with the right support and positive mindset, the body is capable of making great recovery strides. Obviously, the longer you have been ill, the more time and support will be needed for removing offending factors and creating repair.

Finding a cleansing regimen and low-inflammation diet is key. Your practitioner will also see if you are a candidate for chelation therapy to remove heavy metals, as well as how to repair a possible "leaky gut" intestinal lining.

Addressing your body's pH balance is also essential. Most modern stress levels, fast foods, alcohol consumption, coffee, and pharmaceuticals tip us into the acidic domain, which allows all sorts of microbes, yeasts, and parasites to thrive. Lyme and cancers love acidic pH terrain.

Fresh vegetable juices (especially green drinks), a low load of animal proteins, and eliminating sugar, gluten, alcohol, and coffee will help alkalinize the pH. Alkalinized water may also be helpful. Your practitioner will help you address remediating a moldy home, as well as how to use homeopathic nosodes to rebuild your system's reaction.

If tick-borne organisms, especially Lyme disease or mycoplasma, are involved, they do a real "spin cycle" on the body and the brain's neurotransmitters. Dr. Richard Horowitz explains in his MSIDS (multi-systemic infectious disease syndrome) healing model, in his bestselling book *Why Can't I Get Better? Solving the Mystery of Lyme and Chronic Disease,* the mechanisms of how the Lyme bacteria get inside the various types of cells in our bodies, and from there wreak havoc on our various systems. The solution involves rebuilding your depletions, remediating your environment, and tailoring your diet to minimize inflammation.

ROLE OF THE ADRENAL GLANDS

Two small glands, each about the size of a peanut, sit atop our kidneys. They are very powerful in their ability to secrete certain hormones: adrenaline for "fight or flight" rescue efforts; natural anti-inflammation steroids for infections, wounds, and injuries; histamines for allergy responses; and other sex hormones (including estrogen post-menopause). The adrenals help to cue other glands in the intricate endocrine system, to keep balance.

At age thirteen, I decided I wanted to become an endocrinologist. Something about this finely tuned, delicate symphony of glands and their intricate secretions fascinated me. I went to Duke University as a premed student, but changed my mind about becoming an MD in the mid 1970s, as doctoring was extremely rigid and clinical in that era. I became a classical homeopath instead, where I was able to develop patient-practitioner relationships in a way that fit my skills and personality. To this day, I must admit, I have a love of endocrinology. Specifically, the adrenal glands bear enormous respect, in my opinion.

Designed to thwart danger from harming us via infection, allergies, or trauma, these small but mighty glands deserve our attention. They are our guardians and bear lifesaving energy and means of survival. Most of us do not even recognize their functions, where they reside in our body, or how to keep them healthy. In fact, the opposite is true—we push the adrenal glands to work overtime, tax them heavily, and then wonder why severe inflammation, food allergies, and anxiety or chronic fatigue riddle us.

Adrenal collapse or inefficiency has become an American epidemic, and in my clinical experience, is one of the three top reasons autoimmune illness and chronic Lyme disease take root. I will explain the fundamentals of how adrenal gland imbalance plays into these illnesses.

Designed to give you the burst of strength you need in a perilous, life-or-death situation, adrenaline is a powerful chemical. We all know the immediate mental clarity, heightened reflexes, and burst of energy an adrenaline jolt gives when you are frightened, startled, or facing a daunting deadline. You can feel your heartbeat pick up, greater strength, and heightened energy surge.

I recall darting out of the house, child in arms, the rooms filled with smoke, my son's face swaddled in a blanket, our living room in flames, standing on our snowy deck on a cold New England winter's night. My heart was racing as I assessed our trouble and ran back inside to grab the phone and dial 911. We averted death in a house fire, and it was my adrenal glands' "primal rescue" measures that saved us. You know this exact feeling. Thank you, adrenal glands!

Sadly, we push these workhorses daily in a steady continuum we were not designed for. As we gallop to a meeting, multitask managing errands and phone at the same time, work twelve hours in front of an electronic magnetic-radiation mechanism called a computer, these tiny adrenal glands are doling out cortisol and other hormones to help us calibrate and manage. If this push and dash happened perhaps once every two or three weeks, our body wouldn't like it, but we could manage. However, daily stress levels and endurance feats are extremely demanding on the adrenals.

Cortisol is a naturally occurring hormone meant to be secreted in a biorhythm cycle with elevations in the morning helping us to awaken with energy and clarity, then to dim down in the evening, helping us to let down and sleep. Hectic pace, multitasking, stress, sugar and caffeine, highly refined carbohydrate diets, the electronic kingdom barrage, vitamin and mineral deficiencies, and even a natural event, like pregnancy, prompt the adrenals to produce more cortisol. Over time, if they are not continually nourished with the right foods and supplements, or allowed to relax with meditation and deep, extended sleep, the adrenals start to fatigue and eventually can burn out.

Adrenal insufficiency, or collapse, is very common in modern Western culture. I have burned out my adrenals at least three times I am aware of, ending up with chronic fatigue syndrome, Lyme disease, and nervous system problems (neurasthenia). Even to this day, if I work fourteen-hour days while traveling and speaking or get another shocking life event thrown in there, I can feel my adrenals kick in and pump the cortisol, giving me a racy high feeling, enabling me to meet the immediate demands of circumstances but also "jacking me up" too much. Consciously, I start meditating immediately, take special adrenal support supplements and homeopathic "Rescue Remedy," and force myself to get still. Even on an airplane, I will meditate and practice affirmations, helping to quiet the cortisol pump.

When the adrenals pump cortisol and even tiny amounts of adrenaline continuously, an entire daisy chain of associated endocrine gland reflexes occur. The thymus, pancreas, pituitary, and ovaries all get triggered and end up underproducing their natural secretions as the cortisol and adrenaline surges act as alerts telling your body it is in a state of threat (danger). These glands go into self-protect mode, storing resources just in case your body must face a deep freeze of winter or no water or massive bleeding. These are all primal responses our minds and bodies were designed to cope with eons ago.

The limbic stem of the brain, hypothalamus, and our biochemical responses are not going to be redesigned. Our job is to be conscious of our behaviors and our emotional reactions and learn how to nourish and sustain our bodily parts, our minds, and our spirits. Becoming self-aware, self-caring, and addressing lifestyle measures in an accelerated, overindulged, adulterated world is critical. Pharmaceuticals may Band-Aid symptoms, but healthy measures mean addressing depletions, damages, and imbalances.

The symptoms of adrenal insufficiency appear in all autoimmune illnesses and most chronic Lyme disease cases. This imbalance must be tended to as one of the first fundamental steps for healing. Some people may exhibit the opposite extreme, which is overactive adrenal glands, showing insomnia, emotional tension, runaway thoughts, anxiety, GI upsets, or impulsivity. We will look at symptomology for both and highlight lab testing and basic restoration measures.

A very helpful book depicting more in-depth information about adrenal function and burnout is *Are You Tired and Wired?* by Marcelle Pick.

Years of adrenal burnout or insufficiency were referenced as nervous exhaustion, collapse, or hysteria in the ages past. In our current times we instead have clinical diagnoses like CFS, fibromyalgia, anxiety, depression disorders, IBS, and migraines. Paying attention to those tiny, yet powerful little adrenal glands is a game changer for many.

Symptoms of Adrenal Insufficiency or Burnout

- exhaustion on waking and throughout the day
- craving salty food
- frequent colds/flu
- inability to handle stress
- higher energy in the evening (reversed cortisol cycle)
- asthma, allergies
- dark circles under the eyes
- dizziness
- dry skin
- extreme fatigue after exercise
- frequent urination

- painful joints
- loss of muscle tone
- low sex drive
- low blood pressure
- low blood sugar
- poor circulation
- weight gain

Symptoms of Adrenal Acceleration

- Upper body weight gain
- Round face
- Increased fat around neck or a fatty hump between the shoulders
- Thinning arms and legs
- Fragile and thin skin
- Stretch marks on abdomen, thighs, buttocks, arms, and breasts
- Bone and muscle weakness
- Severe fatigue
- High blood pressure
- High blood sugar
- Irritability and anxiety
- Excess facial and body hair growth in women
- Irregular or stopped menstrual cycles in women
- Reduced sex drive and fertility in men

If you would like a close-up portrait of your adrenal function status, some very finely attenuated lab testing via saliva over a twenty-four-hour period can be done. This is far more specific than what endocrinologists typically test for via the bloodstream, as those tests are screening for pathological imbalances, which means the gland has become so far out of norm that you end up with Cushing's syndrome (hyperactive adrenal) or Addison's disease (collapsed adrenal).

A huge spectrum of our population, however, including our children, is showing symptoms of adrenal fatigue or insufficiency. Genova Labs runs a rather impressive array of adrenal (and other hormone) function tests that use a more narrow range of standards versus the clinical standards the average GP or most endocrinologists use. As you improve, the tests can be rerun, marking the return of normal adrenal function. Another supportive book on restoring adrenal function is *The Adrenal Reset Diet* by Alan Christenson and Sara Gottfried.

What so vividly happens when the adrenals oversecrete cortisol for too lengthy a period is that the cortisol flood in the bloodstream triggers assorted brain and glandular responses. The body starts storing fat in the midriff, which is the stress response of the brain facing hardship and survival, such as in a fierce winter or being lost and isolated without food. Also, sleep cycles become brief with easy waking. An edgy, irritable vigilance surfaces, where you are hyper-alert and anxious, then after weeks or months in this mode, the entire body and mind flip-flop, to collapse.

Sleep cycles reverse as cortisol-release rhythms have become distorted, then individuals feel dazed and lethargic in the morning, lope along with a fuzzy mind and no energy all day, to find they perk up after dinner and can't fall asleep until well after midnight. These "night owls" have a reversed cortisol cycle, with the adrenals producing more in the evening, when normally they secrete very little, allowing the brain to slow down for sleep at darkness. With adrenal insufficiency we often see reversed cortisol or, worse yet, no cortisol or immeasurable amounts.

As the cortisol runs haywire, the other secretions of the adrenal become involved. Histamines for allergy response, natural corticosteroids for inflammation, and sex hormones and the immune regulation of the thymus all get affected. Even the pituitary, thyroid, and pancreas can fall off their usual tempo, resulting in all sorts of disorders and autoimmune conditions surfacing in succession.

Typically we find individuals with tick-borne diseases (including Lyme, bartonella, mycoplasma, EBV), viruses, sugar, and heavy metals in their bloodstreams to be demanding steroid production by the adrenals to arrest the inflammation induced. These foreign substances are stirring the inflammation cascade. The symptoms will typically surface at the area of your genetic predisposition. This may be joints (RA), the cranial nerve (migraines), the brain (MS, Bell's palsy, Alzheimer's), pancreas (diabetes), thyroid (Graves' or Hashimoto's), or the gut (IBS, Crohn's disease, colitis, appendicitis, etc.). When the adrenals become taxed by persistent infections and/or toxicity, we see autoimmune-style illness or pseudo-symptoms occurring readily. The adrenal glands take the immediate "hit" from long-term infections, leaky gut syndrome, or any sizable contaminant particles in the bloodstream (candida, proteins, viruses, bacteria), as they are cranking out histamines, steroids, and many hormones to "arrest" this foreign invader. You can take an immediate burden off of these tiny but hard-working glands by cleaning out all the inflammation-inducing foods, petrochemicals, and additives.

A functional medicine doctor or naturopath will have many tools to help you replenish and restore your adrenal gland function. If you are in the revved-up stage of overproducing cortisol, there are lovely herbals to quiet the runaway freight train effect. "Cortisol Manager" from Integrative Therapeutics, adrenal support blended formulas from Mountain State Health Products, and the Pekana brand carried by BioResources Inc. are very helpful. Sleep will naturally restore to deeper and more regular cycles, and anxiety and irritability will diminish.

Your practitioner may also recommend supplementing with vitamin C, B vitamins, salt, and potassium, as well as restorative plants like black currant, licorice root, ginseng, rehemannia, and ashwagandha. Many wonderful formulas are available and truly weave miracles. One interesting helpmate comes in the form of a naturally occurring sex hormone called DHEA (didehydroepiandrosterone). A precursor to testosterone, DHEA is called the "youth hormone," as it helps us maintain mental clarity, smooth skin, energy, and sex drive.

Robust octogenarians in the Mediterranean countries test with high levels of DHEA, which help to keep them vital and joyful, while so many in the more industrious, cloistered climate zones show significantly lower DHEA levels, even in their fifties, with obvious erectile dysfunction, weight gain, and loss of energy and spunk. Supplements in oral or cream form are easy ways to replenish this hormone.

Adrenal burnout is capable of happening at any age; however, teens staying up until the wee hours, overworked attorneys or military in service (PTSD is a strong adrenal cortisol misfire), mothers with many youngsters are all at risk. When the adrenal imbalance occurs, the entire endocrine system is susceptible to toppling into other dysfunctions, as each gland relays off the other. The Graves' disease could have been triggered from adrenal insufficiency, which could have occurred over the recent few years of your new hectic job and rushed meals of takeout food, combined with the fact you have been on birth control pills for a decade or you are unsuspectingly living in a moldy house. If we throw in a tick-borne disease infection or low levels of iodine, bingo the daisy chain of elements clearly creates your thyroid and other endocrine glands to be imbalanced.

Just as the woodwinds must come in on cue and the strings blend harmoniously, if one gland in the endocrine symphony disrupts its glandular and hormonal tempo, the entire song is affected. In other words, as a symphony sounds horrible with a miscue, our body feels and acts just as horrifically when the thyroid or adrenals are roaring in too aggressively or not cuing in on time. This masterful endocrine system is beautiful, finely articulated, and severely prone to disharmony by many external and internal influences.

People with rheumatoid arthritis, fibromyalgia, multiple sclerosis, and neuropathy are showing glaring evidence of totally tapped-out adrenals. These glands have secreted all the anti-inflammatory hormones they can, and have gone into a deficit.

This is why the cortisone/steroid injections and pills of decades past seemed like instant miracle workers for a generation or two, until we realized that these synthetic forms were trashing our kidneys and causing other dangerous side effects, such as "moon-face bloating," and when a patient tried to taper off the medication, symptoms would often escalate dramatically. Additionally, corticosteroids are immunosupressive, meaning they actually allow the potentially existing microorganisms, like Lyme disease, mycoplasma, Chlamydia pneumonia, and Epstein-Barr virus to bloom.

Physicians turn to steroids more cautiously now with chance conditions, but our traditional medical doctors have not yet learned how to "rebuild" the adrenal glands, enabling them to once again produce their own natural steroid hormones and create effective energy output for an individual to function. Adrenal "burnout" is so very common and a direct link to ME, chronic fatigue syndrome, Lyme collapse, Hashimoto's thyroiditis, lupus, Lyme disease, and more in the autoimmune spectrum, as well as other disorders.

The rat-race-paced stress of multitask lifestyles, the grueling marathon of divorces, the aloneness so many of us feel as we try to raise our families on tight budgets and separated from our ancestral generational clans, bring us to a mental focal point of survival thinking. We work hard in the Northern Hemisphere societies. We grind through our busy days and chore-filled weekend, scurrying here and there, juggling too much for our bodies and minds to adequately synthesize.

When do we relax? When do we find daily or weekly idle time to be still, nourish our soul, stay open to the beauty of love or divine presence?

A wise old yogi once said to me, decades ago, "For every hour of the day you spend using your mind in mental focus, you need to allow yourself the same number of hours using your physical body, and also the non-thinking, receiving heart." This stuck with me—and I saw how completely imbalanced my own daily life was—eight to ten hours ensconced in a mental world, merely an hour in meditation and another one or two hiking, sunning, gardening, or such. The Eastern cultures have much more reverence for such harmony.

A thorough naturopath or integrative medicine physician will run a bunch of metabolic profile analysis tests targeting adrenal function, gut biome (your good and bad flora inside), inflammation cascade, genetic markers (23andMe), amino acid levels, heavy metal toxicity, sex hormone ratios, and lots more if necessary. From there a tailor-made restoration regime will be designed, with special attention to the very worthy adrenal glands.

REDUCING INFLAMMATION

There are many aspects to integrate as we work to bring down inflammation. Rebuilding the adrenal glands by supplementing with natural anti-inflammatory enzymes and herbs is a first key step. Another great avenue is the acute-care use of homeopathic remedies specific to your particular symptom picture. Dozens of homeopathic remedies are pertinent for inflammation and pain. A classical homeopath (CCH) is schooled in matching your symptom picture to a specific remedy that can often be like a "golden arrow" in targeting your case exactly, reducing pain readily. Locating a practitioner is best done via the Council for Homeopathic Certification, or the National Center for Homeopathy (both can be found online).

All homeopathic remedies are FDA labeled as "over the counter" (thanks to a bill the Rockefeller family got passed in the 1930s), and can be found in health food stores or online at Boiron.com, Dolisos.com, StandardHomeopathics.com, and others (see appendices). There is a vast array of guides, philosophies, and textbooks on homeopathy at HomeopathicEducationalServices.com. I advise purchasing a few for self-help care at home on common complaints.

Regarding pain management and inflammation as pertains to Lyme disease and autoimmune illnesses, homeopathy provides some common helpmates. Please read the homeopathy chapter in this book to ascertain more on this healing discipline and how to employ the remedies. Homeopathy is a safe, gentle, nuanced, and effective healing art. So finely tuned, some people dismiss its capabilities when a bowling ball clout is not felt, as with pharmaceutical drugs. This is one of homeopathy's founding tenets: "Use the dose that does the least harm." There are hundreds of homeopathic remedies to use for autoimmune/Lyme discomforts. See Appendix: Pain Management.

Many individuals resort to anti-inflammatory drugs and painkillers. In spite of reducing the symptoms, such medications usually only minimally accelerate the healing process. Many people complain of side effects, such as gastrointestinal troubles, as well. There are some natural alternatives available to aid in the healing response to such injuries. One very interesting one is the proteolytic enzymes.

Proteolytic enzymes are proteins that can break down other proteins. These substances accelerate the healing process of injuries such as muscle sprains, torn ligaments, spinal disc protrusions, whiplash, and bruises, and minimize excessive inflammation of surrounding soft tissue in the joints or vertebrae, as well as the gastrointestinal lining. With the pain of fibromyalgia, CFS, lupus, Lyme disease, RA, Crohn's disease, or IBS, they are able supportive healing allies.

These enzymes are readily found in tablet and capsule form. There are two sources, animal and vegetable. The animal sources may be purchased under the names of trypsin, chymotrypsin, or pancreatin. They are usually derived from sheep or cow sources. These essentially are very similar to the same enzymes our endocrine glands release in response to infections, inflammations, and injuries.

Vegetable sources include bromelain (papaya stems), papain (green papaya), and ficin (fig trees). Some enzyme supplements are also made from molds and fungi. Our bodies naturally makes proteolytic enzymes in order to help minimize the inflammation response. Sometimes severe infections, flora imbalances, heavy metals, toxins, or injuries can over-use our natural store of enzymes. The body gets caught in a catch-22, attempting to produce extra enzymes, but not quickly enough. By adding the proteolytic enzyme supplement, the healing process can be accelerated and enhanced, and help shut off the autoimmune inflammatory cascade that has been "tripped." This is a significant player in addressing autoimmune illness and Lyme disease recovery.

Before corticosteroids and anti-inflammatory drugs, such as ibuprofen or Enbrel, became commonplace, proteolytic enzymes were used in prescription form by physicians. When Butazolidin and then Indocin were heavily marketed in the late 1970s, the enzymes were discarded. Thirty years later we realize the long-term side effects that strong corticosteroids and severe drugs like Methotrexate have on our kidney and liver. Some people never recover from the bloating, weight gain, sluggishness, and organ damage.

Looking for a natural anti-inflammatory substitute, without the side effects, is a way to help support the overburdened adrenal glands, and also deliver pain relief. Proteolytic enzymes are truly very effective in this capacity. Clinical trials run with professional athletes using proteolytic enzymes show them to exhibit a much faster recovery rate than those not using them. We also find an injury location to rehabilitate better and not be as prone to restressing, compared to those relying on the pharmaceutical versions. This suggests something of a reconstructive or restorative ability, which NSAIDs, ibuprofen, and cortisones necessarily do not.

These enzymes work best when taken three to four times per day between meals. They help to keep inflammation at bay when employed this way, versus taking them with a meal, whereby they act as a digestive enzyme. A healthcare practitioner's advice may be helpful when trying to determine how much is an appropriate dosage for your circumstances to get started. Most manufacturers state their recommendation on their product, which is a comfortable place to start. There are no known side effects. But, like everything in life, moderation and appropriateness should be exercised.

Many practitioners also favor a product from Germany called Wobezyme PS. However it is not sold to the general public, but an integrative practitioner, or other certified healthcare practitioner, can access it via distributors. Chiropractors and nutritionists are quite knowledgeable with proteolytic enzymes, as they use them often for injuries, as an important adjunct to the healing spectrum. Additional to the support these forms of enzyme create is the complementary use of a good-quality digestive enzyme to be taken *with* your meals, to break down and absorb food and nutrients more completely. Pure Encapsulations has a marvelous one.

The ancient art of Ayurvedic medicine also has a vast number of formulas for reducing inflammation, many of them containing turmeric. Use this in your cooking (delicious with rice or in soups), or in a capsule. A product named "curcumin" is highly recommended by renowned Lyme-literate practitioners and autoimmune specialists as it is very laser-like effective with its bioavailable quality to be absorbed effectively for inflammation reduction.

Some lovely herbal products include rosemary (oleic acid), in their ingredient list. Kaprex, by Metagenics, is a time-honored favorite, as well as some other leading products from nutriceutical food-grade companies. Mountain State Health Products in Colorado carries several wonderful suppliers that your integrative doctor or natural healthcare practitioner can order from.

BioResource Inc., in Santa Rosa, California, supplies incredibly top-grade synergistically compounded homeopathic formulas in the German Pekana brand. The Inflamyar drops and ointment do amazing justice for a runaway pain and inflammation crisis. Professionals can obtain this gentle and deeply restorative line. See their website for details and more aids.

Many talented and clinically attuned doctors and nutritionists have created very helpful natural ingredient products to support the body in creating its own corticosteroids, as well as break the self-destructive autoimmune cycle that has been tripped, inducing our system to go into "overdrive," essentially. We see great products from Dr. Susan McCammish, Dr. David Jernigan, Dr. Lee Cowden, Dr. David Perlmutter, Dr. Mark Hyman, and Dr. Bradley Busch.

Diet also plays a big role in inflammation. Many of us are completely unaware of the negative influences sugar, caffeine, and gluten (part of the protein molecule in wheat, barley, oats, rye) trigger inside us. Whether eating out or at home, simple, pure, organic, local produce, meats, and dairy (if you can tolerate) are the best options for eating. I recall a summer in Brittany, France, when we did a home-exchange with another family. Living in a small coastal sea village near the westernmost jutting point of Le Conquet, my nine-year-old stepdaughter would bike down the hydrangea-trimmed lane daily to fetch us fresh-made croissants and bread. No preservatives or hydrogenated oils there. Wednesday and Saturday rolled out the most scrumptious and color-popping fresh market of local farmers' wares, artichokes, carrots, honey, fish catch of the day, and cheese made from tiny farms of a mere few acres each.

Interestingly enough, the butchers told me the French refused to import American beef, as it was so heavily infused with chemicals and hormone additives. Yes, the delicate flavor of finely sliced local French beef was lovely. Our mass production of huge American farms—with synthetic fertilizers, pesticides, and genetically modified hybrid seeds—takes away both the pleasure and the nourishment of eating.

These are all terrific books focusing on how foods create inflammation inside our body, what to avoid, how to detoxify from them, and some easy, delicious recipes:

Wheat Belly, by William Davis
Nourishing Traditions, by Sally Fallon
Recipes for Repair, by Laura and Paul Piazza
The Sugar Blues, by Mark Hyman, MD
Grain Brain, by David Perlmutter, MD
The Lyme Diet, by Nicola Fazden, ND
The Practical Paleo, by Diane Sanfilippo

The American diet has become saturated with too many chemical additives and processed foods. This is one of the key triggers to instigating the inflammation cascade, as well as preventing adequate nutrient absorption by way of creating a situation called "leaky gut syndrome."

"Leaky gut" means the lining of the intestines has become altered from a silk-like fine mesh quality, which only allows for micronutrient and liquid absorption, to a looser, gap-like quality, more like a fishnet texture, where larger particles can slip through from the gut into the bloodstream. Fungi, gluten, sugar, other protein molecules, and more then free-float in the bloodstream. They are not intended to be there and our body's own immune system senses this, too. So, it kicks into action by secreting hormones, T-cells, cytokines, and more chemicals to attack these invasive agents. This internal "warfare" creates assorted symptoms of the autoimmune illness variety.

We say the body has "turned on itself," as joints inflame, headaches rage, the digestive tract is raw, or optic neuritis occurs. These are samplings of where the wayward molecules that entered via the "leaky gut" have basically landed in your system. Most likely your genetic weakest link has been exposed. Some of us manifest arthritis, others nervous system or mitochondria dysfunctions. A root cause, however, ties back to the offending foods we ingest, over many years' time, which induces damage in the digestive tract lining, and instigates many seismic shifts in biochemistry, immune function, and eventually episodic cycles of symptoms or chronic states.

The gluten story has exploded upon our consciousness recently. Years ago I recall a neighbor being sick because he had celiac disease and could eat no bread or spaghetti or muffins. That felt odd then, but now everyone knows someone who has gone "gluten free." Why? The dominant piece is that genetically, the majority of us are incompatibly "sensitive" to the protein molecule found in gluten. Gluten is found in harvested grains, the most prolific being wheat, then oats, rye, barley. According to *Wheat Belly*, by Dr. William Davis, the wheat that 90 percent of the world now ingests is a genetically modified hybrid variety that now has two harvest cycles in one year.

It is a shorter, stockier plant with a higher starch and gluten content than the taller heirloom, one-harvest type my grandparents ate. That heirloom wheat had a lower gluten content, was locally milled, not sprayed with numerous pesticides and fertilizers.

Celiac disease is an allergy-type response to gluten-containing foods, which induce all sorts of digestive issues such as gas, bloating, diarrhea, IBS, Crohn's, colitis, gut pains, eczema, fatigue, and headaches. Gluten sensitivity includes all these type symptoms to a lesser degree. I did not believe I was gluten sensitive, as I did not notice obvious headaches, GI upsets, or rashes when eating locally baked organic breads. However, when I went gluten free I lost twenty pounds in four months without even trying! My entire metabolism shifted, as well as eliminating fibrocystic breast disease in me! Certainly gluten plays a big role in all forms of Lyme and autoimmune illnesses.

You can reduce systemic inflammation by very closely monitoring your diet. Not a weight-loss diet, but an anti-inflammatory diet. Some of us need to go on a complete detoxification process as a first step of cleansing a huge stew of toxins. The next two chapters address both anti-inflammatory diet and detoxification.

FOOD

When the Americas were first discovered, the European explorers were intrigued by the very powerful abilities of the shamans, medicine women and men, and wise-folk of these tribal cultures. Whether it was in the Caribbean islands, the jungles of the Amazon, or among the North American natives, every community held such a revered and powerful person. When they would chant, dance, spew forth visionary prophecies, heal the sick, and talk to the spirits time and time again, the effect of their powers was quite impressive. These healers had powerful substances to rely upon in order to bring them into these altered states. In their ceremonial rituals they used coffee, sugar, tobacco, peyote, mescaline, ayahuasca, or coca leaves to obtain their visionary abilities and tap into healing energies. These substances were known to be powerful. They were considered to be sacred. They were not consumed by the average person for everyday use, but were saved for ceremonial and religious purposes.

The explorers witnessed that they could instill amazing powers. They were smitten. Besides the gold, silver, and precious gemstones, their sponsors would be overjoyed to claim possession of these other wondrous treasures. As some of these substances returned to Europe, only the royalty, and then the very wealthy, had access to them. Even in the 1600s, sugar was looked upon suspiciously by many and referred to as "poison from the devil." People who ingested it talked quickly and foolishly, sweated profusely, developed rashes and boils, moved around at an accelerated pace, and craved the substance more and more. For more than a hundred years it was feared by some and coveted by others.

As greed for these unusual substances won out over the fear of them, the Spanish, Portuguese, and British implemented ventures to the New World to bring back shiploads of sugar, coffee, and more. We all know how the pirate heists then developed. Importation of these substances throughout the Western world enabled coffee, tobacco, coca, and sugar to infiltrate from the rich to the general populace. Over the generations, the Europeans started consuming these substances more regularly. These powerful and revered substances, originally respected and used specifically in the Americas, gradually became part of the everyday European lifestyle.

Now, all over the world, people consume coffee and sweets to perk up and smoke cigarettes to calm down. These seemingly benign substances actually still do have significant effects on our systems. Beyond their natural effects, cigarettes contain over twenty-three additives, including formaldehyde, sugar, and preservatives; coffee beans are sprayed and treated with many chemicals, and are now often coming from genetically modified beans that have been heavily sprayed with glyphosate (Roundup). Now we are ingesting a melange of ingredients, with even more influence on us than back in the tribal days.

Sugar is a prime source for fungi, yeasts, bacteria, and viruses to feed upon. In fact, by ingesting sugar and high fructose corn syrup, you are basically putting timber on an already kindled fire, enabling an infection and its accompanying inflammation to roar. Researchers find elevated cytokines (biological by-products of inflammation) in chronic tick-borne infections, and all autoimmune illnesses. Stop the sugar! Coffee has some beneficial aspects, but it also makes the system very acidic, and acidic systems are prime breeding grounds for bacteria to thrive and multiply in, and are also prone to growing cancer cells.

An acid body pH is ample breeding ground for bacteria and viruses to multiply in. Some of you will have to take alkalinizing measures, which your treating practitioner can focus on. This essentially involves lots of greens and avoiding key foods. Review the list below to help shape your diet into one that is optimal for healing. Conversely, as we age past fifty, many of us do not make enough digestive acids and our system becomes unable to break down foodstuffs well. Many indigestion issues and intestinal and colon issues and more surface without enough of our natural enzymes manufactured by the pancreas, liver, and gallbladder. Digestive enzymes are a big help in these instances.

FOODS TO ELIMINATE

Sugars

Sugar is one of the worst additives that has entered our food chain. Excessive amounts cause tooth decay and have been linked to obesity, inflammation, and chronic diseases such as metabolic autoimmune illnesses, and type 2 diabetes. Sugars also "feed" unwanted microbial organisms, yeast and fungi. Infectious organisms thrive on sugar as an agar of sorts. Processed sugar does no good for us: it only causes harm. This taste pleaser is linked to so many illnesses. Removing it is critical for healing.

Sugar has many names: beet sugar, cane sugar, corn syrup, dextrose, fructose, high fructose corn syrup, golden syrup, maltose, sorghum syrup, glucose, agave, and sucrose are all types of unhealthy sugar.

Sugar-sweetened beverages like soft drinks, fruit drinks, and punches are some of the major sources of dietary sugars that many of us ingest. A can of Coke is equivalent to ten sugar cubes! Sodas line our grocery and convenience store shelves. Once considered a "treat" item, many people consume sodas on a daily basis, jolting their blood sugar levels and setting up an inflammatory reaction systemically.

Many times we think giving our children a fruit juice is a healthful, vitamin-rich beverage instead of a soda. But most of the juices are not naturally extracted or sugar free. Reading labels is key. Fruit juices containing the word "concentrate" or "concentrated" mean this juice has been extracted from a fruit and heated to make it more dense or "concentrated," and even though water is added back in, this version is a walloping dose of condensed fructose sugar!

Besides sodas, the other obvious sugar-loaded foods to avoid or at least limit include pastries, all baked goods, ice cream, candies, and snacks.

If you have a sweet tooth, opt for natural sweeteners like stevia, honey, or blackstrap molasses to flavor beverages and foods modestly. Natural sugars found in fresh or dried fruits and fruit preserves with no added sugar are also great choices. Not only do they give you the sweetness you crave, fruits also supply you with vitamins, antioxidants, and fibers that you won't find in sugary foods and drinks. Dates, figs, persimmons, kiwis, tangerines, and various types of berries are some of the natural healthy snacks you can enjoy without triggering inflammation from glucose spikes.

Vegetable Oils

Common vegetable cooking oils used in many homes and restaurants have very high omega-6 fatty acids and dismally low omega-3 fatty acids. A diet consisting of a highly imbalanced omega-6 to omega-3 ratio promotes inflammation and breeds inflammatory diseases like heart disease, autoimmune illnesses, and creates a breeding ground for Lyme bacteria, viruses, and cancers to grow. Polyunsaturated vegetable oils such as cottonseed, safflower, corn, soy, and sunflower oils are the worst offenders. These industrial vegetable oils are commonly used to prepare most processed foods and takeaways. Fast-food items are loaded with these "bad" oils and sadly those salty, crunchy chips and crackers often fall in this category, too.

Replace your omega-6 saturated cooking oils with macadamia oil, extra virgin olive oil, coconut, grape, or sesame oils, which have a more balanced omega-6 to omega-3 fatty acids ratio. Macadamia oil, for instance, has an almost one-to-one ratio of omega-6:3 fats, and is also rich in oleic acid, a heart-healthy, monounsaturated fatty acid. Grapeseed oil is a high-grade omega-6 that is *not* an inflammatory oil.

Note that in the olive oil industry, there are three grades, refined (labeled as "Pure Olive Oil"), Virgin Olive Oil, and Extra Virgin Olive Oil. Olive oil is primarily a monounsaturated oil, not a high source of omega-3, and should only be gently heated, if heated at all. We want the "cold-pressed" extra virgin oil variety for the best health benefits. Heated or refined olive oil has lost its healthful properties.

Trans Fats

If you see the words shortening, hydrogenated, or partially hydrogenated accompanying one of the oils mentioned above, you are essentially coating the lining of your blood vessels with oil that will build up and up with more consumption, as well as tax the liver enormously. Labeled as "trans fats," these food additives have been some of the most deadly additions to our food chain in the last sixty years. Prior to World War II, trans fats were relatively obscure.

Trans fatty acids are notorious for their double-whammy effect: they increase the levels of "bad" cholesterol, while lowering levels of the "good" cholesterol, as the liver cannot make any enzyme capable of breaking them down other than cholesterol. Certain individuals, due to their genetics, will immediately experience excessive inflammatory reactions to trans fats, setting up a chain of inflammation throughout their body, from gums to gut to heart. Trans fats also create obesity and resistance to insulin, and lay the groundwork for degenerative illnesses to take place.

Common sources of trans fats include deep-fried foods, fast foods, commercially baked goods, and those prepared with partially hydrogenated oil, margarine, and/or vegetable shortening. They appear in almost all packaged and prepared grocery store items from crackers and cold cereals to granola bars and canned soups. Bread, frozen dinner entrees, salad dressings, and cookies are all common culprits. Read the labels!

Also, please notice that items that list 0g trans fats on the label may still contain some amount of these toxic fats. This is because in the United States, the government allows items containing less than 0.5g of trans fats to be declared as trans-fat free. Commercially prepared peanut butter is one good example.

Dairy Products

Bad News: As much as 60 percent of the world's population cannot digest cow's milk. In fact, researchers think that being able to properly digest milk beyond infancy is abnormal, rather than the other way around. Milk is also a common allergen that can trigger inflammatory responses, such as stomach distress, constipation, diarrhea, leaky gut syndrome, skin rashes, acne, hives, headaches, sinus congestion, and breathing difficulties in susceptible people.

Milk and dairy products are as pervasive as foods containing partially hydrogenated oil or omega-3-deficient vegetable oil. Besides the obvious milk products like butter and cheese, foods with hidden dairy content include breads, cookies, crackers, cakes, canned soups, cream sauces, and boxed cereals. Scouring the ingredient list is still the safest way to rule out cow's milk.

You can substitute goat and sheep milk, which have a smaller curd, similar to human mother's milk in molecular configuration. Our gut can digest and absorb this milk more readily. Greek, Turkish, Armenian, and other Mediterranean cultures have farmed goats and sheep rather than cows for millennia. Their feta cheese is made from sheep or goat milk, unlike the Americanized cow's milk version (read labels even on yogurt and feta cheese store choices!). Kefir and unsweetened yogurt are acceptable in moderation for those who are not allergic to milk. They are easier on the stomach as the lactose and proteins in the milk have been broken down by beneficial bacteria and/or yeasts.

Feedlot-Raised Meat

Commercially raised animals are fed with grains like soybeans and corn, a diet that is high in inflammatory omega-6 fatty acids but low in anti-inflammatory omega-3 fats. Due to the small and tight living environments, these animals also gain excess fat and end up with high saturated fats. Worse, to make them grow faster and prevent them from getting sick, they are also often injected with hormones and fed with antibiotics. The result is meat that you and I shouldn't be eating.

Unless otherwise stated, most, if not all, beef, pork, and poultry you can find in the supermarkets and restaurants come from feedlot farms.

Substitute organic, free-range, grass-fed beef, pork, and poultry. Or skip red meat altogether (see below).

Red Meat

Researchers at the University of California, San Diego School of Medicine found that red meat contains a molecule that humans don't naturally produce called Neu5Gc. After ingesting this compound, the body develops anti-Neu5Gc antibodies, an immune response that may trigger chronic inflammatory response.

The link between processed meat consumption and cancer is even stronger. Processed meat includes animal products that have been smoked, cured, salted, or chemically preserved, such as most deli meats, hot dogs, sausages, ham, etc. While a high protein diet is encouraged for those overcoming autoimmune illness and specifically Lyme disease, make sure to limit red meat consumption especially and choose fresh, organic chicken or fish instead of processed meats. The price spent is irreversible. Organic organ meats are very healthy, as they are rich in amino acids and proteins, necessary to nourish your cells and build back damage to bodily parts. To reduce the formation of heat-generated food contaminants, it is also advisable not to overcook your meat and use moist-heat cooking like stewing and baking more often than high-temperature dry-heat methods such as grilling and frying.

Alcohol

High consumption of alcohol has been known to cause irritation and inflammation of the esophagus, larynx (voice box), and liver. Over time, the chronic inflammation promotes tumor growth and gives rise to cancer at the sites of repeated irritation. Alcohol taxes the liver and kidneys enormously, compromising your ability to detoxify your own body.

Substitute beers, ciders, liquors, liqueurs, and wines with a refreshing and thirst-quenching glass of pure, filtered water. Or how about a cup of anti-aging and anti-inflammatory jasmine green tea? If you find the idea of swapping ethanol for water or tea ridiculous, at least limit your consumption to no more than one drink a day.

Refined Grains

A lot of the grains we eat nowadays are refined. They are devoid of fiber and vitamin B compared to unpolished and unrefined grains that still have the bran, germ, and the aleurone layer intact. Refined grains, like refined sugars, have a higher glycemic index than unprocessed grains, and when they are consistently consumed, can hasten the onset of degenerative diseases like autoimmune illness, cancer, coronary disease, and diabetes. The Lyme bacteria particularly love grains, as they ferment into the sticky-sweet glue they feed on. Cut out grains and starve the bugs!

Products made from refined grains are almost everywhere. The common ones are white rice, white flour, white bread, noodles, pasta, biscuits, crackers, croutons, and pastries. To make things worse, many products with refined grains undergo further processing to enhance their taste and look, and are often loaded with excess sugar, salt, artificial flavors, and/or partially hydrogenated oil in the process. A prime example is boxed cereals, which contain substantial amounts of added sugar and flavorings.

Look for minimally processed grains (if you are not gluten intolerant or allergic to grains). If you are an avid bread or pastry maker, invest in a grain mill to produce your own flour. It will be much fresher than the stale grain found in stores. When buying cereals or other products made from grains, do not take the words on the packaging for granted. Just because the box says whole grains, it does not mean the grains inside are 100 percent intact. The problem is due to a lack of an internationally accepted definition for the term "whole grain." When in doubt, if it does not look close to its natural state, don't buy it. Health food stores usually carry some top-grade whole grain alternative bread and pasta choices.

Artificial Food Additives

Some artificial food additives like aspartame and monosodium glutamate (MSG) reportedly trigger inflammatory responses, especially in people who are already suffering from inflammatory conditions such as rheumatoid arthritis. They are also linked to migraine headaches, asthma, and potentially glaucoma and tumor growth.

Fresh produce, local farm products, free-range meats/eggs, wild fish should be additive free. Read the labels carefully and weigh your risks if you buy packaged crackers or chips or such. If you order Chinese takeaway, make sure you have the option to ask for no MSG. Otherwise, look elsewhere.

Besides limiting the consumption of processed foods, use anti-inflammatory herbs, spices, or natural sweeteners to add flavor to your dishes instead of relying on food additives. Turmeric, cinnamon, ginger, rosemary, and oregano are wonderful spices that reduce inflammation and flavor your cooking.

Fill in the Blank

Pro-inflammatory Agent: Why is this blank? Because it is meant for you to fill in with the food that you are sensitive to. Many people are sensitive to certain foods but are totally unaware of it. Unlike food allergies whereby symptoms usually come fast and furious, symptoms caused by food intolerance may take a longer time to manifest or they can come on quickly, too. Consequently, when symptoms of food intolerance do appear in a delayed fashion they are often brushed off as common minor ailments such as tiredness and headaches. But repeated, long-term exposure to food that irritates can cause inflammation and lead to chronic disease.

A food sensitivity reaction can come on quickly just like a food allergy reaction. The difference is not in the speed but in the mechanism of reaction. An allergy is an "antigen-antibody reaction." So if you react to a substance other than via antibodies, it is not an allergy, but a sensitivity. Examples are MSG and sulfites. These are intolerances not mediated by antibodies. This is an important issue when selecting a lab test to look for allergies or sensitivities.

Common food triggers include gluten, milk, nuts, eggs, strawberries, bananas, and nightshade vegetables (tomatoes, potatoes, onion, eggplant). Contrary to common belief, it is possible to develop an allergy to the foods that you eat often.

If you suspect that a particular food may be responsible for your food-intolerant response, try avoiding it completely for three weeks and monitor yourself. Are certain complaints subsiding? At the end of the abstinence period, reintroduce the food to your diet. If you are in fact incompatible with it, you should be able to notice the difference in how you feel easily. Typically within forty-eight hours of reintroducing the food you will note a symptom such as a headache, sinus congestion, gassy belly, bloating, or joint pains.

PALEO DIET

The paleo diet can be hugely helpful for reducing inflammation in cases of autoimmune or Lyme illnesses. The paleo diet is limited to an assortment of food groups that go back to the pre-farming days when our lifestyle was that of hunter-gatherers—mainly grass-fed meats, fruits, vegetables, nuts, seeds, eggs, and healthy oils. The paleo diet cuts out all grains, dairy, refined sugar, and anything processed.

The human body is designed to have high-quality animal proteins with lots of amino acids and essential fatty acids and good-quality protein in its muscles and glands. Organ meats are particularly helpful and have been treasured by civilizations for eons, with their generous amino acid and truly good fat content. We require good, high-quality fat to nourish the nervous system, eyes, and immune function.

The paleo diet encourages generous amounts of greens, berries, and root vegetables, which have abundant minerals. Polynesians like taro root, the Africans yams, the Latin Americans maca, and the Native Americans ample berries. These vegetables and berries are very alkalinizing and deeply nutrient rich, especially in antioxidant levels.

The other essential asset of this diet is the emphasis on high-quality good omega-3 fats or oils. If you look back over the centuries, all of the indigenous cultures found wonderful food sources for vitamin D and "good fats"—herring, salmon, coconut, avocados, organ meats.

The diet basically eliminates all the grains and carbohydrate-high vegetables that readily convert to starch and sugar, leading to inflammation and a breeding ground for all sorts of bad microbes and fungus. As a person's blood sugar levels start to yo-yo, we get into cravings and eventually the pancreas and adrenals become taxed, and leaky gut syndrome develops. Sticking to the paleo diet can reduce inflammation and create a healing environment in your body. A couple of great books on this subject are *Practical Paleo* by Diane Sanfilippo and *Against All Grain* by Danielle Walker.

GOOD FATS VERSUS BAD FATS

There is plenty of confusion about what types of fat are good or bad and how they affect our health. Once upon a time we said no to eggs and butter and yes to margarine, which is essentially hydrogenated oil. Now we understand that eggs are balanced out with a natural lipotroph in them that breaks down the cholesterol they contain. Eggs are back in (but choose organic, please)!

The writing of Mary Enig, in her well-honed book, *Know Your Fats: The Complete Primer for Understanding Fats, Oils, and Cholesterol*, backs up a great deal of what I will explain here. Look for it, along with Sally Fallon's *Nourishing Traditions*, on traditional cultures and the critical slow-cooking method, and how to live a long life.

Saturated fat in its natural form comes from animal sources, such as butter, lard, and animal fats in meat, poultry, and eggs. There are also natural fatty oils, such as fish oil or vegetable oils, like olive, palm, or coconut. Then, there are the newer chemically derived "trans" oils, such as partially hydrogenated or hydrogenated soybean, corn, "Crisco," and linseed.

Saturated fats in their natural forms do some very important nutritional work for our bodies. They nourish the brain and nervous system, they keep inflammation down, and are precursors to much hormone production, particularly those involved in stress reactions and reproductive function. Women with low body fat (below 12 percent) have a hard time conceiving, struggle with a difficult menopause, and often have irregular menses. Healthy saturated fats also boost our immunity and keep us warm in winter. Vitamin D from herring, mackerel, and organic cream fall in this category.

The human body needs some saturated fat in the diet, even though dieticians and the medical establishment have yet to embrace this fully. The heart, kidneys, adrenals, and lungs actually rely upon this fat as their natural energy source. Stored fat is know as glycogen, and converts to glucose (sugar) when needed for stamina, immunity, metabolic function.

We look at the French with their ample, rich cheeses, and note low rates of arthritis. The Scandinavians love their fatty smoked salmon and creams. They rate as one of the healthiest regions of the world by the World Health Organization, partly because they are more likely to ingest foods from local sources, which are neither GMO nor adulterated.

The problem over the last sixty years is that people in the United States have been consuming huge amounts of the wrong form of saturated fat, and from tainted sources. The result is internal chemistry gone awry for so many Americans. The liver has gone into stress mode and is pumping out cholesterol (a natural body fat) by the bucket load. The body then provokes a situation of "bad" HDL and LDL findings. The contemporary prescription is to cut back on animal fats (meat, eggs, butter) and yet the rates do not go down. The next step is synthesized, pharmaceutical medication to balance the cholesterol levels, which further taxes the liver. Obesity and a myriad of health complaints dot much of America's population, all based on consumption of the wrong saturated fats! Somehow we have "accepted" that 50 percent of adults over forty in the United States are on cholesterol-reducing medications!

Some critical information needs to be disseminated swiftly and broadly to help arrest the seriously catastrophic dilemma our culture now faces, all since the 1950s. As the food industry has spent its last forty-five years promoting processed and adulterated foodstuffs, they have literally been feeding our whole society poisons in the forms of hydrogenated oils, which are added to most every packaged shelf item you can buy. I find it close to impossible to buy a cracker, cereal, loaf of bread, canned soup, or other item that does not contain hydrogenated oils, unless the item is specially labeled as organic. Most of us who are dialed into the poison of hydrogenated oils shop in health food markets or the organic section many grocery stores are slowly beginning to house. The Whole Foods Market grocery store chain is making its presence in major suburban and urban areas, helping to introduce pesticide-, hormone-, hydrogenated oil-, and chemical preservative-free foods to our populace.

The core principle is this: natural fish oils, such as omega-3s found in coldwater fish (cod, mackerel, ocean salmon), are excellent for the heart, brain, and immunity. So are other omega-3 vegetable oils like olive, coconut, grapeseed, borage, flax seed, sesame, almond, and evening primrose. We want these oils to be of the highest grade possible, and not heated when extracted from the nut or seed. "Cold pressed" is what you want to see on the label. Organic means the crop was not raised with chemical fertilizers or pesticides, or GMOs in the United States. Labeling from overseas is not as clear, if you are Internet shopping.

When an oil such as corn, soybean, or safflower has the word(s) "hydrogenated," or "partially hydrogenated," next to it on the ingredient label, you need to put this product back on the shelf. Essentially, hydrogen has been added to the extraction process as this oil was being culled from the vegetable source. Adding hydrogen makes the oil more of a stable agent, enabling it to not go rancid quickly. Rancid oils or fat (butter) taste awful and harm us. This effort enables our huge American food industry to produce millions of products with very long shelf lives. That is why bread and crackers and cold cereals, baked goods, and chips are still "fresh" a year later and bear a distant expiration date. But, just as that hydrogenated oil is not disintegrating on the grocery shelf, it is not breaking down or being properly digested inside your body.

In fact, our stomach, liver, gallbladder, and intestines do not have the actual enzymes to do this. So instead, that hydrogen-molecule-modified oil runs around your bloodstream, eventually clinging to artery walls and building a layer called plaque. This plaque narrows the blood vessels, crowding your blood volume, which forces the vessels to have more pressure exerted on them, like an overinflated balloon or garden hose, and bingo, you show up with elevated blood pressure, high cholesterol, too many triglycerides (obvious fats/lipids) in the blood, and eventually heart disease, blocked coronary arteries, and either a heart attack or need for bypass surgery or a carotid artery cleanout.

Saturated fat in its natural form exists as animal fat in meats, poultry skin, eggs, butter, cheese, milk, oily fish (mackerel, cod). Lard and bacon grease are also examples. Some of this saturated fat is needed by the nervous system and brain, as well as the endocrine system for hormone production and immune system function. Generations before us lived with less heart and liver disease, with moderate amounts of these naturally derived saturated fats in their menu. They are not deadly in moderation, especially if they are organic.

Organic meats and poultry are so much safer and healthier for you and your liver/heart/cholesterol levels than the hydrogenated oils in bread, packaged dry goods, and salad dressings. Organic animal products are somewhat pricier, but have no antibiotics and steroids in them. It is cheaper and healthier to cut out the packaged dessert cakes and croutons and eat organic chicken or hamburger. (Non-organic lamb, by the way, is usually less fatty and less chemically treated than other non-organic animal meat.) Even organic chicken fat, used for pan greasing or recipes, is healthier than any partially hydrogenated oil.

Besides the danger of hydrogenated oils, it is important to avoid fats that are used in frying. This high-heat method of using oil damages the structure of the molecules, essentially making them "free radicals," or carcinogen status. They are difficult to digest and of course tough on the liver, again prompting the liver to secrete more cholesterol. French fries, potato chips, fried fish, etc. are all this type. Rather than deep frying, I prefer to quickly and lightly sauté with a good olive oil or coconut oil.

Good old cod liver oil is chock-full of vitamin D (immune booster) and natural anti-plaque building basics. The omega-3 fish oils are essentially a similar form. They are heart healthy, and a good boon to all of us, including children with nervous system problems like ADHD, Tourette's syndrome, autism, learning disabilities, autoimmune illness, and the rampant inflammation of Lyme disease, since such fats nourish the nerves and brain.

Good fats are very important in all autoimmune illnesses and with tick-borne diseases. This special food group does powerful work in relieving inflammation, the root player in pain and paralysis of nerves (Bell's palsy, MS, speech impediments).

Also to remember is that the tick-borne organisms, *Borellia b.* in particular, eat the fatty lining of our muscles, nerves, and organs. That is their food, and why an MRI will show indicative erosion spots on the brain, optic nerves, and myelin sheaths. Again, these organisms are gobbling up the essential fatty acids that nourish our brain transmitters—serotonin, dopamine, gaba—and a person readily experiences depletions at this level, which include horrid symptoms like anxiety, depression, OCD, Parkinson's tremors, ALS nerve paralysis, and neuropathy.

When microorganisms are involved in your autoimmune case or Lyme case, a regular diet alone will not rebuild these massive fatty acid depletions. High-quality supplements, like flaxseed, borage oil, and evening primrose oil, are critical to restore neurotransmitters and heal nerve damage. I love the homeopathic remedies hypericum and kali phos as well; they nourish the nerves.

Remember my philosophy—detoxify the system, rebuild all depletions and damages, and kill the "bugs." Working with an integrative medical doctor, or certified clinical nutritionist, or naturopath makes the protocol easier. You can carefully select your food choices, though, and cut out all bad fats and build in good fats.

GOING ORGANIC: READ THE LABELS

With the tremendous onslaught of chemical agents in our lifestyles today—from the air we breathe to the building materials and fabrics in our home and work spaces—our bodies are required to maintain a heavy workload of detoxification processes. Such a burden on our system has effects over time, primarily evidenced with the voluminous increased incidence of chronic diseases in our culture, compared to generations past where chemicals were less present. Since we have some control over our food selections and products in our home, paying attention to ingredients can be a constructive measure.

As many of us today attempt to improve our health status from autoimmune and Lyme diseases, we realize that clean, pure food is a key component. Dietary guidelines have shifted in recent decades regarding matters such as food groups, fat content, and protein vs. carbohydrate proportions. An issue that rings home to almost all food-conscious individuals, however, is the subject of food additives and what we consider to be natural, homemade, and organic food choices.

You may have noticed that within the past few years food labels now show a breakdown and percentage profile of proteins, carbohydrates, saturated fats, cholesterol, and sodium. This new labeling law is a big step forward in helping us monitor our intake in these categories, and a healthful step for all of us.

Almost any packaged food item found in today's modern grocery or convenience store, however, has preservatives, coloring, flavoring, or stabilizers to "enhance" it in some way, or it has been sprayed with pesticides. Plus, animals are fed growth hormones to bulk up their muscle mass and make for a more generous-sized animal. These hormones and chemicals make their way through the food chain into our own bodies. Americans are so much bigger and "beefier" in size than our relatives in the 1950s and '60s. Look at group photos of Americans in the 1960s—they generally look a few clothing sizes smaller than we are today. The growth hormones and such have taken their toll over time.

The majority of food additives are chemicals or synthesized items. The food merchandising industry has tampered with what we eat in order to make it more presentable, attractive, quicker to consume, or longer lasting as it sits on the grocery shelf or in your cupboard at home. The frank realization is that food really does not have to be this adulterated. We really can have healthier, less chemically laden, more nutritious foods, if big business would change their objectives and we could have state or federal incentives to promote the return of local, organic farms. Food is more nutritious and tastier when it is purer and fresh. In fact, backyard organic gardens or even small "raised" veggie beds on a condo rooftop or community garden patch can bring you cheaper and certainly fresher produce!

Chemicals in our food are typically not good for our bodies. Some are milder than others, such as carrageenan (seaweed by-product found in ice cream) or acacia gum, a thickener. Conversely, the hydrogenated oils, sodium acetate, MSG, and dyes tax our liver and digestive organs immensely. The poor liver has to work like crazy to break down and rid our system of these chemicals. The liver is one of our blood's primary filters and unlike an air-conditioning unit, it cannot just be replaced periodically. Wise practice is to take care of our organs and protect your gut lining from additives that induce inflammation. Many preservatives and pesticides induce this.

A constructive way to go about keeping your blood cleaner and in turn your body healthier is to try to look for foods devoid of chemical additives. Reading labels in the store is the first step. The less you see added, the better it is for you. Eventually, you will find brands, like Aunt Millie's tomato sauce or Paul Newman's salad dressings, that have just one or two "lesser" additives. Turning to a health food store, a local organic farmstand, or a food co-op are other options, as health food stores strive to carry items that are as organic as possible, and often local. The newer commercial Whole Foods Markets are in most major cities now, proudly bringing us organic, chemical-free foods.

The labeling "natural" can be tricky. Some items, such as potato chips, may contain only potatoes, salt, and oil, thus making its ingredients more than 70 percent chemical free, which is the rating necessitated by the FDA for something to be labeled as "natural." Yet, the oil used can be hydrogenated, and essentially worse than eating lard! So, be careful and read the ingredients on the "natural" foods, which may also contain lots of corn syrup or sugar, which are natural, non-chemical items, but can wreak havoc on your body.

When a food is labeled as "organic" it must pass stricter standards. The core issue is that it must be chemical free in its processing. So, an organic cracker is made from grains grown without chemical fertilizers, pesticides, or preservatives. Additionally, the other ingredients (oil, egg solids, seasonings) are likewise obtained in a chemical-free fashion, too. Organic cheese is made from milk from a cow that ate only pesticide- and hormone-free grain. However, natural cheese could be made and packaged without chemical additives and preservatives (making it natural), yet the cow that produced the milk was fed hormone- and antibiotic-laced grain, thus it is *not* organic. Organic is generally the classification to ascertain chemical free at all levels.

Eating solely organic food is a wonderful goal. It was how America ate prior to WWII. Organic foods tend to be pricier, as they require more work to produce and are produced in lesser quantities, making less bulk and in turn higher prices. However, I am seeing price trends dropping, and joining a food co-operative enables a community group of citizens to buy items (rice, butter, ketchup, oats) in bulk quantities and then divvy up the amounts together, bringing prices down if you buy half a case of applesauce jars or several pounds of rice. We do that in our community with success and camaraderie!

Here are some guidelines I recommend, if it is not affordable for your household to go totally organic. If you can only choose one food category to eat organic, it should be the animal products. These items contain some form of animal fat (meat, fowl, dairy), and it is the fat molecules present that transport chemicals. So, non-organic milk, cheese, or hamburger contain all the growth hormones (steroids), antibiotics, and pesticide residues fed to the animals. These enter your body too, and account for all the voluptuous young teenage girls we now raise, who are essentially heavily estrogen laced, via our dairy, meat, and chicken food chain. Such estrogen dominance leads to a rash of gynecological issues as we enter our adulthood (endometriosis, ovarian cysts, cancers), and in men it creates lower sperm counts, erectile dysfunction, and loss of muscle tone. Meat is often pumped with dyes too, to enhance coloration. Many European countries ban American beef and poultry from being imported.

While the average person may not suffer immediate detrimental effects from food additives, there are many individuals with food sensitivities. Reactions to MSG, sulfites, and dyes are some examples. Other people have reactions to yeast, gluten, corn, eggs, or soy. Knowing the ingredients is crucial in such instances. If you are on a restricted diet, it may be worthwhile to save the ingredient label from a product and contact the manufacturer for a complete itemization of ingredients. You should explain the necessity due to your health condition or allergy. These ingredients of lesser amounts can then be identified to you. Items in a proportion of less than 2 percent are not required by FDA labeling law to be listed. Some of these substances, even in minor amounts, are problematic for certain people, however. Asthmatics in particular are sensitive to sulfites, found in red wine, dried fruit, and grain products.

For the average health-conscious individual there are some other key labeling ingredients to be alerted to. Sugar comes in the disguised forms of corn syrup, corn sweetener, malt, and sucrose. Breads, crackers, soups, ketchup, and cereals often have disguised forms of sugar. Nutrasweet and aspartame have their controversial aspects, too. Stevia, a natural plant derivative, is the safest alternative to cane or synthesized sugar. Raw honey and molasses are preferable sweeteners for teas and cooking.

We discussed the matter of eliminating the intake of partially and fully hydrogenated fats and oils earlier, which is critical in reducing elevated inflammation and cholesterol levels. A high-fat diet is associated with weight gain, certain cancers, liver troubles, chronic gastrointestinal issues, chronic inflammation, and a sluggish lymph system, which relate to impaired immunity in many people. Vegetable shortening is also troublesome. These substances are food preservatives, giving the item a longer shelf life. Even though they retard spoilage, they are incredibly difficult for the liver to process. When searching through labels you will find this adulterated form of oil in literally thousands of food products. It is frightening to discover how much of this detrimental oil we unknowingly ingest. Shopping becomes discouraging, as finding a "pure" bread or cracker in the grocery store is close to impossible.

Once you have taken a month or two to master finding organic meats, poultry, and dairy, the next step is produce. All commercial grocery stores carry mass-farmed vegetables and fruit that are shipped to us from distant states and countries and are expected to stay fresh and colorful on our shelves often for weeks and months after they were picked. Some were picked when still green and are lacking in the peak vitamins and minerals. To stay "good looking" they have been sprayed with preservatives and were likely fed hefty chemical fertilizers to grow big and were misted with insecticides to not be decimated. This chemical stew meets your mouth, mucous linings, and innards. We get sick inside with assorted GI inflammations, leaky gut syndrome, pancreas, liver, and other conditions that involve the organs needing to assimilate it all. Apple cider vinegar soaks of all produce in your sink can extract some of the chemical "glaze," but apples often are sprayed with a wax too hefty to soak off and strawberries, grapes, and non-skinned fruits are very vulnerable. Really think about starting your own garden beds!

Though it could take a few months to get into organic shopping, the final cornerstone is the carbohydrate area. All good grains—brown rice, kamut, millet, cornflower—can be found in health food stores and I have the good fortune of a discount "Lots" store carrying Bob's assorted packaged grains and legumes. Put your antennae up and you will find these items and organic gluten-free breads too!

Again, if you cannot tackle a completely organic diet, at least managing the meat, fowl, dairy, and produce is significant. Read your labels and make lists of your favorites. Have your children taste test with you for the yummiest but least sugary items—they are great little food detectives for sensing out chemicals, as their bodies are less tainted and "gunked" up!

AMAZING AMINO ACIDS: BRAIN CHEMISTRY AND MORE

There are twenty-two known amino acids found in protein foods. Animal proteins such as meat, poultry, eggs, and fish contain ample sources of these vital nutrients, while vegetable sources that contain protein, such as legumes and grains, carry some but not all of the twenty-two. It is quite important to eat proper food combinations at a meal (rice and beans or lentils and yogurt) to obtain the full amino acid and protein balance, especially if you are a vegetarian. When we skimp on our protein intake a host of irregularities can surface. In fact, many nutritionists link the overly available high-carbohydrate/low-protein diet of modern America's children to many of the learning disabilities and weak attention span classrooms are so commonly riddled with today, as well as obesity, elevated blood pressure, and allergies. Readjusting our children's breakfasts to contain generous amounts of protein (versus the flimsy breakfast cereals many subsist on) could bring about a dramatic shift for the better for our children. This means eggs or organic yogurt and bacon in the morning.

A complete protein contains nine essential amino acids: tryptophan, lysine, methionine, valine, leucine, isoleucine, phenylalanine, threonine, and histidine. With these present in our diet, the others can be internally manufactured. These essential nine, however, must be present in our food, as our bodies cannot manufacture them. An adult requires between 50 and 100 mg per day of complete protein.

Like fat, protein has gotten a bad rap in our society over the last few decades. Consequently, many people have eliminated meats and fat from their menu. If eggs and fish are being consumed you are most likely getting some sources of the essential nine amino acids. If you are following a vegetarian diet it is critical to adhere to good food combinations—don't try to subsist on a heavily processed carbohydrate regime of pastas, breads, and baked goods. Whole grains (millet, quinoa, corn) and legumes (beans, lentils) are necessary to obtain your amino acids.

Amino acids are involved in the regulation of our brain chemistry. Brain chemistry controls our moods and mental well-being. With depleted amino acids, we end up with imbalanced brain chemicals and a variety of emotional and physical symptoms. In trying to keep this information simple I will discuss the major four primary amino acid/brain chemical imbalances commonly manifested. Remembering that we need all twenty-two aminos to be happy and healthy, depletion in any of these four essentials leads to the following troubles. If you would like to learn more on this fascinating subject I recommend reading *The Diet Cure* by Julia Ross. It delves into constructive detail and advice on these matters and more, including binge eating, anorexia, alcoholism, anxiety, depression, and bipolarity.

When we are low in dopamine (our natural caffeine), feelings of depression, lack of energy, lack of drive, and poor focus occur. This is where conditions like attention deficit disorder and progressed illnesses like Lyme disease, MS, and Parkinson's disease come into play. The amino acid regulating dopamine is L-Tyrosine.

Those of us with low endorphin levels often feel sensitive to emotional and physical pain. Crying easily, we try to find ways to feel "good." Comfort foods or craving rewards, or "numbing" treats, are recognized behaviors. People who are addicted to exercise or who turn to pleasure-sensation drugs or even bulimics are often examples of endorphin deficiency. D-Phenylalinine (DLPA) is the amino acid most strongly lacking here. Again, the autoimmune diseases are rife with this issue; fibromyalgia, CFS/ME, lupus, MS, Lyme, and RA stumble with this depletion in spades!

GABA, the body's natural Valium, is responsible for making us feel relaxed and peaceful. Symptoms of anxiety, stiff and tense muscles, inability to relax, and a "burnt out" feeling signify a GABA deficiency. I suggest all Lyme and autoimmune disease cases have GABA levels studied.

When we are low in serotonin (5HTP) a myriad of complaints ensue. Depression, low self-esteem, obsessive thoughts/behaviors, irritability, insomnia, panic attacks, SADD (seasonal affective depression disorder), and physical ills such as fibromyalgia, lupus, CFS/ME, thyroid problems, IBS/Crohn's, and TMJ develop.

The recommended dosages of these amino acids vary according to the individual. Some people actually need more than one of these four major cornerstones to balance out their brain chemistry. It is advised that you seek out a healthcare professional (naturopath, nutritionist, etc.) who has worked with them before, to target your specific needs. Many people find relief within hours or days, others may have to be on the program awhile. Once you regain a good amino acid reserve you will not have to continue to take these supplements, but rebuilding them is a significant contributor to regaining quality of life with Lyme and autoimmune diseases.

Several specialty labs are saving lives by delineating these deficiencies. NeuroScience, Genova, and RealTime Labs helped us pinpoint my very skewed amino acid issues. In fact, taking glycine would stop an anxiety attack for me in a mere twenty minutes, while multitudes of SSRI drugs only made me worse!

Anyone suffering from drug addictions, OCD, phobias, anxiety, depression, eating disorders, or severe stress should consider exploring this avenue, as help may be at hand here. Remember that tick-borne microbes and other organisms essentially bring about inflammation of the brain lining and spinal column, inducing all sorts of biochemical reactions, our neurotransmitters get thrown off-kilter very easily, and amino acids leach rapidly. Even some of the pain management medications for RA, fibromyalgia, migraines, and more will fiddle with the neurotransmitters and amino and essential fatty acids. Hence the good support of borage, flaxseed, and fish oils for rebuilding the brain. Lyme bacteria (*Borrelia b.*) and one of the parasite co-infections, bartonella, move rapidly into the spinal fluid and tap the brain and nerves, as well as the fascia lining of the muscles. Borrelia survives on eating the fatty layers and lining of the body—fascia, mylenin nerve sheaths, and other joint and heart linings. Besides the obvious pain with these tissues and parts damaged, the brain fats are gobbled up and our neurotransmitters become altered—hence the mood swings and all sorts of emotional issues in formerly very normal and emotionally healthy individuals (like me!).

I recall my late mother saying I was the most well-adjusted, happy, and confident teen and college kid—to see me deeply depressed and racing with runaway anxiety problems was confounding and heart wrenching for us all. And, I healed with the able help of amino acids, essential fatty acids, EMDR therapy for trauma induced from chronic illness, and lots of sunny vitamin D. Seek testing and help. Healing is in your orbit!

THE PROBLEM WITH PLASTICS

Many in the field of natural medicine have held reservations about the prevalence of plastic products in our lifestyles, most specially a prime culprit used as the wrapping material for many foods. Known as polyvinyl chloride, or more commonly, "cling wrap," health-conscious individuals have been worried about the effects of these chemicals leaching into the food they protectively wrap. The chemical by-products found in these plastics adversely affect our endocrine system, particularly our hormonal balances. They are known as "estrogen disruptors."

Fifteen years ago England followed the European Community's Scientific Committee for Food's recommendation and has outlawed the use of the chemical configuration found in the cling-type plastic wrap we still use here in the US. "Endocrine disrupters" are chemicals that mimic estrogen and estrogen-like chemicals in our bloodstream. The result is that the body believes it has adequate or even excessive amounts of estrogen present, and consequently doesn't necessarily produce what it naturally needs to in order for proper hormonal functioning to continue. What transpires is a daisy chain of hormonal imbalances for both sexes. Breast and ovarian cysts, endometriosis, uterine fibroids, infertility, PMS, fibrocystic breast disease, reproductive cancers, low sperm counts, erectile dysfunction, prostate enlargements, birth defects, emotional disorders, and in turn a host of other endocrine problems (Hashimoto's thyroiditis, Graves' disease), and a trigger to adrenal malfunction can ensue. Informally known as estrogen dominance, these estrogen mimickers are potentially threatening our population in many ways.

The latest generation of young girls are commencing their menses at ages less than the more historically typical thirteen-year-old mark. Nine- and ten-years-old menarche is frequent now. Our population notices significant difficulties in conception rates, with infertility affecting one in six couples, we also have mass obesity, and estrogen dominance is akin to pregnancy, wherein excess weight is "padded" onto the hips, stomach, thighs, and breasts. Alongside these substantial issues, we are all intimidated by the huge increase in reproductive cancers amongst both males and females. Many have wondered what is jimmying our reproductive system so. A major contributor may have finally been identified: these endocrine disrupters found in plastic wraps, which touch meat, poultry, cheeses, produce, and baked goods.

The plasticizer in problematic cling wraps is known as Bis (2-ethylhexyl) adipate, or DEHA for short. It is the component that gives these polyvinyl chloride wraps their cling quality. According to the Natural Resources Defense Council, recent studies indicate "that DEHA has been studied in a number of species of rodents, where it is shown to interfere with male reproductive function in all species.[1]" Whole Foods Market has asked manufacturers of cling wrap used in their stores to identify which products contain DEHA.

Consumers Union tested several national-brand cling wraps for DEHA levels. Some were Glad Clear Crystal, Duane Reade, Foodtown, Saran Wrap, America's Choice, and Reynolds Plastic Wrap. Reynolds came out with the worst DEHA levels, and the others were only marginally better. No labeling requirement currently exists as to

[1] http://www.nytimes.com/news/style/eatting-well.html

notify the consumer if DEHA is present in the cling wrap formula of the product.

Try to purchase meats from a grocer who will wrap them in traditional butcher paper. Choose cheeses off of a wheel and wrap them in paper. Try to purchase your produce in a store that does not wrap it in plastic wrap, and put it in brown paper bags instead (bring your own, if you must). If your meats or cheeses are in plastic, remove them immediately, scrape off the outer layer in cheeses, and what you can of meat, and rewrap in paper. In our household we now use cellulose baggies for storing veggies, or wax paper for lunch food. Use glass or ceramic bowls, covered with aluminum foil or wax paper, for food storage. It's back to a 1940s household.

Certain plastics leach more estrogen disruptors than others. The "firmer" the product, the less DEHA. Water bottles are particularly dicey, as they often are left in hot, enclosed cars or backpacks, where the heat encourages the release of the chemical. (Plastic containers heated in the microwave are high-risk for this reason as well.) The best water bottles are glass or stainless steel. We reuse and refill bottles from ice tea and other drinks.

Use a saliva test to assess the three types of estrogen in females: estrone, estradiol, estriol, plus progesterone, DEHA, and testosterone. Men can have specialty hormone profiles done as well. The surge of erectile dysfunction in seemingly healthy fifty-something men has skyrocketed (hence the thriving Viagra and Cialis industry). Loss of muscle mass, premature hair loss or graying, fatigue, lower libido, and weight gain plague too many formerly athletic, virile, strong middle-aged men. The estrogen dominance is clinically tossed about as "low T," a colloquial expression for hormone imbalance. The plastics industry has damaged generations.

An imbalanced endocrine system, as we have discussed earlier, is a huge factor in setting up autoimmune illness and Lyme disease, as well as varied states of emotional issues and "brain fog." Get your hormones checked. Have bioidentical corrective ones made for you, to rebalance your chemistry, lose weight, reboot the immune system, and reduce reproductive diseases as well as all the illnesses in this book. Rid your home of cling wrap and plastic bottles, and reuse your glass products. Keep jars or buy glass containers to store leftovers in. Then tackle your cosmetics and children's toys.

Do your research. Be informed. Beware of plastics!

ELECTROMAGNETIC FIELDS

As a classical homeopath, I am trained to identify an individual's constitutional type, or blueprint. These constitutions come in many different forms. Some people are solid and stable and very earthbound. Others are fine-tuned and reactive and sensitive to many influences in their life, from foods to stress to emotions. My master teachers from Europe with more than forty years of experience, have conveyed that years ago the majority of constitutional types were more stable, solid mineral types, prone to general "aging" illnesses primarily. They got creaky and tired, but not "infirmed."

Our observation currently is that many more people, particularly today's children, exhibit finer-tuned constitutions. Allergies, asthma, learning disabilities, and poor sleep are infinitely more common among modern children. In our homeopathic analysis, their nervous systems are more sensitive or raw, making them more susceptible to fluxes and reactions from many of life's constant bombardment of stimuli. Theories abound as to why. One of the major ones pertains to the influences of electromagnetic radiation fields.

Electricity has become a constant in our lives over the past century. With almost every home being equipped with a refrigerator, television, stereo, microwave, washer and dryer, home computer, WiFi, and game console, the amount of high-voltage A/C and the electromagnetic energy frequencies we rely upon is quite strong. Questions are being raised as to the seriousness of the electromagnetic energy they radiate and the effects on our health.

We realize that accidental high-level exposure to electric currents causes electrocution. But, Dr. Dietrich Klinghardt, Sophia Medical Institute, also pointed out in his interview on "Lyme Light Radio" that low levels of constant electromagnetic fields can impair health. Individuals living near high-voltage power lines suffer higher cancer rates, particularly leukemia and Lyme disease. Some sensitive adults, and often children, whose beds are near the incoming household electric lines and cable or satellite, note sleep problems, poor immune resistance, and fatigue. He has many remedial concepts to try.

The appearance of portable mobile cell phones and smartphones in the last decade has exploded! Twenty-five years ago, when I moved to a backwoods home a mile up a dirt road, my Long Island safety-conscious mother panicked over my isolation and potentially being trapped alone on an icy country lane. She insisted I have a new-fangled car phone and mounted one in my aging jeep as a Christmas gift. I used it in emergencies only.

Now, five-year-olds play games with cell phones, held mere inches from their heart and face. Some of us talk for hours every day on our smartphones, making business calls and connecting with loved ones. The EMF radiation is frankly pouring directly on you. We are constituted as energetic beings. Body of bones and organs and cells, we vibrate in our unique visage and frequency. Energy medicines, like Reiki, homeopathy, Rife technology, and shamanic healing, understand the frequency patterns we each bear, and that symptoms are expressions of vibrational frequency disturbances.

Cell phones plunge right into your body with a non-compatible frequency. Repeated exposure can upset your cellular and organic function. Studies in Russia pinpoint this damage. Please do not sleep with cell phones in your bedroom. Do not carry them in your pockets all day long. Think seriously about this radiation you are absorbing!

Your body is naturally attuned to its own energy patterns. Oriental medicine pays close attention to these energy meridians and dis-ease, via the system of acupuncture. Exposure to strong electromagnetic fields can affect us, as evidenced by many more of these "nervy" constitutions being born into the world, and suspicious links to many chronic health problems. Research has not yet pinpointed what electric frequencies and amount of exact exposure are critical to particular health problems, but studies are suggesting a correlation (Dr. Dietrich Klinghardt, Sophia Health Institute).

We cannot see electromagnetic fields, but technical equipment is available to measure them. Some companies exist that provide test equipment for sale or rent. They can easily be used to screen your house or office, to determine which appliances or locations are emitting high levels of EMF radiation. From there you can make some changes, by replacing leaky microwave seals, and turning off the modem at bedtime. Aluminum shielding can be put up in a net over your bed to thwart exposure.

All electricity coming into the house and the appliances should be checked to see if they are properly grounded, thus reducing EMF radiation. Sit at least six feet back from the TV, and unplug when not using. Battery alarm clocks are preferable to digital illumination ones. Electric blankets wreak all kinds of havoc. Use them to warm the bed and then unplug for sleeping, since sleeping with them has strong influences on our body's energy field. Some of us have chosen to eliminate as many questionable appliances—such as microwaves, cordless phones, or the Internet—as possible from our homes, in an attempt to reduce unneeded exposure to EMF radiation. Certainly, removing them from the bedroom is a must. See Sophia Health Institute's website (www.sophiahi.com) for examples of how to reduce EMF exposure in your home.

This new area of health awareness suggests a reevaluation of how we may need to live. Until more information is discovered, caution is suggested. In this day and age of high convenience and fast-paced living, many seemingly innocuous agents may cumulatively combine to create a virtual stew of chemical and radiation exposure. Unfortunately, we cannot live in the benign innocence of generations past, and expect to live long, healthy, illness-free lives, where fresh air, regular sleep, and good food could be counted on to produce good health. These elements have all become tainted in recent decades. Conscious living is essential for all of us, even in our beautiful, and somewhat healthier, small towns and farms.

MOLDS

Houses, apartments, condos, offices, schools, and most any indoor facility can harbor various forms of molds or fungi, which can lead to myriads of health problems. Some people are very sensitive to such molds, while others are not affected at all. It is a matter of resistance, such as seasonal pollen allergies, cat dander, or ragweed are. Some of us bear a genetic "flaw" that creates the susceptibility. Tests from 23andMe Labs can pinpoint such a flaw, and others, called "snips."

Symptoms of mold reactions run the gamut. Indoor mold allergies however, do not typically present in the same obvious fashion as air-borne pollens and grasses or even dust mites do. Molds wreak a weird kind of havoc, which leaves a person wondering just "what" is making them feel so unwell, without any really telltale allergy symptoms. The runny nose, sneezing, and heavy congestion are atypical.

Dry eyes, somewhat itchy, along with a "fuzzy" head, headaches, chest tightness, or even asthma are most common. Skin rashes, post-nasal drip, repeated colds and coughs, irritability, anxiety, and exhaustion are all feasible. Loose stools, GI sensitivity, muscle weakness or aches, and depression sometimes show up in individuals. Severe cases will even show pronounced illnesses like fibromyalgia, migraines, chronic fatigue syndrome, MS, or nervous system disorders, like ADHD. Doctors are left baffled as to what the person is plagued with.

In recent years, some media attention has shown us horrid instances where the dangerous indoor mold stachybotrys atra killed some individuals, causing others to have serious health problems, enough to merit ripping down sections of their homes, tearing off roofs, or even tearing the whole house down in a few cases. Insurance companies and health organizations became involved.

Humid southern or tropical conditions are where molds grow most easily, and the dry deserts and high plains of the southwest or west are the safest bets. Seattle, New England, and other rainy spots are prime moldy locales as well. Interestingly enough, the northern tier of the United States, Canada, and Europe show the highest MS and Lyme disease rates in the world. Could mold toxicity from rotting, damp, old wooden houses and barns be setting up breeding grounds and damage, along with vitamin D deficiencies?

Old earthen basements with wet spring conditions are lush breeding grounds for basement mold. Ice damming on roofs, and houses closed up six months of the year can create a mold/fungi terrarium effect, with hidden molds sprouting and being "held in" with a closed-up house and frozen or snow-blanketed roof. The molds release spores and we breathe them in unknowingly. The spores are what cause all the health problems. Even decaying autumn leaves will trigger mold allergy reactions in a large section of the populace.

Obvious molds come in the form of mildew or bathroom molds, found in showers and tubs. Mildew gives off a moldy or musty odor in damp areas, such as closed-up rooms, closets, laundry hampers, or behind furniture or heavy curtains.

The most common non-odorous molds that abide in our homes are penicillum, aspergillus, monilla (yeast). Testing is available to determine what the mold/fungi levels are in your home or office, plus identifying some of the specific ones. A simple self-test kit is available through www.nationalallergy.com. There are also all sorts of allergy cleansing aids, such as air filters and hypoallergenic bedding.

If you are suspicious of an indoor mold causing you health troubles, your space may need to be remediated. Some people will have to move to a new office or home if it is a major mold infestation, but most cases are addressed by redoing a particular bathroom or roof. Strengthening the individual's resistance to the mold/fungi internally is one of the major steps to take in all cases, as well as cleaning up the toxins the molds may have dumped in your system. This is a *huge* area of chronic autoimmune illness and Lyme disease syndromes. Mold damages within our body are one of the foundational pieces why some cases progress so direly or do not recover.

Naturopathic physicians, homeopaths, nutritionists, or integrative physicians can help you with this. The adrenal glands, lymphatic system, and immune systems (thymus gland) all need boosting, with specific herbs such as black currant, licorice root, and others. Mold detoxification needs to be done in your body, too. This means low-yeast diets, which eliminate breads, mushrooms, and vinegar, and emphasize yeast fighters such as kefir and garlic. They need to be adhered to for a solid six months or more.

Many wonderful natural aids like black walnut extract, oregano oil, Pau d'arco, and caprylic acid are fungal and yeast fighters. Some great formulas are available in the health food stores or through practitioners. Prolonged cases may need a couple of rounds of an antifungal drug like Nystatin or Ketokonazole, along with the herbs and diet, to jump-start the healing process. Many incredible products and homeopathic nosode formulas with the aid of a qualified practitioner can help you detoxify your system from the bogged-down inner swamp the molds have induced as well as heal the damage. The Pekana line from BioResources Inc. is stellar!

The other important step is simply to air out your home. Opening windows, fans, and air circulators can all aid or prevent indoor mold problems. When purchasing a new dwelling or office I would run an air-test-kit sample, just the way we test the drinking water, if you are sensitive to molds. Look for spaces with dry basements, sunny locations (not shaded), and new roofs.

All autoimmune illness and chronic Lyme infections need to be examined for mold toxicity. Dr. Ritchie Shoemaker's work on this subject, *Surviving Mold*, is brilliant. In addition to environmental "mold load," once you become affected, the damage may never be repaired unless you get the proper nutritive supports or homeopathic remedies. Likewise significant candida, systemic yeast infections, wreak havoc within, setting off all sorts of GI issues, cognitive problems, reactions to scents, chronic fatigue, eczema, and more.

Molds are part of our environment, even in nature. The essential piece is finding out if you have been damaged from exposure, and how to repair and live better in symbiosis.

THE NEED FOR DETOXIFICATION

Think of your body as an individual ecosystem—the skin the outermost layer, with miraculous functions, systems, and musculoskeletal structure housed within. We have long heard, "the body is a temple." We need to care for our own personal ecosystem with fine attention.

I marvel how fluidly our organs and glands help us adjust to weather changes, noxious fumes, a bleeding wound, or invasive pathogen. We become stricken with bronchitis or food poisoning or the shock of a beloved's death, and our systems recalibrate and support us, always aiming to return to homeostasis or balance.

When ill with autoimmune illnesses or Lyme disease and co-infections, an individual perpetually cascades through rotating sorts of symptoms. The inflammation cascade, hormonal imbalances, endotoxins produced, and assorted depletions set off so many discomforts. One of the four cornerstones to address for full illness recovery is the essential work of detoxification. Just as important as killing off the "bugs" of underlying infections is opening up our given systems of elimination, allowing for thorough drainage of the toxic stew that poor diet and environment and endotoxins cause, as well as the "die-off" (or herxheimer reaction) of particulates floating in the bloodstream and cellular tissues as bacteria, viruses, fungi, parasites, and heavy metals.

Back to basics time now with this biology class refresher. We rely upon the liver, bowel, kidneys, skin, spleen, lymphatic system, and the mucous membranes for cleansing pathways. Some of us in natural medicine refer to the skin as the "third kidney," as the sweat glands and pores eliminate fluids. Most integrative medicine doctors, naturopaths, and homeopaths often start a Lyme disease and/or autoimmune case (as we did with me) by focusing on supporting the liver, kidneys, and spleen immediately, and commence cleaning out debris, accumulated toxins, a sluggish liver and bowel, or retained fluids. By "opening" these pathways with the aid of homeopathic liver, kidney, and spleen formulas and herbs like milk thistle, red clover, cleavers, and marshmallow root and/or supplements such as glutathione, activated charcoal, and alpha lipoic acid, many individuals note brain fog, acid reflux, fatigue, migraines, and assorted muscular and joint pains reduce within a four- to six-week period. These gentle detoxification aids are reducing the burden your brilliant ecosystem has been laden with.

The research of specialist Dr. David Jernigan (Hansa Health Center) has highlighted that a key reason that individuals feel so ill, weak, nauseous, and brain-logged with Lyme disease is that the bacterium causes a massive amount of ammonia accumulation within. Our brain in particular goes into a sort of "numbness" or foggy-minded, apathetic state from the ammonia overload. Dr. Jernigan advises that the most effective means to reduce the ammonia buildup is with activated charcoal capsules (a favorite of my grandmother's generation), and the special properties of a plant indigenous to North America's heartland, the Compass plant. See the website HansaCenter.com for more information on this plant and its uses.

As antibiotics, herbal antibiotics, and energy frequencies (such as the Rife machine) are introduced to kill off the borrelia, molds, mycoplasma (RA and Lyme), and coinfections, there are often very few or no side-effect symptoms if our detoxification channels are open and running efficiently. It is important to keep checking in with your practitioner and to maintain your detox regimens throughout treatments, to aid in curative work. Periodically, symptom clues can guide your practitioner to a spleen, liver, or kidney support adjustment. The most sensitive people need fine-tuned adjustments.

Before I highlight some at-home, practical detox helpmates, let us note what a herxheimer reaction is. Named for two syphilis experts, Dr. Jarisch and Dr. Herxheimer, it was noted that a worsening of symptoms, such as fever, chills, headache, tachycardia, hypotension, muscle pain, skin lesions, and anxiety, occurred after administration of antibiotics or antimicrobial herbs and even homeopathic nosodes.

This J. Herxeimer reaction is a reaction to the endotoxins released by the death of harmful organisms in the body. Lyme disease, bartonella, mycoplasma, Epstein-Barr virus, and syphilis can induce the "Herx," as the body is unable to release the heat-stable proteins from spirochetes' death, creating much inflammation internally. Severe cases require IV fluids. Supporting our natural detox pathways can keep "Herxes" to a minimum.

Some believe the treatment is *only* working if they note a herx response, but this is not true. A strong herx response essentially means your detoxification pathways are sluggish or blocked. A wiser choice is to take a "time-out" from the "killing" protocol, reevaluate and support the detox pathways for a couple of weeks, feel clearer and stronger, then return to the attack tools. We want a good defense posture, meaning detox is working well, and not to rely totally on offense attack agents. Detoxification and attack protocols must work in harmony.

Another caveat of very significant note is the recent illumination of some certain genome markers, or genetic mutations some of us possess, which perhaps set certain individuals up for very dire autoimmune and Lyme disease catastrophes or very prolonged journeys to wellness. The work of Dr. Ritchie Shoemaker presented at the Boston 2012 ILADS conference by Dr. Wayne Anderson, is a brilliant educational piece on just exactly why some of us (myself included) succumb to Lyme disease and autoimmune states so severely. Visit ILADS.com to view this genius work and video.

Dr. Shoemaker highlights that some people house a genetic detoxification flaw called MTHFR marker, which leads to elevated homocysteine levels and inflammation problems, linked to heart disease, autoimmune illness, chronic pain, and detoxification burdens. If you have this genome, you will have a very difficult time detoxifying via your liver on your own. Your body needs firm support. Sometimes intravenous infusions are necessary. These are often the people who struggle miserably for years or decades, until a savvy practitioner figures this out. The toxins are making you feel worse than the medications.

Naturopaths and homeopaths are well skilled in employing detoxification measures. Integrative or functional medicine physicians have learned such tools too. Make sure the practitioner you select embraces the philosophy of detoxification and rebuilding depletions.

The common supplement agents for detoxification fall in two categories: the binders and pushers. Binders are activated charcoal, bentonite clay, milk thistle, chlorella, and green drinks. The pushers are alpha lipoic acid, apple pectin, glutathione, and homeopathic formulas.

Pushers help release toxins from cellular space, muscle fascia, connective tissue, the nervous system, and excrete through the liver, gallbladder, bowel route. We therefore want a good bowel transit time, and no constipation. If toxins such as yeast, bad bacteria, or estrogen dominance accumulate in the bowel, the lining gets irritated and more porous, allowing these offenders to permeate back into the bloodstream. This reverse process is termed "leaky gut syndrome" and many, many chronically ill Lyme-stricken and autoimmune individuals are caught in this muddy crosscurrent. Coffee enemas are an old Ayurvedic practice to help promote good bowel transit time, bind, and pull toxins out, and clean up a leaky gut. Please seek practitioner guidance on this procedure and all liver/bowel cleansing "flushes."

The kidneys respond well to herbal teas and homeopathic formulas. Using a far-infrared sauna, biomat, Rife kidney cleanse frequencies, and aerobic exercise that makes you sweat for only twenty minutes (don't go overboard and tax the adrenals) are excellent kidney/skin aids. Lots of pure water is to be consumed daily. Flush!

Not to be overlooked is the lymphatic system, often *extremely* overburdened and inactive with couch-bound cases. The lymph nodes make white blood cells to deal with infectious microbes. The dead white blood cells accumulate and are filtered out by the spleen, a large organ under the lower left ribcage. The lymphatic system only moves the lymph fluids along with our body movement and circulation, or with the aid of reverse gravity. Staying upright or horizontal does not propel lymph. We then become plagued by lymph stasis, which leads to congested mucous membranes and makes you feel foggy-headed, bloated, and very fatigued or "heavy." Certain viruses, like Epstein-Barr, tax the spleen enormously. We want to get the lymphatic system moving and draining.

Viable methods include:

Skin Brushing: A Swedish technique using a natural boar bristle brush (obtained in health food stores or online). On dry skin, the dry brush is used in long strokes on lymph pathways, promoting sluggish fluids to move and stimulating the lymph nodes. You brush five to ten strokes on the inside of the arms (elbow to armpit), inner thighs to groin, and sides of the neck (ear to shoulder), all directed toward the heart region essentially.

Lymphatic Massage: Certain massage therapists are trained in specific lymph stasis techniques that help break up lymph accumulations.

Rebounding: Small mini-trampolines (approximately three feet in diameter) are excellent to promote lymph circulation. Please be gentle; the knees and back can be injured. No more than five to fifteen minutes of rebounding is necessary. Benefits are obtained even by keeping the balls of the feet on the trampoline and just softly bending the knees and sort of "pumping" versus jumping.

Inversion Tables: Actually going upside-down is a means to move lymph. Children hanging from monkey bars or doing somersaults or headstands keep their lymphatics moving effortlessly and pass through infectious illness quickly. Static, vertical adults rarely go upside-down except in yoga classes and such are rarely moving lymph. If you have been bed- or sofa-bound, trying to hang upside-down or do an inversion apparatus will make you feel extremely nauseous, headachey, or sick. Below is a gentler, yet useful measure to employ instead.

Slantboarding: A sturdy, closed ironing board works perfectly. Place a brick or similar solid item under one end of the ironing board. Lay on the board, with your feet at the brick end, so that your head is lower than your feet. Remain three minutes in this "reversal" posture, then slowly get up. Some people feel nauseous or dizzy if their lymphatics are very congested. Repeat this posture daily until you can build up to ten minutes without side effects. Then move the ironing board on top of two bricks. Again, start with three minutes and work up to ten daily. Eventually you can escalate to propping the board on the bottom step of a staircase, then the second step, etc. You never have to get completely inverted with this technique. Working at a two-brick or such level of inversion is very effective, even over months of application. Some sit-up boards have adjustment notches in their setup. This can be another version of the ironing board setup.

Homeopathics: Mountain Health Products, BioResources' Pekana line, and Vinco Labs all make a spleen/lymph "drainage" liquid formula that helps promote good spleen function. Talk to your practitioner about these products. They were very helpful for me.

In summary, detoxification is a crucial piece of the Lyme disease and chronic autoimmune illness recovery equation. Many cases plateau or never really totally cure due to the toxic overload a body is submerged by. Do not overlook this important piece. It truly is the turnaround quotient needed for many of the long-suffering, chronic cases, children and teens included.

THE ROLE OF EXERCISE IN MENDING

Exercise enhances the function of so many systems of your body and also elevates your mood. Exercise increases endorphins levels produced by the brain, and those very feel-good happy neurotransmitters called serotonin, GABA, and dopamine!

When we have chronic conditions that impair our mobility, like fibromyalgia, Lyme disease, CFS, RA, or MS we do not move around much. The lymphatic system gets sluggish, which means it cannot clean out the dead blood cells and make room for the new ones. We feel more toxic, more bogged down, and lethargic and do not want to do anything at all! But movement and exercise are key. A well-running lymphatic system is essential to healing, and is closely tied to exercise. The lymph nodes swell up and produce white blood cells when a microorganism enters our bloodstream, whether it is through the mucous membranes of the respiratory tree or a urinary tract infection or a blood-borne condition like Lyme disease, HIV, or hepatitis. All these white blood cells, plus the fighter cells that the thymus makes, need to be flushed out of the bloodstream. That is the job of the lymph (a sloggy fluid), which then moves into the spleen, the organ sitting to the left of the stomach under our ribs. The problem is the lymphatic system will not propel the lymph fluid along if we are lying down or sitting still. It needs circulation and also inversion—reversing gravity—to move.

Children who do somersaults or hang upside-down from monkey bars and go on swing-sets are naturally propelling their lymphatic systems along nicely. Inversion postures such as "downward dog" in yoga also do the same. Not all of us feel well enough to start a yoga class or hang upside-down from monkey bars! In fact, I do not suggest it if you have been ill. However, a very useful old naturopathic technique that is safe and easy to do at home is called slantboarding, and this helps the lymphatic system drain. See the detoxification chapter.

For those of you who have been wheelchair- or bed-bound like I was, the next literal step is to start walking. I recall the day I felt this deep awareness that I could "walk my way to health!" I had been bed-bound for over two years and could barely make it to the bathroom and back without help. But, I had started treatment for Lyme disease after having been misdiagnosed for five years with chronic fatigue syndrome, fibromyalgia, and Epstein-Barr virus. My boyfriend and I practiced walking down the small corridor of my house back and forth two or three times in a row. It was the dead of winter, but I was determined to get moving. I also started doing yoga postures lying down in my bed to start building up a little strength in my muscles. Within a week's time we made it out the back door of my small house around the side yard and into the front door! Soon enough it was down the driveway and back and eventually my little Welsh Corgi joined us on the trip, and we began trying the cement block sidewalk of the street I lived on.

Though it took approximately six weeks, I went from bedridden to being able to walk a mile. I must say my spirit started to grow in magnitude with each stride I took and as I watched the season start to change before my very eyes while my dog Lucky and I would take our daily walk. I felt an enormous sense of accomplishment, pride, and actually renewed levels of health coming to me—my mind felt clearer, my energy was improving, and my digestive tract was even functioning better.

Sometimes it takes a lot of willpower to get going, especially when we have been ill for a very long time and have very low self-confidence, and maybe feel insecure about how we look or how little we can do. This is where perhaps getting a yoga or tai chi DVD, or just starting with short walks in your neighborhood, can really bring about that momentum you need.

Eventually, you will gain the confidence to join a class somewhere or sign up at a gym. I was an athlete all my life and being bedridden and so sick for so long was really demoralizing. But when I was able to conquer that mile walking with my dog, and eventually get in the local pond and start kicking about on a child's swim noodle, I realized that my body was going to rehabilitate. Though it took me a couple of years, I was able to swim a mile in open water and now I can dance and do most any activity for hours on end!

Exercise is very vital if you need to improve your sense of confidence, well-being, and immune function and reduce pain and inflammation. When we get twenty or thirty minutes daily of aerobic activity we are improving so many aspects of our physical function as well as our emotional mood. Our ancestors used their bodies in this fashion for eight or ten hours in a day—such a stark contrast to how sedentary most of us have become!

I can recall my grandmother in the 1950s still scrubbing laundry on a washboard and hanging it on the line, and doing all sorts of garden work, in her eighties. She was never sick and lived to a healthy eighty-nine. My paternal grandfather who lived to a hundred walked everywhere, was a physical fitness "nut" in the 1920s and '30s before it was popular, and swore by a fresh diet that was loaded with garlic and onions and foods in the cabbage family. He never had an antibiotic until he was eighty-nine years old! He used his body liberally all day long in his delicatessen and was at the epitome of a "sharp tack" well into his late nineties. They both lived active, non-sedentary, physical lives. There is a lesson in this—we must look to exercise and motion as a means of rehabilitation. Turn on some music and dance a little in the living room!

Get up and start moving, even if it is down your hall and back as I did in those early days. Every step you take is a stride into your better future.

CULTIVATING HARMONY: YOUR SACRED SPACE

Our home, or living space, is often referred to as one's sanctuary, nest, or castle. This dwelling, which provides us with the common needs of shelter and security, in most cultures of the world also embodies a place of refuge, peace, and tranquility for us. In our hurried lifestyles many of us have skimmed by the importance of maintaining a sacred space of our own in our home. Instead, we feel stressed about upkeep, unkempt quarters, and clutter.

The Eastern cultures in particular, make obvious gestures to maintain a counterbalance from the rigors of the busy outer world by creating a placid energy inside the home. Tibetans hang a colored door curtain on the threshold, as a reminder that you are leaving one world and entering another. Shoes are removed at the door in Japan, replaced with silken slippers. Besides keeping the space cleaner, one is leaving the energy of the streets behind. Their living space is often done in whites and neutral tones, devoid of clutter, and neighbored by a reflecting pond, water fountain, wind chimes, or a neat garden. The five primary senses are each attended to intentionally, in order to find inner balance and harmony.

Many of us here focus on making a home comfortable or decorative by focusing on furnishings, paint colors, flooring, curtains, and gardens.

Some of us are happy with our results, others are not. Many feel they try to make their homes neat, attractive, and comfortable, yet it feels useless, endlessly strewn with children's toys, sporting equipment, winter boots, junk mail, and miscellaneous everything that always somehow manages to find its way into your living space! Almost as soon as you rally and get everyone to pick up, the mess is back. What to do?

I, too, struggle with this dilemma. But, in researching the ancient Chinese art of Feng Shui, or balancing of energy flows in a given space (i.e., home, office, bedroom), I have learned a few worthy tips. If you have resolved yourself to thinking, "I hate being a constant slave to picking up or nagging the family, I hate the frustrating clutter," it is possible to find some emotional and physical harmony for everyone, without having to gut the entire house or throw out all possessions. Here are some points to help cultivate harmony in your dwelling-space—an important step in de-stressing your life, quieting your racing adrenal glands, and allowing peace, comfort, and nourishment to take seed. This will enable you to "let down" and permit the parasympathetic system room to step in and promote restoration. Living at sympathetic nervous system dominancy brews illness.

The first critical piece is to find ways to comfort each of your five senses—sight, sound, touch, smell, and taste—in your living space. If you can tackle one room in your home, great! If not, you can integrate pieces in different areas, such as refreshing lavender water in your bathroom to splash on after a shower, a cheery paint color in your kitchen, a snug throw in the TV area.

I chose my bedroom, incorporating all there. A soothing all-white room now has a mocha wall and a soft, cottony bark-toned quilt satisfying my need for earthy colors. Scented candles provide aroma, with the perfect cotton sheets against my skin. I hung delicate wind chimes out the window for melodic sound and finally removed all the knick-knacks—extra magazines, books, photos—to make it all less cluttered. A nice cup of ginger tea and I am feeling blissful.

The other integral component is finding a tranquil space in your home that is meant for your spirit to feel at peace. Not a place of doing, but a place of just resting and being still. Not a place meant to sleep, do work, cook, but a place to just be. Easier said than done. If you can incorporate the five-senses theme here, fantastic. You will help your brain's ancient limbic stem align to the elements and find the very important "sense of place" we all need.

The simplest idea is to claim a chair just for you and move it to a special spot that you like. Put it near a sunny window or in a corner of a quiet room. Make sure you find this item comfortable to you. Then, surround the proximity of that spot with any colors, posters, curtains, or smells that make you feel calm and relaxed. If a tropical beach stirs that mood for you, then hang a travel poster of a Caribbean island. If the color green or blue brings you peace, go get a few yards cut from a bolt at the fabric store and drape it over the chair, wall, or curtain rod. Light a candle or incense of vanilla or another calming aroma. Play a soothing tape of waves. Claim this spot as your own and enrich it with your feelings of comfort and safety. Remind the rest of the family that it is "off limits."

Try and visit this spot daily, even if it is just ten minutes spent gazing out the window. Make sure you clear your mind, put away the "to do" list, ignore the phone, the laundry, the world for those moments in time. If you can find a feeling of tranquility in this spot after frequent visits, then you are achieving some inner peace and your spot is growing in its personal value to you. You are centering and gathering, building up your reserves, letting go, and accepting the art of being. The emotional, physical, and spiritual benefits will be bountiful.

I do believe these kinds of spots can be claimed outdoors, too. Some of us find great relaxation at the beach or out fishing. I myself find deep forest glades or outcroppings with a view on a mountaintop to be particularly serene for me. I get very still and can feel deep levels of understanding and perception forming. People who are avid gardeners create beautiful spaces within their own yards.

Find your own sacred space. Do not be afraid to imbue it with items that matter to you—a bluejay feather, a shell, your child's poem. We are finding ways to create harmony within and without. These balance points are primal and necessary. Healing begins from the inside.

THE INFLUENCE OF THOUGHTS

Thoughts often are like winged birds. They fly through the mind—random, transient, moving. Do they settle on a branch nearby and we take notice? Do we work with certain thoughts, making them into something useful? Or do we let thoughts move on through, vanish, like the rapid trajectory of a crow's flightpath? More difficult yet are the fixated thoughts—the obsessive, non-productive ones that are locked in our brain's cycle-sphere of overanalysis.

Thoughts have merit. Clear, clean, directive thoughts prompt energy to create and manifest, or inspire us to communicate to another, make a choice, or remove us from danger. The being must be conscious, however, and cleansed of clogged mental and emotional byways, for when these clogged "arteries" persist, thoughts can deteriorate into confusion or worse yet, compulsions or neuroses. Irrational decisions, mood swings, insomnia, or haywire energy can overtake us when we get stuck in the mind and are unable to balance it with the heart.

Beliefs hold a union between thought and desire. This is where the mind and heart marry. A belief is all of our own doing. We experience a situation, see a tragic accident, suffer a devastating relationship loss, or, more positively, taste the pride of a task well done or an athletic quest won. No matter how simple or very grand our experience has been, we internally derive a conclusion that we embody as a belief:

"I won the 5K, which felt wonderful. I want to do it again. I'm born to be a victor."

"I lost my tender, beautiful daughter. Now I am broken, unseen, too fragile to love again."

"I saw a magenta sunset and my spirit felt at peace and in awe, bathed in natural beauty. Nature has a profound effect on me. I need more space for nature in my life."

Each of these experiences have evoked a feeling, which prompted a thought. The thought became a "window through which we see the world." A belief, in turn, was concluded. From that belief we hold an energetic stance, and that stance is projected from within, outward, through the open window, and toward beings we encounter and the environment we inhabit.

We must think wisely. More accurately stated; we must think purely. The powers of our beliefs are profound. Our psyche, the neurochemicals we create, our body's own physiology and health, the people and circumstances we attract or repel, all are downstream results of our belief process.

Conscious intent, clear thought, and emotions felt fully yet allowed to move through and away from us are essential processes to living a life of higher good, greater comfort, more fulfilling love, abundant pleasure, and true companionship.

When we establish our beliefs we in turn create a grounding force. Belief holds power. Say a belief statement of your own out loud, such as "I am kind." Sense how you feel within, by uttering these words. Where in your body do you sense energy or focus? Note this. Do you feel a glow, an opening in your heart, a smile on your lips? Try another belief statement: "People with lots of money are greedy." Once again, move inside yourself, sense within. What kind of energy do you note? Is there a tension in your chest, a downward sinking or pit in your belly? Or perhaps an angry voice in your head?

Our thoughts, our beliefs, and our body are all entwined. The powers we possess are vast. Thoughts and beliefs are what inspire, direct, stymie, heal, motivate, or ruin us. The process of waking up to this dynamic is profound. And most magically and truly beautifully, we can literally turn our lives around by changing our beliefs.

Beliefs are like prayers. They reach from our core heartspace, unite with the power of the mind, and ultimately transcend the physical body, through our crown chakra into the divine conduit. When we unite with Spirit, we call it Higher Power (God, to many). Higher Power is infinite and totally available to us, with practice.

OUR OWN INNER HEALING PATHWAY

"Pathway" suggests a trail to me. Not a blazed, trampled one, but instead one that is evocative and maybe even secret or discreet. Likewise, a pathway gives me a direction. It suggests a way to go; a known route to a destination. Those marked hiking trails up mountainsides maintain distinct progress, as step by step you ascend to the summit, worn roots and knobby boulders passed over by others before you. The path is reassuring—in fact, it is an intricate map of sorts.

I have guided us through the marvelous systems of our body, illustrating the symphony of the endocrine system and the vast network of the nervous system, its delicate dendrites, sending impulses across fibers as we elect to move an arm or unconsciously take a breath. These bodily system pathways still marvel me with their faithful workings and interplay.

A pathway of particular interest and great regenerating capacity is the invisible one working between our mind and body. This pathway was diminished for decades by twentieth-century doctors, as they chalked all illnesses and recoveries to physical measures. Why would a mind be involved in physical processes? This blip in modern-era medicine will likely be recorded as merely a "disconnected" moment in doctoring, as for thousands of years prior, the mind and spirit were entwined with healing, even taking in great reverent religious tones in Europe of the Middle Ages.

At the dawn of the twenty-first century, we witness the growing understanding that our emotions and thoughts actually very much do interconnect with our physiology. Though hospital surgeons remain removed from their patients' daily care, the nursing staff pays very keen attention to their post-op charges, working with great nurturance and attention to keep their spirits positive, coaching for a swift recovery and more optimal return to well-being. Nurses intimately know the feelings of their patients, how vulnerability creates fear, pain evokes distress, isolation creates depression.

The endocrine system appears to be the known bodily system that interplays continuously between mind and body. Anger can raise your blood pressure, worry cause a knot in your stomach, grief a lump in your throat, and too much of a workload can create tension in your neck and shoulders. These are just the most obvious acute manifestations of our emotions triggering physiological recourse.

When we recognize that chronic illnesses carry an emotional footprint, too, doesn't that make you curious to explore the pathway to the origin? My interest is certainly piqued.

The section ahead on the Seven Energy Chakras conveys the assorted emotions piggy-backing with the specific bodily symptoms. The entire human body is not randomly designed. Joy and sorrow favor the lungs, indignation the gallbladder. Metaphysics studies this interplay. Coming to understand these interrelationships puts an extremely different posture on doctoring, as there are more influences to effect change and cure than just externally directed modalities. Humans bear inner powers and use of the mind is a prominent player.

Take a look at each of the seven chakras in the map section. Here the essential interpretations are illustrated. Much of this chakra information is centuries old. The ancient healers of worldwide cultures follow these threads. It is empowering to learn how to activate the energy of each chakra site and in turn promote more energy flow or the effect of balancing runaway energy in your bodily systems.

The art of stillness, creativity, will, affirmation, intention, meditation, and prayer all have intrinsic roles. These personal powers are natural and free and all yours. You do not have to pay someone for these healing services, you merely must practice them faithfully and with care, because reinforcement on a daily basis is what will translate to cellular change at the physiological level, enabling you to transform a condition, state, or symptoms.

You have the power. My job is to orient you to the pathway. Just as the map of a hiking trail serves the hiker, these pages will help guide you on the mind-body pathway. Igniting this circuit is not that difficult once you understand. The work is in finding clarity within yourself, making a commitment, and persisting with daily practice. The model I base the chakra healing methods upon came from the direct teaching of my spiritual mentor, Dr. Meredith Young-Sowers. Part V delves into the material with great depth.

PART V

The Map

THE MAP

This portion of the book is designed to help you visually assimilate the information and to help as a guiding tool.

We understand that the human body is composed of nine major functioning systems that contain an assortment of parts—organs, glands, tissues, and bones. These systems are housed in alignment with seven essential energy sites called chakras. The chakras have been discussed for millennia. The average person cannot see these energetic sites, which operate like funnels and are about the size of an orange. But energetic and spiritual healers are trained to see or read chakras, and to help shift energy when the funnels become blocked.

We are all familiar with energy sensations, like being jittery when anticipating something. That is emotional energy. It can translate into our body parts, as the chapters ahead will communicate. We also have energy fields on and around our body. You are familiar with the sensation of someone standing too close to you for comfort. This person's auric energetic field has entered yours. The same holds true for being aware when someone steps up to you from behind. They have entered your auric energy field. Our being senses several feet away from our body.

The seven energy chakras can be influenced by external energetic or physical occurrences, internal emotional states, geopathic stress, acute infections, overwork physically or mentally, and even sometimes by psychic influences, such as "attack" from non-benevolent people or groups. Our beings sense at multiple levels, more than just physical touch, and all of these sensations interplay. This is a chart to give us the layout of this energetic grid.

This map outlines the chakra sites by color and the coordinating bodily system associated with each. Primary metaphysical emotional qualities are written alongside the chakra as well as the companion organ system. This is a map of orientation. The upcoming chapters will flesh this material out more thoroughly and explain how we work with our systems internally.

Accessing particular mind-sets or using personal energetic practices like prayer or affirmation will help activate or balance the energy of a chakra and in turn translate to vibrational shifts, which can relay to our bodily functions.

THE PHYSICAL BODY

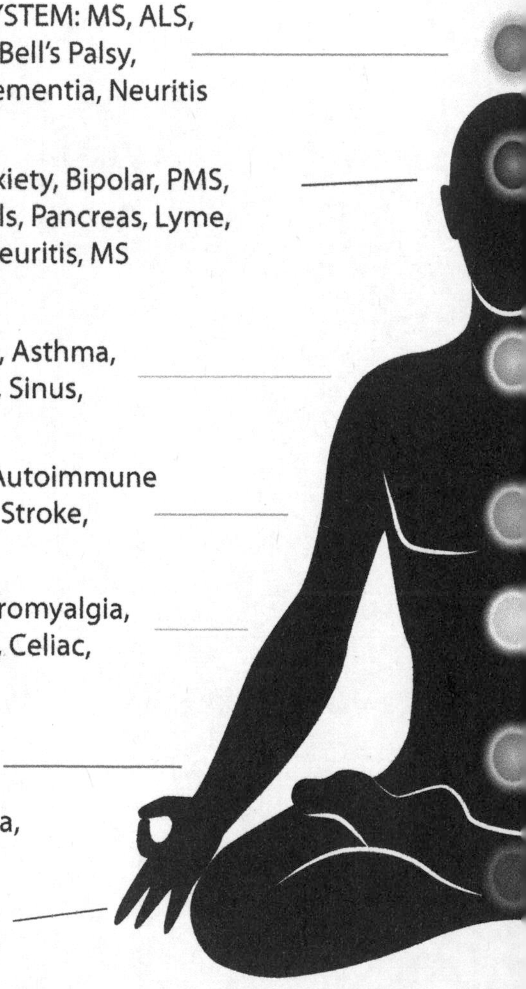

BRAIN AND NERVOUS SYSTEM: MS, ALS, Lupus, Lyme, Migraines, Bell's Palsy, Neuropathy, Seizures, Dementia, Neuritis

ENDOCRINE: Depression, Anxiety, Bipolar, PMS, Menopause, Thyroid, Adrenals, Pancreas, Lyme, Lupus, Fibromyalgia, Optic Neuritis, MS

RESPIRATORY: Neck Pain, Lyme, Asthma, Bronchitis, Air Hunger, Thyroid, Sinus, Tinnitus

HEART AND SPLEEN/LYMPH: All Autoimmune and Lyme Diseases, Heart Issues, Stroke, Pericarditis

DIGESTIVE AND MUSCLES: Fibromyalgia, CFS, Lyme, IBS, Crohn's, Colitis, Celiac, Gallstones, Diabetes, MS, ALS

URINARY AND REPRODUCTIVE: Miscarriage, Infertility, Fibroids, Kidney Stones, IC, UTI, Skin (Eczema, Rashes, Hives), Lyme, Lupus

SKELETON: Joints, Bones, Spine, RA, Lyme

THE MIND-SPIRIT BODY

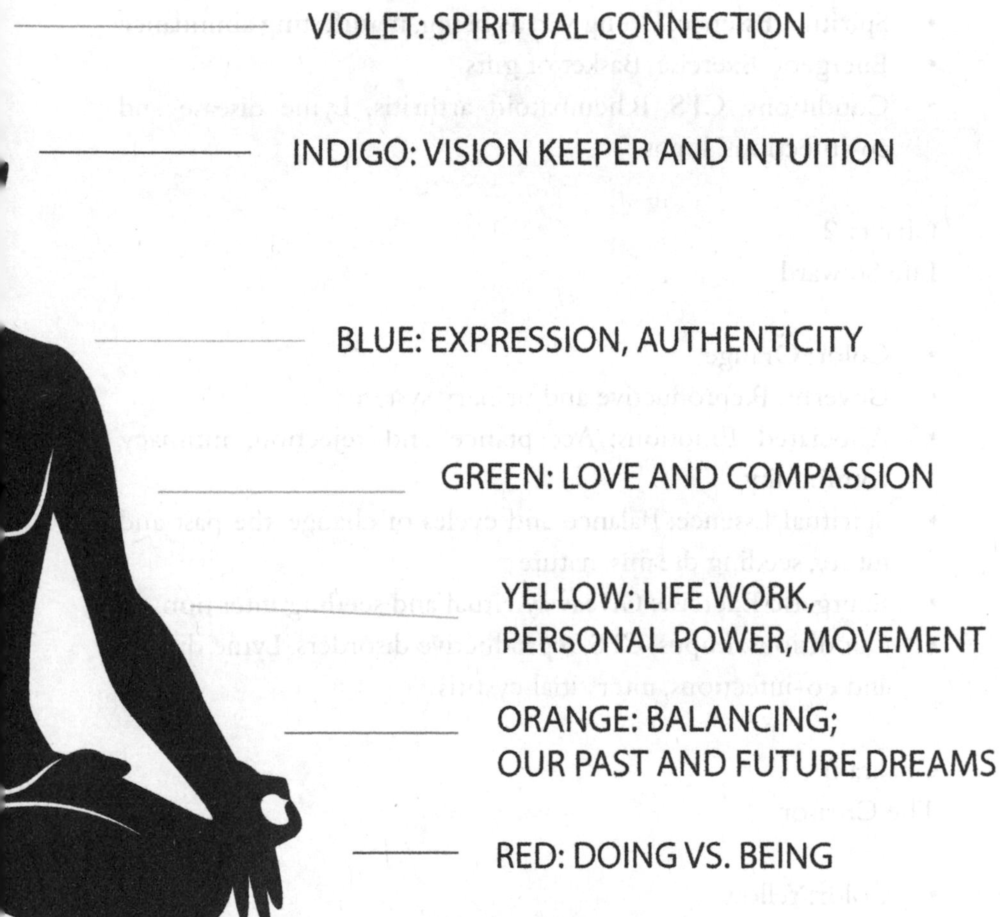
VIOLET: SPIRITUAL CONNECTION
INDIGO: VISION KEEPER AND INTUITION
BLUE: EXPRESSION, AUTHENTICITY
GREEN: LOVE AND COMPASSION
YELLOW: LIFE WORK, PERSONAL POWER, MOVEMENT
ORANGE: BALANCING; OUR PAST AND FUTURE DREAMS
RED: DOING VS. BEING

Chakra 1
Root Chakra

- Color: Red
- Governs: Skeletal system
- Associated Emotions: Groundedness, security, familial bonds, serving others
- Spiritual Essence: Doing versus being, manifesting abundance
- Energetic Exercise: Basket of gifts
- Conditions: CFS, Rheumatoid arthritis, Lyme disease and co-infections, lupus

Chakra 2
Life Steward

- Color: Orange
- Governs: Reproductive and urinary systems
- Associated Emotions: Acceptance and rejection, intimacy, community
- Spiritual Essence: Balance and cycles of change, the past and future, seeding dreams, nature
- Energetic Exercise: Giveaway ritual and seeding intention
- Conditions: Lupus, CFS, reproductive disorders, Lyme disease and co-infections, interstitial cystitis

Chakra 3
The Creator

- Color: Yellow
- Governs: All digestive organs and muscles, connective tissues
- Associated Emotions: Personal presence or confidence, creativity, drive, and willpower

- Spiritual Essence: Contributing our work to the world, assimilation and production, trust
- Energetic Exercise: Movement with intention
- Conditions: IBS, Crohn's disease, fibromyalgia, MS, ALS, CFS, Lyme disease and coinfections

Chakra 4
Heart Center

- Color: Green or Pink
- Governs: Heart and circulatory system, spleen, and immune system
- Associated Emotions: Love, passion and compassion, jealousy, betrayal, abusiveness
- Spiritual Essence: Love, body, mind, spirit, boundaries
- Energetic Exercise: Cupped hands
- Conditions: Arrhythmias, MS, CFS, lupus, all autoimmune illnesses, Lyme disease and coinfections

Chakra 5
Peace Maker

- Color: Blue
- Governs: Respiratory, ears, neck
- Associated Emotions: Joy, sorrow
- Spiritual Essence: Authenticity, accountability, exchange
- Energetic Exercise: Breathwork, chanting, humming, song
- Conditions: CFS, asthma and respiratory problems, Hashimoto's thyroiditis, Lyme disease and coinfections, ALS

Chakra 6
Vision Keeper

- Color: Indigo
- Governs: Endocrine glands
- Associated Emotions: Clarity, open-mindedness, disillusion, confusion
- Spiritual Essence: Reality versus fantasy, perception, intuition, emotional intelligence
- Energetic Exercise: Meditation and focused visualizations
- Conditions: Endocrine disturbances (thyroid, pancreas, adrenals), diabetes, hypoglycemia, Lyme disease and coinfections, fibromyalgia, CFS

Chakra 7
Crown Chakra

- Color: Violet or White
- Governs: Brain and nervous system
- Associated Emotions: Devotion, reason, ethics, guidance, safety
- Spiritual Essence: Authenticity, spirituality, big picture in life, wisdom
- Energetic Exercise: Prayer
- Conditions: ALS, dementia, Bell's palsy, migraines, neuropathy, MS, Tourette's syndrome, Lyme disease and coinfections

PART VI

Mind-Spirit

MIND-SPIRIT

"Our task must be to free ourselves . . . by widening the circle of understanding and compassion, to embrace all living creatures and the whole of nature in its beauty."

—Albert Einstein

This section is designed to bring us in concert with the Self as a whole being. We will look more closely at the interplay of the energy chakras, the conditions typically manifesting in certain ones, and the energy to work with in each site, as well as specific "practices" to help break blocks or recalibrate imbalances; traditionally called "symptoms". Though we are moving into the realm of metaphysics, many of you will deduce that this feels "normal" to you or not so difficult. In fact, some of you may feel these chapters are a reminder or perhaps a structured format to help you get some routine and discipline going in your daily life; to help you take care of yourself, move ahead in your work or from illness, or even to start teaching to your children.

One of the exercises I teach in the pages to come, actually was spawned by my late father, a magician at working with intention and visionary manifestation. These are my favorite pearls of wisdom to share with you. Though they came "hard earned" to me via illness, these missives blend beautifully in the mayhem world-place of living in modern times. May their teachings bring you realization and resource.

The model in this section is a reflection of the work I was trained in by Dr. Meredith Young-Sowers, co-founder and director of The Stillpoint School of Integrative Life Healing. Thousands have benefited from the Stillpoint model of healing. Please read the powerful foreword for more insights from Dr. Meredith Young-Sowers.

THE INNER TOOLS WE BEAR

Healing involves more of what we don't see, what happens in an inner realm, than what we actually do see on the outside. Beliefs, feelings, and intuitions about ourselves and others as well as belief in higher power all align as factors in our healing. There is no one set way that works for everyone. Each of us must tap into or resonate with a belief system, a healing modality, or certain practitioner that matches our likes and dislikes, our sensitivities, fears, power, and trust. Each new day we are blessed with a fresh canvas to draw upon. Make it your own painting.

Healing energy is always available to you. Being the "exceptional patient" is always your choice. You have much more influence upon your body and spirit than any medicine or person. It is up to you to tap your powers and also thwart the negative words, attitudes, or assumptions of an outside person, poor diagnosis, or circumstance. We all know exceptional people—the thrivers who arch their way out of a ghetto upbringing, stage-four cancer, or an abusive marriage to shine in new ways. This can be you, too.

When your body is struggling, you are being given an opportunity to examine your past behaviors or harbored feelings and embedded patterns. Often we dwell on shame or betrayal or guilt or resentment. These thought forms brew disharmony and affect our biology. Allow yourself some time to reflect on your past and acknowledge the "wrongs," but ultimately you must let go and not fight the past, but instead allow your spirit the encouragement to move on with life.

This is when the healing begins. We embrace hope and breathe in joy and the precious gem of potentials and of new beginnings. Like that preschooler's blend of wonderment and timidity, many of us question the step toward a new direction or a place of unfamiliar ground. In an odd way, managing your given symptoms and illness routines gains a familiar, though painful and burdensome, gestalt over time. Most of us fear change, yet it is life's constant. We must let go of the "familiar illness" to embrace healing.

Just as the preschooler crosses the threshold of discovery, finding playmates and an alphabet and tools to navigate a bigger world with, as you embrace the vaster world of spiritual energy and available healing, you too will gain confidence and step up to the plate of growth and transformation. You too will gain new tools and language.

Healing asks us to tend to our spirit if we wish to mend our body. As my mentor, Dr. Young-Sowers, taught me, there is a "healing rainbow" that connects our spirit with our physical body and thinking and feeling mechanisms. When focusing our mind in unison energetically with our spirit and body we align with divine love. In this way we reach up and above, flowing through our Seven Energy Chakras, out our "crown" and into "God's hand"!

In order to create this healing arc we must practice specific energetic "exercises" to both cleanse and engage each chakra and generate fluid movement in our energy fields. The more positive energy we can create with our thought patterns, emotional awareness, lifestyles, behaviors, and ability to let go and open our hearts and spirits to change, a new future, the greater the promise for profound healing. By actively engaging in your own healing and working on generating more positive energy, shifting occurs and new cells are born with a new healthier imprint.

Your destiny summons you. Will you answer the call, pick up the phone, enter the dialogue, and say yes to healing? The great masters equate true healing with enlightenment. Enlightenment can be a momentary experience, while true healing is meant to be permanent. Engaging the "rainbow arc" is our quest, akin to a holy grail.

Modern times have sanitized vision quests and pilgrimage walks of sanctimonious cleansing. We carry many emotional and mental burdens on a daily basis. The sacred church hour, Sabbath day of stillness, and alone time for prayer have evaporated within the past fifty years for so many. Spiritual neglect has climbed. Tending to the spirit and heart are essential if we desire healing.

My healing journey began at a spiritual retreat weekend. Others experience immediate miracle "cures" via encounters with living saints, touching a holy relic, potent prayers being answered by divine grace. The underlying theme is a deep desire for transformation and an urgent willingness to let go of the past.

Most of us find true healing occurs over a span of time, with devout practice and adaptation, as we make adjustments and find new balance. We need to become responsible about embracing our process, understanding that with time and guidance and fortitude, like any pilgrim on any true quest, the modern-day plague of chronic disease can be removed. And it is the spirit that desires to grow in love and care of self that will meet the challenge head-on with angels of mercy under your wings. For you are not alone, the unseen is just as real as the seen, and sickness and healing are the deepest embodiments of the eternal lesson.

We have explained the concepts of health and disease, why we get sick, the raw truth that our food chain and habitats have become polluted, and the philosophies of assorted healing disciplines. We have charted the bodily systems and their correlation to acupuncture meridians and the Seven Energy Chakras. By now, matters illustrate that as human beings we are important and resilient and occasionally we need assistance to obtain wellness.

My message of spirituality woven into serious conditions, like autoimmune illness and Lyme disease, asks you to dig deep. Exploring your feelings and habits and past history as well as your hopes and dreams are all out on your table now. The energetic restorative skills helping ignite your mighty mind-body healing pathway need to be honored and practiced routinely.

Until you can replace those old, illness-coded mental, emotional, physical, and psychic record grooves with newer, more positive ones, you will play the same old tune. But, with practice you can retune your mind and body to a higher, more optimal vibration and healthier life.

Now, in this section, let us explore each of our fascinating energy chakras, the systems they physically correlate to, as well as their emotional counterparts and the very real spiritual essence within each. These chapters all include an energetic restorative practice or "exercise" to begin in order to gain personal influence over your health, well-being, and transformation from one place of illness to a growing path of enlightenment. My wish is that you prosper and grow with these understandings and self-help tools.

SUFFERING AND REBIRTH

Illness is capable of inducing true suffering. Relentless or excruciating pains are consuming, ripping our attention away from our daily life, a conversation, the ability to concentrate or even go to work. Suffering from illness can embody more than pain—we may experience deep fatigue, heartbeat arrhythmias, incontinence, malaise of depression, and more.

From the endless pain of fibromyalgia, or the bedridden incapacitation of advanced MS, or the erratic swings of a bipolar disorder, suffering often becomes our tablemate. Families and caregivers experience our suffering, too. Resentments, displeasures, even emotional abandonment or abuse can develop in a relationship or family when chronic illness becomes a constant.

Before the advent of modern medicine, extended family dwellings were more common, and the woes of the infirm or elderly were more accepted. Many individuals were available to help, so caregiving tasks were rotated and accepted as part of life and family duty. Today, because fewer people grew up in an environment where caregiving was part of the daily routine, suddenly having to witness the suffering of another and be part of the healing process can feel like an overwhelming burden.

My suffering during a ten-year Lyme disease trial was decimating. It stripped me of everything I valued and worked to create. Bedridden for three years in collapse and pains, my well-crafted career, beautiful home, and vibrant marriage washed away. So did many friendships, my nuclear family, my financial savings, and my self-confidence. Suffering became more than physical. The emotional despair, the mental anguish, and spiritual tragedy overwhelmed me. I know these states are not unique to my story—they range worldwide and can be induced from illness or war or famine or bankruptcy. The instigator is not the crux, the greater issue is our reaction to suffering.

Life presents us with endless lessons. Our journey is fraught with challenges from the day we are born. We are also graced with the wisdom of our elders and many great teachers and friends. We may feel deeply alone and isolated at times, suffering putting a magnifying glass before us. But the larger perspective suits us well if we understand that suffering is actually a truly powerful teacher.

C. S. Lewis said, *"God whispers to us in our pleasures, speaks to us in our conscience, but shouts to us in our pains. It is his megaphone to rouse a deaf world."* Illness has a strident way of garnering our attention. Suffering is like a five-alarm fire. Living in a myopic way of self-ambitions, or what the Buddhists term "ignorance," we get distracted from the true purpose of our life path. Modern living holds many placebos and temptations that pull us away from thoughtfulness and a heart of clear intent. When we experience suffering, our senses are heightened and we may be forced to confront our self and our lifestyle.

Suffering also strengthens us for future tasks. It makes us more sensitive to the pains of others. Suffering helps us to let go, cleanse our old patterns, and purify for a new beginning. Suffering is part of life's school of experiences, teaching us patience, fortitude, humility. Suffering helps us gain inner strength. We become more tender and open, one of life's deepest objectives. Suffering may seem cruel, but in the truest depths, it expands our souls. We learn to let go.

Pain, loneliness, burdens, and feeling overwhelmed all lay heavy coils of dark energy upon our beings. We tighten, we retreat, we get angry, we get drunk, we get sick, we harbor resentments, and most abysmally we die a little every day. Feelings and circumstances may truly be dire moments in our lives. Fear, loss, and betrayal evoke true states of inner discord and distress. Physiological and spiritual components entwine, making us feel miserable.

Life is an ever-evolving dance of adjustments. Rarely are things static, and when they are so for too long, we get bored and go slack. A key factor is allowing ourselves to unwind, let go, exhale out the tension, the worries, the responsibilities, the fear, the darkness. It is important to remind ourselves that we are a microcosm in a far-greater whole. Our suffering may be real, but there is so much beauty and light and love surrounding us, and we can absorb all such mystery and let our smallness and our individual suffering be erased by the light surrounding us.

Each day the sun rises, bathing the environment in color and glory. Each evening the dark descends and envelops the happening in onyx. We can be reminded that always the light emerges and we can use that light to bathe in, to fill our beings and senses with. This daily reminder and rhythm is one of value. Honor the light and the darkness. Find a way to release your burdens and embrace even the smallest ray of light into your heart. A budding flower, a faithful pet's joy, or a good bowl of soup feels good! Take it!

Suffering makes "saints" of common people as they master patience and hone away the needy emotions of greed, envy, possession, disdain, self-pity, and delusion. The lessons gained and the rebirth from the outcome of suffering are akin to Lazareth's. We arise resplendent and awakened, a new being and a cleansed spirit. Faith is a call to trust God or the universal higher power and not the life-sustaining props on the earth-school plane. We become so dependent on many sources: homes, people, jobs. Suffering asks us to examine and seek our inner treasures.

Suffering ultimately is a harrowing passage, and when the enormous task of patience is mastered and the emotional demons stripped away, the reward is revealed in a rather unsuspect way. An entirely new life opportunity, talent, or individual is revealed to you. For when we embrace the root of suffering, we find the attachment is that of desire.

Buddhists phrase suffering as the attachment to desire, and that by mastering the need to cling on to desires and the associated emotions, we in turn achieve a self-awakening. Our desires, emotions, and thought patterns define our behaviors, which, in turn, translate to our authenticity and place in the world.

Greed, hatred, grief, and delusion drive us to hold on or cling to negative thought patterns and involve the sympathetic nervous system stress response. As communicated before, our endocrine, nervous, and immune systems get caught in a vicious loop. Illness perpetuates, especially the self-destructive mechanisms of the autoimmune relay. The suffering then escalates beyond reason. We feel "out of control," our body running haywire in all sorts of ways.

Suffering through illness is potentially a gateway to move beyond your literal, tangible, seen world and venture into the dimension of self-awakening and personal transformation. Coming to live in mindfulness is the very first step of our appropriate nature, to break free from the entrapments. The path of suffering is something besides the limitations and withdrawal it induces—we face a journey. The journey is yours.

CHAKRA 1 (ROOT CHAKRA): THE ACT OF BEING

Gratitude asks us to be still for a moment or more, to sense within, to honor. When we give thanks, we embody the gesture of appreciation. This small act, this quiet internal posture or our outward expression of gratitude delivered to another being, place, even a job we hold, or the mere fact that we are alive today or free of pain, enables us to step away from doing or achieving or pushing ourselves in some way.

At this moment, when we acknowledge what we are grateful for, that gentle turn within allows us to actually adjust our energy store. The striving, caretaking, achieving, organizing modes are momentarily stopped. The yang drive quells and when honoring the yin, or appreciating our ability to receive, we restore our well waters. Being present in gratitude is a quietly powerful gesture of deep sanctity.

The ability to receive is not so easy for many of us, especially in an achievement-oriented culture like in the United States, where we teach our toddlers to count, and climb, and write, and build Lego kingdoms. By age seven our children have turned their left brain hemisphere on to high-speed drive and they can recite states and capitals, presidents' names, and compete with others on the soccer field. And, somewhere along the way, we hopefully remind them to say "please" and "thank you," use their indoor voices, and to share their feelings, not shove the annoying kid in the neighboring seat to the ground.

I truly believe we are really trying as parents and teachers and guardians to help youngsters to be good people. Often this very structured achievement allows something, however, to slip between the cracks—imagination.

My mother, blessedly in hindsight, did not believe in structured time for us kids in the 1960s, beyond the six-hour school day. She encouraged us to ride bikes, invent recipes, sew, and ramble like wildcats in the woods of the bygone estate land beyond my house. My moss garden under the old sycamore was so soft, dappled summer light reflecting off shining bits of mica. Sprays of starlight filled the night sky as my best friend and I slept on heavy Hudson Bay blankets in the meadow, and were deliriously filled with giggles and the scampering thrill to catch fireflies, with our nimbus nets sweeping gaily in arcs. I loved to watch the fireflies blinking in the jar beside our heads in the soft, humid heat of August.

Many decades later I still am truly most at home in the outdoors. Daily, I distance-swim at the local pond, deep green waters luring me forward as I stretch and kick, all limbs propelling me like a mermaid, as my stepdaughter says. And, every single swim as I return to shore,I float on my back and gaze above to the sky. Sometimes it is crystal blue and sun-filled, other days cloudy and low.The twilight sky shows sherbet-colored sunsets, or at night a sliver of a crescent moon as I faithfully swim. But, the ritual I partake in that is most joyous is the ending spell when I float and turn my conscious attention to the practice of gratitude.

As I float starfish-like, limbs out wide, I offer my thanks for what I appreciate in my life. These moments of reverence are mine. And I am still and very awake. And I receive. I receive the sunshine or the cloudcast and I also receive the bounty of the incredibly lush beauty of all the elements surrounding me. All my senses are fed in these still moments.

And beyond these very feelings, I sense something bigger. It is the universe, the hologram of living. I am aware of my complete insignificance as one tiny, singular human being amongst billions on this planet Earth, and simultaneously somehow I am calibrating, too, that I am significant. For my waking hours are mostly spent in contributing to the art of living—by caring and creating, doing, and teaching others.

In these serene moments of quiet on the pond waters, akin to those firefly nights in open meadow sleep-outs as a child, I am feeling grateful. And in feeling grateful, my spirit shows respect. This respect allows me to stay open. Openness permits me to find an inner balance point. That balance point is the truest Zen of life. For when we allow our spirit to be free like that, to not be pushing and striving, like the seven-year-olds on the competitive soccer field or the ten-year-old's quest to recite presidential lineup, we give amplitude to our brain's right hemisphere—the imagination side, the spatial side, the receptive side. It is here that the healing energy resides.

The healing energy we can tap into internally, not derived from an external drug or potion or prop, but is turned on from within, is accessed from this balance-point, the still place of gratitude and the ability to receive. As I offer my respects for good health, my happy child, a safe home, and wondrous work, I, of course, am deeply grateful for the freedoms nurtured in my childhood. No matter our age or status of health or illness, the practice of gratitude allows us to receive, and in turn to begin our healing.

Chakra 1 asks us to examine our balance between doing and being in life. As a society, we are ramped up to carry out tasks, achieve victories, lend our energy to events, children's activities, manage chores, and take care of other's needs. Some of this is very normal and part of being human and in relationship with others, our community, and society. But there is just as much need for us to be as there is for us to do. The ability to receive translates to abundance. For, in receiving, we hold and gather. We find a grounding rod in this vessel bearing abundance and fertility. Abundance grounds us, makes us feel valuable, and brings an inner peace that cycles around again, allowing us to once again give and share.

The spiritual masters of any society or religion are very adept at being. Via prayer, meditation, and mindfulness these individuals are moving at a slower pace and bear a certain carriage that reflects as grace. People gravitate to them with ease, sharing both their burdens and gratitudes. Spiritual masters also imbue vast healing auras. Their very presence is calming and healing. The most enlightened live in deep gratitude.

The relationship between doing and being are the metaphysics for chakra 1. High-achieving, industrious personalities who seriously apply themselves in life are often prone to disorders such as all forms of arthritis, "water on the knee," joint pains, tick-borne diseases, connective-tissue autoimmune disorders like lupus, and injuries. How many of us multitask, are running from a past hurt, or just are uber-responsible, and never take a moment to be still?

Your illness is asking you to transform. You are being asked to examine your ways of doing and being. Multitasking, hamster-wheel lives, and high-stress loads churn out cortisol from the adrenal glands and turn the sympathetic nervous system on to a high-wire frequency that if allowed to run at that pace over time (meaning weeks and months) we set up a cavalcade of neurotransmitters and hormone production that is worse than popping amphetamines. Soon, our biochemistry is imbalanced, immune function flip-flops, and the panoply of triggers outlined in Part I tumble like a matchstick tower. The result is symptoms and then disease. Becoming chronically ill is not random; our inner life is at play.

Awakening to the presence of here and now, to the magic of our experience, to the lucidity of our spiritual being is a gift like none other. Life's distractions, the noise of traffic, voices, electronic bombardment, our whirling thoughts drive us away from the self—the essential clarity and purity of our inner voice and knowing. Instead, we tumble recklessly at a steady, but blinding, pace through the day, determined to master the hours, and the rigors of job demands, commitments, children's needs, sustaining food and shelter. Many of us cannot help this, so we believe. We are merely caught up in the demands and pace of our current societal tempo.

Being aligned to the core silence of our self is hard to maintain. This requires conscious commitment, mindfulness, and often an agreement with your partner, mate, or family. A week rambling on the beach, a weekend lost in the bedsheets with a lover, an electronics-free evening in front of a crackling fire are the rare pleasures bringing us home to our self, and are so very nurturing. How much energy do we put into others, our jobs, and the busy-ness of doing versus the all-too-precious act of being? Just being still, with our self, in the gesture of receiving instead of expending, skims by all too easily. And, in these precious interludes of quiet and beauty, we can take a few moments to offer our gratitude.

Energetically this chakra site and our bodily systems correspond to the dual nature of doing versus being in life. The yang process of being active and moving about is one side, and the other is the yin art of just being, stillness. The greatest lesson I learned in my ten-year Lyme journey was the patient process of living in stillness, the ability to become totally motionless, reflective, accepting, and being alone in silence with myself.

This was incredibly difficult for me to master. It took me an entire decade to master the sacred space of stillness, and to actually come to honor me, Katina Makris, for just being me—not the homeopath, the nurturing mother, the fun-loving friend, the adoring wife, the creative cook, or the adventurous athlete. No, all that had to go. Those were "ways" I knew myself, "ways" I gained familiarity or confidence in relating with others.

Lyme forced me down deeper than all those external manifestations. It made me search within, to accept, to contemplate, to distill and get very small and centered. And, honestly, only then, after years of inner work, did I eventually come to really know who I was, what made me valuable to me—not to others, but to me.

And then, after many self-affirmations and blessings, as well as gratitude, working with chakra 1, was I able to turn and face the world again and open and expand and rebirth in new ways. Ultimately, if we can take this journey within and learn how to be, to embrace our own precious qualities, then we shift these energetic holding patterns and change happens, first emotionally, then energetically, and finally at the cellular level. This chakra rules the bones, skeleton, spinal column, joints. All issues here need inner attention.

A simple exercise to help balance chakra 1 and practice gratitude is a variation on a teaching from Meredith Young-Sowers. Called "Basket of Gifts," this practice is loved by thousands and invokes our ability to come to value our own self and nourish the first "root" chakra.

CHAKRA 1 EXERCISE: "BASKET OF GIFTS"

This energetic healing exercise helps us restore balance and harmony to our root chakra numbered 1.

So many of us overextend ourselves, giving our energy, service, and care in endless ways in a very busy lifestyle. Learning to tend to our own inner state of being, and receiving energy and restorative order is not so easily or regularly done. In fact, many of us tend to neglect ourselves at this energetic level. It seems more instinctive to value putting our attention and efforts on others than on restoring our wellsprings.

This lovely exercise is a way to help us come to value and cherish our own being and qualities we possess and maybe even need to cultivate. This is a very simple practice but reaps great rewards. In short order you will begin to fathom the energetic shifts it propels to reflect and value your own self.

Get out some lined notebook paper and a pencil or pen. The exercise is to be done spontaneously without any focused thinking. Start randomly writing down on each line qualities you value or appreciate about yourself. They can be completely simple aspects such as "friendly, good cook, organized, thoughtful, creative, athletic, patient," etc.

After you have written as many qualities down as you possibly can, whether it is one side of the page or five pages long, get out a pair of scissors and snip each line out individually, kind of like the strip inside a fortune cookie.

Now fold up these strips of paper and put them in a basket or bowl. This is your basket of gifts. Each day take a random strip of paper out of the basket. Read it. This is your gift that you want to honor today. Throughout the day please take a moment here and there, to internally acknowledge and express self-gratitude for this quality. In doing so you are starting to shift the energy that you always extend toward others onto your own self. Put that strip of paper into a separate bowl that will serve as a reservoir for all of the strips of paper as they accumulate there in the days and weeks ahead. Eventually, you will have worked your way through your entire basket of gifts. Then it is time to recycle from the reservoir bowl and just start the process all over again. If at any point in time you resurrect new or other qualities you appreciate about yourself add them to the basket.

This may sound like a nonsensical practice but actually it is very lovely. It is not so easy to look at ourselves in the mirror with appreciation. We tend to find flaws, which set up negative thought patterns and beliefs. Basket of Gifts helps us come to value our inner riches and helps us ground in that first chakra of receptivity. It is not uncommon that as we help our inner self shine with self-appreciation, we soon start to draw people into our lives that reflect the very qualities we are now coming to value in our own self. This is called creating abundance and is very essential in restoring this chakra site, and relates so intrinsically to people that are having issues with joints, the skeleton, and taking steps forward in their life literally and metaphorically.

CHAKRA 2 (SACRAL CHAKRA): CYCLES OF CHANGE

Because every relationship is made up of unique individuals, there's no easy formula for getting them "right." We meet one another in so many different forms. Are we friends, co-workers, neighbors, business partners, lovers, spouses, parents, siblings, mentors, students, athletic teammates, muses, spiritual allies, enemies, or some duet that doesn't fit neatly in any category? Connection is often challenging, but it is part of the human instinct. Our hearts and minds and spirits need companionship and most ultimately love. The urge to merge is innate.

We must not forget that at the core, each of us is a spiritual being. Yet instead of cultivating this inner place of beauty and refinement in each of us, with quiet time in nature, playing an instrument, or daydreaming, we are trained to turn on our left-hemisphere thinking, analytic mind, as well as strike hard to meet externally imposed standards and expectations, which are often seen as "goals"—good school grades, athletic awards, and favor from our parents. As we mature, we still end up seeking approval from friends, spouses, bosses. Striving to be a good person is not a bad quest, but balance is what will bring health and happiness.

We try to win approval from the people in our lives, but we're also walking around with all kinds of emotional scars. Pain and trauma cause some of us to retreat inside ourselves. We shield our hearts in attempt to avoid more hurt. Or, conversely, a combative, aggressive behavior is bred, and an angry, assertive, controlling stance manifests. Most of this is unconscious, a form of self-defense and personal protection. "Fight or flight" is an instinctive human reaction, whether we are a preschooler or an adult.

The key is to learn how to remain open, yet not become a doormat and be stomped upon, nor an orchestrator who always "runs the show." Remaining open to another being, what they bring to the table, or how you interconnect is the magic of human relations. Living with acceptance, compassion, and the wonderment of co-creating makes for beautiful harmonies, and is one of life's great teachers.

The art of "letting go" is necessary if we want to live in balance within our own self, and also in harmony with others and even the natural world. The second chakra, housing the urinary system (kidneys, bladder, urethra), and reproductive systems (uterus, ovaries, vagina, or prostate, testicles), asks us to be able to "let go." We release impurities and toxins in the mighty filtration of the kidneys and urinary fluid, as well as in menstrual flow or male ejaculatory emissions, as well as emotions we harbor.

Chakra 2 is a balance point of culling our inspirations and dreams (ovaries, uterus, prostate) and bringing them forth, by birthing (female) or delivering (male) into the world, and the converse of shedding, or "letting go." It is also our space of true intimacy. Closeness, tenderness, care, and honesty are fostered here. Mother and infant, husband and wife, best friends, creative work partners—such intimacy is life's treasure and intended to be sacred and honored.

The human being, like other mammals, goes through natural cycles, just like the seasons. Seeding, cultivating, harvesting, shedding. It is a wise person who takes the time to sense and honor their innate rhythms, noticing and responding when she needs an alone day, and respecting the need for regular periods of exercise to keep balance. But, ultimately we must live in concert with others, too. This is where our emotions can become tricky, and if held onto too tightly, we fester and brew ovarian cysts, kidney stones, lupus, reproductive cancers, and more abnormalities. Learning to be aware of what we hold onto is essential for this chakra. Our culture has taught us how to build and amass, but not how to release. Letting go of our past, a friendship, a home, or a child is excruciating for many of us. We gravitate to familiarity, comfort, our attachments. How de we let go with grace and also plant new seeds, accepting new beginnings?

Chakra 2 asks for balance between the past and future. Like the moon cycles, tidal changes, and rhythm of the seasons, our reproductive organs and urinary system represent the give and take, the ebb and flow, the past and future. We are looking at seedlings of tomorrow here, the energy of hopes, dreams, aspirations. What can we shed to make room for new energy to enter? How can we abandon fear and welcome a new beginning?

I spent a week in a prominent Boston hospital in July 2014 for surgery for a "suspicious" kidney tumor requiring a massive operation—it required slicing through my ribs, deflating a lung, and lopping off a growth and part of my kidney. Blessedly, I was in the rare ten percentile carrying a benign tumor. Still, the surgery was intense, and my convalescence arduous. The nursing staff who cared for me were angelic beings, filled with tenderness and great dollops of encouragement. No matter how I writhed in pain, or moaned over a week of unshampooed hair, the loving hands that helped me bathe and the ardent belief that I would heal up beautifully and blossom anew boosted me onward. When nurse Colleen insisted on day two that, though doped up on Dilaudid, I would stand and walk to the nearby chair, I felt like she was asking me to climb Mount Everest.

"I can't even breathe or turn over," my croaking voice murmured.

"Honey, you can do this," sturdy Irish-stock Colleen chirped as she levered the head of my bed slowly upward, me wincing at each degree of ascent.

"Hold my hands." She grasped them firmly. "Look me in the eyes, Katina, lift your eyelids. Come on, honey. Breathe."

"Oh God! I can't, Colleen. It hurts so bad! I'm too dizzy." My entire right side had been sliced open, a twelve-inch incision, drains, sutures, a collapsed lung. Teetering at my bedside edge, I felt like fainting.

"Use your legs, Katina. Come on, girl. You are strong, a swimmer. Let's do this. Look me in the eyes. You are going to stand. One. Two. Three. Exhale." Her tough love held me fast.

Leaning on Colleen's forearms, I pushed upward, the room careening, my heart flipping about, pain searing, and, I smiled, though gritting my teeth in pain.

"You did it! You are up! First, giant step," Colleen crowed, strawberry complexion flushed as she too exerted herself to help steady a wobbly 5'8" me. "Let's sponge you down, clean the sweat from your skin."

Swift, sure hands bathed me, blue johnny gown a crumple on the floor. Colleen was my encouraging guide. In her I trusted. We inched to the huge leatherette lounge chair. Sitting down was another torture; pumps, IVs tugging and hurting so bad. And Colleen coaxed me on.

"You are doing great, Katina. Just sit here and breathe for thirty minutes. Slow, deep breaths, not shallow." She placed the red call button in my right hand. "Buzz if you need me. Concentrate on being well and doing what you love. You are starting your steps towards mending." I nodded in a daze of opiates and surgical shock, and still I heard that miraculous word, the word I'd earmarked for my manuscript: Mending.

"Yes, I will mend," I smiled up to her. Sparkling blue eyes lit back at me. "You go, girl!"

And so I sat there, the sunny July day glowing outside my enclosed hospital room. My beautiful home and son were two hours north of me in New Hampshire, my favorite swimming pond patiently awaiting my return. I contemplated both the abysmal situation I was dealing with, and the potentials of my future.

The thirty minutes felt like six hours. Each breath brought razor-like pain. But a quiet image surfaced, too. In my mind's eye I saw my fragrant garden back home, hollyhocks climbing, peonies draped in pink, daylilies bursting in orange riot. Those lush gardens called to me. Surprisingly, not to be tended to, but to remind me of a precious something—the cycles of life and the stewardship of my own mending. The fertile blooms of summer mirrored my own lush future. I sensed this vision and its glory. I internally told myself, "Katina, you can be glorious again. Do not give in. Believe in your mending."

And now, in the late days of October, cold soil amid my fingertips, my right flank slightly stiff, but certainly mending four months later, I am in the conscious process of planting tulip bulbs for the bloom of next spring. I place twelve chunky bulbs ensemble, knowing their ruby glory will cheer me next May and nature once again reminds me of life's great teachings. I cannot help but feel grateful for my body and mind's cooperative workings.

In order to witness the bloom in life, reach the success point, mend from a surgery or illness, or garner an important job, we must simply start with that very first step—planting the bulb. Seeding the dream. Honoring the wisdom of cycles, and our ability to move forward with intention. I pat the turned soil over the tulip bulbs. Attentively I anoint them with my dream: "I will be 100 percent recovered when you bloom in May. My body will be functioning perfectly post-op, with great vitality and I will be bringing my creative work to the world in abundance and joy with great success."

As I stand up, from kneeling posture, I recall Colleen and that first horrid rise from my sickbed to standing. Now I rise from the earth slowly but on my own, and on the mend. We are resilient beings, and we cannot hide from our abilities, nor our shortcomings.

I had kidney surgery. The organ of cleaning impurities housed a wayward clump of cells; a fatty tumor encased with blood vessels and surrounded with a hard shell. It popped out in the surgeon's hands. I released pieces and patterns of my past. Old energies, history, "junk" from a once-rampant Lyme disease infection. In the twilight haze of post-op opiates I dozed and drifted, my life scrolling before me like a time-warp in my third eye. Earnestly I worked on saying good-bye to my tendency to be a "mother hen" and to clutch at family members or my mate. I saw my former husband in silhouette and said farewell to him psychically. The deep sorrow I wallowed in after he left me for another woman eclipsed my creative ability. I needed to let go in post-op in order to birth my new self. I saw him walk away into the darkness, his back facing me, and somehow I let myself float free, alone, slightly scared but also unfettered. My lineage to be a devout mate and mother was threatened. I had to accept the challenge to be unattached, a new feeling for me, in more ways than one.

The metaphor did not go unnoticed with me. Chakra 2 embodies our cycles of renewal, seeding our dreams, birthing our creations, sharing intimately. We shed the old and conceive the new. Toxins release, old patterns die, creations take form, we make bonds.

Like all aspects of mending, I needed to face just what was being asked of me in this invasive surgery, and now, on the cusp of a new beginning. My independence and ability to practice balance, *not* in relationship to another, was up for grabs. Planting my "bulbs of spring to come" is a ritual of sorts. Rituals have their purpose. They are like cairns of intention. Rituals focus us and bring consciousness to otherwise random acts of living. I brought my mental focus in to a narrow point of *seeing* myself healthy, active, and freed from physical pain and over concern for others. My ritual embraced a new version of me.

Chakra 2 encompasses the urinary and reproductive systems. Much fluid and flow happens here. Stagnation, repression, lost dreams, or holding on to hidden feelings or poor relationships are examples of blockage. Think about this. Are you in your flow? How do you find or keep your rhythm?

Is it exercise, dance, an art form, making love, journaling, or initiating a project that keeps you fluid? Our beings crave the give and take, the coursing of our life energy. We do not want to let it "pool" or stagnate or get stymied. We all have our "holding patterns."

Balance is critical for health and happiness. Full throttle (interstitial cystitis) or holding back (ovarian cysts, prostatitis) are warning signals of second chakra imbalance—we have lost our flow, let go of or suppressed our hopes and dreams. We must never let them die. Remember that vibrant, exhilarated, young, supernova person we knew in youth? There is a piece of that energy in you, too. Let's find it, claim it, draw it forth, just as Colleen drew me out of that hospital bed and my lush summer gardens called forth, reminding me to plant my bulbs with care for the blooms of spring.

CHAKRA 2 EXERCISES: "THE ART OF LETTING GO" AND "BULBS OF SPRING"

A cleansing exercise for Chakra 2 that helps us free up blocked energy, or balance runaway energy forms, involves a little writing and getting clear on a few matters. Using fire or water is effective here, too. What we will do is take a reflective turn inward to discern just what you want to let go of and release from your current status or past. We will write it on paper or sketch it. Then we will consciously burn the paper and images, or set them afloat on a stream, a river, the sea. Let us begin:

Take a few minutes to center yourself. Close your eyes, put your mind's attention down in your chest, on your heart. Breathe slowly and deeply and follow your breathing with your mind's eye. Relax.

Put your hand over your heart if it helps you center. Then, ask your heart this question: "What do I need to let go of?"

Just sense what comes to you. An image? Feeling? Past circumstance? Do not question this, just accept the insight. Now jot it down or do a quick sketch. This nugget of wisdom is yours. We will set it off, to sail away from you, in a bit. Right now let us complete the cycle here, in this chakra of changes, rebirth, hopes, and potentials.

Close your eyes again and draw back into your heartspace with your breathing. Feel your core self. Smile at your own self, the way you would to a child. Loving tenderness is important; it helps keep us open and caring. Now ask yourself this question: "What do I want to bring in?"

Do not think, just allow your expansive mind to accept whatever image, feeling, or words pop into your mind. This is authentic. If nothing surfaces, just keep breathing and ask yourself the question again.

Once you have gleaned a pearl, write it down. This will be your bulb of spring to come. We will work with this in a moment.

Part one involves letting go, part two allows conception to occur. Like the menstrual cycle, the release of semen, or urinary flow, or an animal shedding its winter coat, we are naturally designed to release and let go routinely in life. As busy, productive human beings we forget about this rhythmic circuitry we run. No wonder our bodies can harbor kidney stones, fibroids, eczema. The balancing act of treasuring our intimate bonds while simultaneously letting go of harmful comments, neighbors, or lost dreams is challenging.

Getting clamped into a pattern or holding on tight to our current situation, like me in the hospital bed, is easy to do. Colleen shook me free, like turning the soil. Mentally and emotionally, we need to remind ourselves how healthy it is to let go of our past, or a relationship, or behavior. Not everything or everyone serves us well, nor forever. Certain people, places, houses, jobs serve us well for a while, then change is in order. Release and renew.

Writing or sketching are fabulous ways to release creative energy. We will do this in a timed fashion, and in a free-form thinking or planned state. Set a timer for fifteen minutes. Get yourself in a comfortable spot with paper and pen, or colored markers, paint, or pastels—any medium is fine.

Take your sentence or word of what you want to let go of. Look at it. Read it aloud. Turn on the timer and just write like mad, free-form, no structure, paragraphs, etc. Or color, sketch, smear pastels around. Remind yourself that this is what you are releasing. If many pages, canvases, whatever are needed just run with it. Your spirit, heart, mind, and body are in great joy right now, finally being given permission to let go! Bravo!

Once you have completed the timed piece, look at or read your work. Some of it will surprise you; parts of it will be brilliant, and other facets rather curious. Do not judge. Hold on to it for a couple of days if you like for "processing," or take a photo of it all. Then, you must fully release these pent-up feelings, thoughts, energy forms. Light a fire, or go to a body of water. Consciously say good-bye to these old parts of you, or a relationship that showed its face. Place these papers, or cut-up pieces of them, in the fire or water, and say good-bye to what was impeding you. A huge array of feelings could arise. Do not be alarmed. This is all part of moving trapped emotions and energy. Know that you are safe and guided and fine. You are initiating healing. Talk to a friend or counselor in the days that follow if processing helps you. I believe in your strengths.

Now, let us take the pearl of "What do I need to bring in?" Do this later in the night or the following day. We are garnering your wise counselor's intuitive wisdom and initiating progression toward your more healthful future and balanced relationships. This is your bulb of spring we will plant.

Look at and read your sentence aloud. Each of your dreams and hopes can be unique: "I want to dance again like when I was twenty-five." Or "I need a talented integrative medicine doctor," or "the perfect mate." Perhaps you conjured, "No more illness, and great energy." Our dreams take many forms.

Again, take out the papers, pens, colored pencils, a guitar, whatever. Set the timer to fifteen minutes. Do not think. Close your eyes, say the sentence once again, open your eyes, and start writing, sketching, playing chords. Allow yourself the freedom to be spontaneous, playful, uninhibited, non-structured, no right or wrong. When the timer dings, review your spirit's expression. Usually a great resonance surfaces for many of us in this exercise. Or we feel a natural "Ok, that makes sense." Some of us are perplexed by what just surfaced. Try hard to not judge.

This time keep your creation. If you like this exercise, feel free to use it again and again. I find that often individuals burdened with years of pains, illness, or feelings of being misunderstood need to do the "letting go" exercise many times over. There is great catharsis in this, as you free up so much blocked energy that your very astute body and mind have been trying so enduringly to hold. Give permission to let go—release.

One caveat: stay with the fifteen-minute time frame. Running into hours of such expression often moves from right-hemisphere intuitive and non-thinking emotions into analytics, rationale, and left-hemisphere judgment and discernment. This healing exercise is not the time and place for this.

"The Art of Letting Go" and "Planting the Bulbs of Spring" are powerful tools. Honor your "Bulbs of Spring." Read them daily. Create a small gesture of respect for one of your "bulbs," such as a trinket or photo representing it. This small talisman will help you cultivate your bloom to come, and shift the mind-body healing pathway to "on."

CHAKRA 3 (SOLAR PLEXIS CHAKRA): WILL AND INTENTION

Health was once our birthright. The majority of us thrived with robust vitality, budding minds, adventurous escapades, agile limbs, speed to run and swing, and imagination a most joyful occupation. Our dreams and desires could percolate and gestate, bubble like dancing brooks as we chattered to a friend or sibling about a future to come. I love this beautiful creativity and freedom of youth. How many images of "what I will be" when I grew up pranced through my soul.

Then, the energies dampen. Too much didactic memorization, dumbed-down school systems, and overburdened households allow leakage and eventually a moldy malaise to film upon a young mind and spirit. The joyful enthusiasms and careening potentials get shelved as "lost dreams" or "maybe one day I can learn to paint, or build my own home, or be a ballerina."

By our thirties it is the rare soul in Western society who is living their passions, loving their world, brimming with vitality. When we meet this person, well, we love them! Vibrant, smiling, open-hearted, these "flames" of desire lift up a damp mood or spirit bogged with illness. Their energy is contagious.

Contributing to the world in a meaningful way brings us pride and fulfillment. When we feel the give and take, whether it is in a one-on-one work situation, as a carpenter to homeowner, or a teacher to a student, or at a broader scale, as a musician playing his personally crafted songs to an audience, we feel valued. The exchange is real and dynamic and empowering. The human factor of honest appreciation for our creation and contribution breeds a growing confidence internally. The positive feedback, or pride in your service or product, helps propel you to cultivate your craft or contribution. When fostered with will and intention, the process flourishes and we develop strength and personal presence, and our third chakra hums happily.

We all are born with desire and curiosity and passions. As youngsters we explore and soak in information readily. Creativity bubbles freely, and all those images of what we will grow up to become are perfectly appropriate fountains of potentials, for we are still forming and stretching. How beautiful the soul is, however, who continues to imagine and create and contribute their life's work with the world as a more mature adult, like Benjamin Franklin in his seventies, still fostering inspiring inventions and contributions! We do not need to damp down and merely ignore our creative juices or precious hidden jewels of potentials.

We have a very potent inner power called will. This sometimes fierce, but typically useful tool unites with determination, and more specifically, a razor-sharp motivational skill called intention. When we understand how to use intention, we can actually generate huge energy shifts internally in our physiology, and truly propel cellular change and energetic states, often overnight!

Strength, determination, and will are internal mind-sets and commitments to our selves. By putting our focus on the energy of determination we use our mind, stir the powerful energy seated in our core or solar plexus of the third chakra, and embody strength within.

When you sit still and pay attention to the feelings you summon when you claim determination, or set a goal, notice what your body experiences internally. I feel a clear, rock-hard energy solidifying in my gut, like I am dropping my energy downward and within, a gathering of force, essentially. This type of internal shift ignites the powerful third chakra, as well as the productive muscular system of our bodies. Determination is an effective example of igniting the mind-body pathway, to both manifest energy within and produce it for movement and function. Determination makes us race 5Ks, get out of bed on a rainy day, or will ourselves into wellness.

It is wise to pick a clear intention to commit to, with strong determination when we want to achieve something. From my perspective as a recoveree from chronic illness and severe depression, as well as a practitioner of three decades, all the illnesses highlighted in this book revolve around wounds, stories, and imbalances in the third chakra, and our misuse of or lack of engagement surrounding our personal confidence, will, creative productivity, and your individual contribution to the world. Questions of, "Am I worthy?" "Do I have personal power?" are core issues with autoimmune illness and Lyme disease. So many of us lay weak and in pain, and truly feel "gutted."

Many of us have turned over our personal power and ability to navigate through physical ills and emotional discomforts, finding a limp sense of willpower or ability to engage our own creativity. Seeking resource from outside ourselves, and trained by TV ads and Big Pharma, and lacking our grandparents' "horse sense" about self-care and lifestyle, many modern Americans are dependent on doctors, drugs, and other sources to "cope with" woes and burdens.

But, coming to understand that we actually have an inner calibrating tool called willpower, and the ability to set an intention and move forward in your day with that living, breathing, mindful process is a masterful ally. When we are chronically ill, most all of us have lost our "center" and our course of direction, the ability to "gather" oneself, and to move toward a healthy tomorrow. I know I did. Three years I floated on sofa and bed, my career gone and no hope I would work again, or dance, or drive a car. Suicidal thoughts took form. My father willed me to "hold on," to fight that dark space and despair. Loss of our sense of self and hope is decimating. Our lives go nowhere but down.

Now we will learn how to set intention, ignite willpower, and reclaim personal power. Chakra 3 focuses on all our digestive organs and our muscular systems. There is much movement necessitated, as the peristaltic activity of the digestive tract propels ingested food along its course. The pancreas and gallbladder release digestive enzymes, insulin, and bile salts. The stomach maintains a balanced pH, and the small and large intestines absorb nutrients and release by-products and toxins. The mighty liver is a huge filter, extracting impurities and cleansing our bloodstreams. All these organs function automatically and "feed" our body, while energetically our muscular system keeps us upright and enables us to "move" forward in life.

Until experiencing fibromyalgia, myesthenia gravis, Lyme disease, MS, muscular pains, or being hobbled by a muscular injury, most of us take our muscular system for granted. How very important our muscles are! They help us move, just as peristaltic activity propels food along. They empower us to take strides and not stagnate.

Sitting in this "solar plexus" of numerous organs and glands is our hara, or chi—the energy center behind our umbilical cords or belly buttons. So many of the martial arts draw attention to breathing deeply and gutturally grunting or growling on the exhale, a powerful tone. Football teams do this too, before taking to the field. Warriors on horseback roared a war cry. All these "power" chants for your energy, or chi, drive right into the solar plexus and core zone of chakra 3—the true great reservoir of will, determination, and courage.

Recovering from chronic Lyme disease necessitates very strong emphasis on moving the blocked energy of chakra 3. All the autoimmune illnesses carry a similar theme with this power center. The individual has lost their center. Their ability to absorb and digest their intention, to put out their personal contribution or work in the world has been lost, undervalued, or ignored. Many are "soldiering" through life, or have "let go" into a void, often having lost their will to create something new, meaningful, and what meets their purpose. Learning to value your self-initiative and nourish your creative endeavor or work will shift the energy of this chakra. The "gut" is a profound well of immunity, personal power, and the ability to move ahead.

A conscious breathwork exercise with a chant is very restorative for all these cases of CFS/ME, fibromyalgia, lupus, RA, Lyme, and the others. We bring great concentrated focus down into the belly, and fill up the weakness or "gutted" feeling that so many experience. Restoring the wellspring of chakra 3 was lifesaving for me. Let us practice the exercise.

CHAKRA 3 EXERCISE: MOVING WITH INTENTION

Close your eyes. Get in a comfortable, solid position. Start by taking a long, deep breath. Then exhale it forcefully through your mouth with the sound "HO." Let the HO exhale really trail out to the tail end. Repeat this. Inhale deeply, then exhale fully to HO. Start a cycle of rhythmic breathing like this, repeating approximately ten times. Feel yourself filling the core or your belly up on each inhale, and forcing all your energy out on the exhale. By repeating this practice, with the toning of HO, you are building up your core energy or chi. This is so essential when chronically ill, and a time-honored way to balance chakra 3.

Next, let's work on setting intention and unifying willpower. Without a shadow of a doubt, willpower is one of the top three emotional qualities that needs to be fully engaged in order to conquer any illness or serious life catastrophe. When we lose our will, or it becomes pale, we flounder or often die. How many stories do we recall of a spouse passing in short order after the death of their beloved lifelong mate? Many of us feel weak and house-bound with illness because no one has told us that full healing is possible. That negativity triggers many to lose hope, and then willpower decimates.

I sense willpower myself as a strongly laser-like focus of my mental attention placed on a certain outcome of intention. When you think of a willful child, you can visibly recognize the set of their mouth, the steel in their eyes, the strength of their muscles as they "dig in" regarding what they aim to do (or not do!), and focus fiercely. That stubborn four-year-old is suddenly very powerful and "hard to handle," even for a mature adult! Hold the picture of that willful child in your mind's eye.

Embodying will is very helpful in igniting the restorative energy of chakra 3. We use a Stillpoint School exercise called "Moving with Intention." You will get clear on a goal or intention you wish to achieve, craft a statement about that intention, and then move—walk, swim, do tai chi or such—with that focused mental image while verbally uttering the statement. This way we engage body, mind, and spirit. When practiced over weeks or months, you will begin to note transformation.

So, let's find your personal pearl of insight regarding your life's work or creative contribution to the world. As usual, we will use our internal wisdom. Close your eyes, put your hand over your heart. Breathe slowly and deeply for several breaths, dropping your mind's eye's attention down into your heart. Feel the breathing and bless your spirit and thank your mighty heart.

Now put one hand on your navel area. Drop your mental attention down to the gut. Just say an internal hello to this intrinsic digestive system, all your muscles, and your invaluable core power. This is a reverent gesture, and may feel odd to some of you at first. Just accept your body and spirit in its strength and in its weakness. Be present with yourself for a minute. Keep breathing.

Now we ask a question, and, like before, just receive whatever impressions, words, feelings appear to you. Your gut instinct is very real. Read this question out loud if possible: "What will help empower me to move ahead in my life?" Jot down the image, words, feelings. As always, each person finds a unique pearl or answer. Read this out loud to yourself. Feel free to sketch or make simple notes.

Now let us craft this into an intention statement. Perhaps you heard the word "peace," or an image appeared in your mind of you tending to a flower bed? Or something altogether different, like moving from your dwelling space? Let's use "peace" as the first example. Your intention statement is:

"In peace I will move forward in my life."

Or,

"By tending to a garden I will move forward in my life."

Or,

"In moving out of my current residence I will move forward in my life."

See the word "will" in all these statements? If healing is a key desire for you to embrace in moving forward in your life, add that word to the statement, e.g., "In tending to a garden I will heal and move forward in my life."

Now seed this image in your mind's eye. Say the statement and start walking, even if it is from your bedroom to your kitchen, or down your driveway. Ideally engaging this mind-body pathway is best achieved when you can "move with intention" for several minutes at a time, or multiple times throughout the day.

When I was bedridden, I would just do this practice each time I got up and crept to the bathroom and back. Eventually, I attempted walking out the back door of my home and around to the front door, dangling on the arm of my boyfriend. And, I willfully cemented my image in my mind's eye. Eventually, I walked a block, then several, finally a mile was conquered at six weeks, and the day I swam a half mile in open water at the pond, I knew I would never be bed-bound and undermined by chronic illness again! The "Moving with Intention" statement is very powerful. You are engaging the mind-body pathway, with kinesthetic movement and mindful intention. If you are wheelchair-bound, just try this by clapping your hands or wiggling your fingers or feet. Any movement is a starting place.

You too can claim this birthright! Willpower and personal pride in a job well done are within your reach.

CHAKRA 4 (HEART CHAKRA): THE HEART'S DESIRE

Loving-kindness and compassion involve our heart center and ability to share love. Those who shutter their heart cannot extend their energy and ability to connect to another being, no less show empathy, equanimity, or compassion. When the heartspace is held back, a person resides within. They are alone in many ways. Some may find a vein of expression perhaps with a pet, tending to a garden, or with children. Yet, the risk of adult connections or stretching beyond singular relationships to groups, mankind, or humanity feels scary. A full heart arises when we relate and share with another being. Letting go of our restraints and fears is a primal step in growth.

Past hurts, trauma, betrayal, too much structure or rules causes one to retreat and withdraw affection, connection, and compassion. The heart "rusts," making for brittle feelings, rigid joints, stark communication, and often, irritable, angry, or cruel behavior. Or we become over-defensive and leery, our immune systems run amok. When the heart is restrained, Chakra 4 energy is imbalanced and disorders of every type arise—cardiovascular issues, immune weakness and autoimmune disorders, and many emotional troubles. Unhappy and unhealthy suffering begins because your defenses have been constructed like barricades.

Chakra 4 involves our heart and circulatory systems, including all the veins and capillaries, as well as the immune system. The large spleen, under our left ribs, is the reservoir collecting all the dead white blood cells our lymph nodes produced to battle an infectious agent. The lymph and cardiovascular systems are working constantly for us. All autoimmune illness, Lyme disease, and infections have central issues involving chakra 4.

The essential energy of our heart chakra is love. Love for those dear to us, love for our own selves, love for mankind. It is from our hearts that we live. When our hearts stop beating, we die. Living from the source requires being honest with yourself. We can all live in comfort and peace if we free our hearts from judgment and fear. And still, we must feel secure in our relationships—we must balance openness with judgment and discernment over whom we allow in to the most vulnerable aspects of our selves.

Judgment involves critique. We need good judgment when driving a car, walking along a rocky hillside, or entering a foreign country where we don't speak the language. But, judgment as a main player in relating to another living being limits our capacity to connect, to love, and to experience life from a true place of fellowship. In judging, we put up walls, retreat, hold a defensive stance. Even in relationships we must learn to discern yet also balance with fluid exchange.

To live in love is nothing short of ecstatic. We are designed to share and care. Most find it easy to be open to a baby or animal; their innocence, sparkling eyes, and playful spirits enchant us readily. We engage, we smile, we adore them. In these moments together, we feel joy inside; our hearts beat happily. The brain makes endorphins—feel-good hormones of oxytocin and dopamine. The experience is beautiful.

Falling in love with another human being brings on a similar cavalcade of feelings. This person who fascinates you, captures your mind, your heart, and your sexual chemistry blows open any shuttered windows of your heart. Instead, our spirit rushes toward them; sometimes cautiously and in small gestures, other times in a wild torrent of willingness. This urge to merge, to share and care, like the encounter with baby or puppy, opens the heart in abandon.

As a society, many of us have cloistered our heart energy. We open up and live in such freedom only in select circumstances. The pressures and tensions of modern life have accelerated our daily tempo to one of hectic pace, endless tasks, projected grievances, and animosity toward even our chosen partners, family members, and neighbors. It takes daily conscious attention and effort to pull down the shielding and choose to communicate with others with openness and honesty. Awareness and practice to hold to the path must be followed. It is so simple to slip back into a former pattern of reserve and communicating from a shuttered heartspace due to fear and wariness. The autoimmune diseases are examples of being overdefended. We were betrayed or hurt to such a degree that we do not trust our own judgments about others. Energetically, this coding has made us misinterpret friend and foe.

Living in love is our birthright. The big, plump heart we are born with is a powerfully hardworking muscle, pumping even while we sleep. We typically forget to acknowledge its endless work, keeping us alive, helping us run up a hill or dance fluidly with grace. We recognize when it's not right—beating off tempo, gripped in tension, flailing in a heart attack. It is wise to give your heart some appreciative attention, an internal thank you, a hand placed over your heart as a gesture of recognition and applause.

By tuning in daily, in this quiet way, besides displaying reverence to the mighty physical organ, we are able to emotionally remind ourselves to live in love, from the posture of a giving, listening, honest, and trusting heart. Try it; you will be amazed and grateful. The smiles, the truer conversations, the abundance of joy showered on you in return is immediate and true. We become filled with energy and beauty and joy from the world and the living beings around us. And in turn, we live a fuller and happier, healthier life.

We can be kind by opening a door for someone or picking up their medications when housebound, saving them that effort and stress.

Loving-kindness asks us for interplay. A communication is involved. It may be a nonverbal form, such as a hug during a teary bout, a warm, cooked meal fed to a bedridden friend, or even words of understanding or sympathy told to one in distress. We can show ourselves gestures of loving-kindness by drawing a hot bath on a weary day or placing a vase of fresh-cut wildflowers by our bedside table. When we care, we engage our heart. This beautiful organ, pumping our blood and goodwill tirelessly and faithfully, is designed to share feelings of love. Self-love, interpersonal love, and love for mankind.

The loneliness of illness, a betrayal, abandonment, divorce, a lost job, or a troubled child causes us to pull inward. We clamp down on the flow of our love and tighten our heartspace. Anxiety, depression, anger brew when our heartspace and flow of loving-kindness are suppressed. The heart rusts. Learning to recognize this very action, the awareness of such restriction, is the first step in restoring ourselves to balance, happiness, and health.

In congruency with our heart and circulation are the walls of defense. Good boundaries help us keep wayward strangers, mooching friends, or abusive co-workers from harming us emotionally, physically, or financially. The circulatory system is buoyed by the support of the defense system, the lymph and spleen are our fortress and warriors. Living in the pure love of an open heart makes for a fully enriching life. Ideally, we strive for this bliss. The co-communion of honest and open relationship bears deep compassion and passion. And, we need to adequately protect our own self and those we love. Our immune system is the metaphysical reflection of this mind-body conduit.

Paying attention to where a wound in your heartspace came from is essential for healing. **Chakra 4** is the central of the seven tiers. Ultimately, our wounds, grief, betrayal, or abandonment need to be examined for the energetic blocks to be released. You may already know what wound "triggered" you to lose heart or become so rattled that you lost your trust in your own judgment of others. This is the crux of the deepest healing required to overcome chronic disease. What has shuttered my heart, and why has my ability to self-defend/discern turned inward instead of outward? Why have I become so confused by betrayal and misrepresentation from someone I trusted, that I can no longer trust my own discernment? This position perplexes the immune system, setting it into overdrive, whereby our natural "fighter" cells start to attack every cell, foreign invaders as well as our own natural organ, gland, and nervous system cells. Let us take a journey within again to our wise counselor and ask these very questions. You bear the answers.

CHAKRA 4 EXERCISE: CUPPED HANDS

Close your eyes, center yourself, and follow your breath as we have learned to do. Take three or four steady breaths and draw your mind to your heart. You are now tuned in. Feel its beat and honor its strength. Say thank you to this patient organ and the neighboring spleen. Now, ask yourself this question; await a sensation, image, word. Let it dawn. Do not judge, just accept: "Why have I closed my heart?"

This is very profound information. Take it with care. Jot it down. Sense your reaction. Recognize any reactions you may have. Next, ask the second question: "Who or what caused me to not trust my judgment/discernment in a relationship?" An image, a flashback, a gut reflex, a sentence may surface. Write it down. This is vital. We have touched the very deepest crux of why your healing has been limited or partial. These self-awareness points are gold for you, more potent than medicine or modalities. Take them with reverence, even if the word or image seems tangential to you. My instincts tell me you have gleaned an essential message that you sense is accurate. Your inner wisdom is real. Your heart is very wise. Bless it in gratitude.

If it feels helpful, do some journaling or sketching about any of what arises. This may help you process a wound or pattern, or merely the fact that you are gaining ground in honoring your intuition. It may take you several days to process this information, or mere seconds. We are all unique. Talk to someone if you need to.

Now, let us practice a gesture of loving-kindness to help feed your heart chakra and alter the ill-running energetic patter, so your immune function can return to normal. This exercise was taught to me by my spiritual mentor, Dr. Meredith Young-Sowers. I love the nurturing quality of it.

Take your two hands and rub the palms together, like you are trying to get warm over a fire. Then close your eyes and hold your hands with palms facing each other, and fingertips not quite touching, so that there is a cupped space between your palms. Sense the energy vibrating between your palms and fingertips. What does it feel like? I sense warm champagne bubbles. Now rub your hands together again and repeat the posture. Imagine the face of someone you love dearly, in your mind's eye, between your palms. What happens next for you?

Most of us feel our hands starting to separate slightly, as if the glow of their loving presence expands our energy field and love.

Now let us do this a third time. Rub your hands, resume the slightly prayer-like hand position and now see your own self between your palms. What happens next? Sense this and jot it down. You are imbuing your own "broken heart" with self-love. This is a very powerful life-restoring energetic healing exercise. Practice it daily.

If you feel the need to mend an emotional or spiritual wound between you and the person that hurt you enough to topple your immune function into disarray, practice this exercise with their image between your palms. If your hands do not "expand" in the warmth of healing touch, do not be alarmed. You can instead ask your Self, God, your guardian angel, to bring healing and love to them. This is a profound and massive energetic use of loving-kindness directed toward a rift, old wound, and damaged immune system and heart. You are beginning to identify and repair an energetic wound and negative mind-body rut that in good chance has tampered very significantly with your health. This is one of the most important exercises that Mending will teach you. Take it to heart and practice it daily.

In closing we need an affirmation statement you can recite to help promote optimal function to the runaway immune system. Coming to trust your own judgment about others you choose in relationships, as well as to trust your ability to self-defend when under "attack," is vital.

Craft a simple line to recite that feels comfortable to you, such as: "My ability to live in love is great, and I am able to judge who threatens my well-being accurately. My body and spirit do not need to overdefend me. I am safe."

Feel free to modify this. The essence is to trust your discernment in relationship choices and to not feel the need to overdefend (autoimmune illness/Lyme), or conversely give up and drop all attempts to defend and become a perpetual victim. Constant "infections" or "chronic illnesses" manifest when we feel so vulnerable and fearful.

Take good care of yourself and your precious heart and spleen. Loving you comes first. Repairing cracks and gaps and shattered hearts can create an even stronger, more lion-sized capacity to live in passion and compassion.

CHAKRA 5 (THROAT CHAKRA): AUTHENTICITY

A steaming summer day in New York City, lugging suitcases out of the cab on West 34th Street, I lumber down the escalator favoring my ginger, strained back, into the bowels of Penn Station. Reared on Long Island, as well as having lived in Manhattan post-college, I am intimate with this thronging city, the aggressive pace and unhinged dangers lurking every second.

My parents taught me to be "street-smart" and savvy, even as a young girl—never wear a shoulder-strap purse, dangling ready to be snatched. Walk in the center of the sidewalk, not the edge, for chance of a wayward car surging over the curb. Don't talk to strangers, only shopkeepers or people you do business with. Be alert at all times, do not dally, get in and out of subways and cabs quickly. The list continues.

The purpose was safety in one of the world's largest cities, filled with potentially many tricksters, thieves, and predators. I was skilled in proactive, self-protective antennae, and simultaneously, there is the gregarious banter of New York's street-circus; the parlance of catcalls and flirtations from construction workers, deli-counter clerks' vibrant humor, the often incredible talent of street musicians! On one hand be wary, on the other hand soak in the magic of momentary, passing encounters.

Amid the constant swarm of several million people on these streets, a palpable thread of realness is felt. Madison Avenue opulence at one level and homeless street people at the other. How often I saw my dad give his loose change to a legless Vietnam vet on a skateboard at his Wall Street subway stop. I, in turn, in my twenties, learned the names of the three homeless people on my city block uptown, donating an apple or my pocket change, too. Human connections are real. In a city like that—one that operates at full throttle—you learn how to navigate around trouble and with cooperation.

On this sticky June day in 2012, I had been residing for more than twenty years in a rural New England hamlet, a distant cry from my big city roots. In town for the annual Book Expo, I was physically and emotionally exhausted from three days on my feet and talking business endlessly. Frayed, with my five fused vertebrae (old horseback accident) aching, managing Penn Station and the Amtrak train connection Northbound felt overwhelming.

Rolling my suitcases down the packed, low-slung, familiar corridor I emerged into the thronging hub at the level above the tracks, commuters and travelers dashing and darting in close to hundred-degree heat. I scanned the huge overhead board for my train and track number, feeling like I might wilt any second.

Teetering into the Amtrak lounge, a bunch of ganged-together metal and leather waiting room seats, a friendly eye caught mine—an Amtrak porter! A godsend! We exchanged hellos, my train number. Could he help me?

"Yes, ma'am. Of course I can help you. It is my honor." Bright smile across ebony skin. Marcus and I began an instant NYC kind of business-at-large conversation. In a matter of minutes, however, we were inquiring into one another's lives.

"How many years have you been down here in the station, Marcus?"

"Thirty-eight, ma'am. Busy every day of my life."

"Well, you must like this job to be here that long, in such hard conditions. I can only imagine being here all day in the hundred-degree weather in summers and below freezing in winters, plus the millions of people commuting."

"Oh that's true, but I get to meet special people like you, too. The ones filled with light and love. Not everyone is cold and shallow."

His remark caught me off guard. How observant this man is, I thought.

"Thank you. You are very kind, Marcus. Tell me about your family and where you live."

From there I learned that his five grandchildren live in Patterson, New Jersey. Marcus noted how beautiful it must be to live up in the countryside, the way I do, with cows and quiet and lakes surrounding me. He was correct; my environment is bucolic.

Marcus minded the clock for me, he reversed the escalator and escalated me to my train, so we could avoid the snare of all the other bustling passengers. In short order my new friend had me seated in a prime air-conditioned car, my bags stowed perfectly, and most palpable, he wove a very protective energy around me in our twenty minutes of communication. I felt truly seen, heard, respected, and taken care of by Marcus. He was a gem!

We talked about my work in natural medicine, I gave him some advice for his wife with asthma, we discussed the truth that people thrive on loving what they do in life by being authentic and open, instead of being robots on a hamster wheel. It was a heartfelt communion between two strangers never to cross paths again. And, the great beauty in this fleeting exchange held meaning for us both—we each saw and heard one another without filters or preconceived notions. Our good-bye was filled with radiant energy and gratitude.

That gift of human generosity stayed with me the entire six-hour ride north, as the graying cityscape morphed to townships and eventually to amber dusk at a track change. I watched goldfinches swinging from reeds in the marsh and the sky turn to flaming orange. I reflected on the busy work of my big-city excursion and the pearl of grace Marcus showed me in his true authenticity. I was reminded of my dad's lesson: "The common man resides in all of us. Be real and you will never be let down in life."

I feel grateful to have had a role model in my worldly and simultaneously authentic father. Nothing feels better than when we interact with another human being and we sense how truly authentic he or she is. Honesty, openness, really being seen, heard, and accepted at face value by another—whether a stranger in a train station, or a friend we have known for years—allows us, too, to remain authentic to our own selves.

An authentic voice and an authentic ability to listen are true virtues of relationship with Self and others. Chakra 5 embodies this core principle. When we shy away and don't speak our truth, clamp down our pure feelings or opinions, or react to another's words, tone, or even their "cold shoulder" of disengagement, we are breaking the natural flow of our own authentic Self.

We react easily as human beings. We are "pack animals" as a species, designed to function best physically, emotionally, and spiritually when in concert with others. Affection, conversation, combined efforts, and mating help us thrive. Statistically, solitary people do not live as long as those in community. And, in our communion with one another, remaining authentic to our ability to communicate honestly and clearly, without malice, manipulation, or defense, is an example of an authentic voice.

The act of truly listening to another, not judging or shutting off to them, and at times "mirroring" their statements, especially when they are distressed, allows for shared space and a bridging or communion of spirits.

My authentic conversation with the Amtrak porter on the swelteringly hot New York City day was a perfect example of human authenticity. We each did not allow preconceived perceptions or judgments to prevent a conversation, nor treat either being with disrespect. Both "open" and able to hear the other and be curious enough to allow our spirits to commune, as all humans are designed to do innately, the exchange was fulfilling, though transient, and remarkable for its realness.

The root of all happiness is joy. Joy is the positive emotional state residing in **Chakra 5**, ruling the respiratory tree. Sorrow is the stymied, blocked energy state of Chakra 5. Grief, disappointment, and suppressed emotions bottle up in this energy center over time if we do not allow ourselves to express them. Natural moments of sorrow and frustration and even just confusion are normal. We need to communicate these feelings to another when they arise. That is our pact of being a pack mammal, as humans.

But, we become schooled as youngsters to have a "tough upper lip," or "don't take up too much of my time with your feelings." We are told "boys don't cry when sad or hurt or scared" and "girls shouldn't speak up about feeling underestimated, or express anger." We all recall being told to be a "good girl" or a "good boy," meaning do not make waves with your words or actions, clamp down your feelings, be seen and not heard.

Two generations back this was de rigueur. Adults had full authority, children were to follow rules, orders, often be robots and even were beaten and spanked. Many admirable people were raised to be capable and generous adults, in spite of these customs. Respectfulness was the reward these undertones did breed. The baby boomers as parents flipped the other way, giving their children many freedoms—especially of self-expression (a good practice)—yet sometimes no boundaries or limits were modeled. The side effect seen is young adults we know who are emotive, often overreactive, and a bit out of touch, at times disregarding our fellow humans' need for consideration, privacy, or for sensitivity to appropriateness in relationships. Too many reactive opinions can fly about—hurting others easily—and certainly damaging the beauty of authenticity. Egos run large, emotions play out in wanton excess, and vulgar reality TV shows are popular.

I illustrate these inter-generational dynamics because the middle ground is likely where we can live with the best level of personal self-respect, honesty, and authenticity of word and spirit. Neither the dampened, ignored child nor the overindulged, freewheeling child is optimal. However, elements of each are required to maintain that balance point of fluid self-expression; neither laced with destructive emotional charge nor squandered to the point of shutting down.

How do you cultivate authenticity? How can you listen calmly to another with an open lens, feel safe, and communicate back to them with your honest, pure heart and voice? How does that Penn Station exchange happen for me or you every day, all day?

We can shift and awaken the energy of a blocked or imbalanced respiratory tract, and the accompanying states of sadness, sorrow, depression, frustration, and isolation, or even feeling too shy to be yourself in public, at a party, giving a speech, bringing up a grievance to your mate or boss. Finding your voice is a beautiful unfolding.

The energetic exercises to begin the shift are simple: humming, singing, chanting, and breathwork all allow us to generate movement physically in the throat, lungs, larynx, sinuses, and ears. Just changing the "holding patterns" with these vibrational acts will commence breaking up old ways.

We know the power of singers, the reverence cantors and chanters held in religious houses of worship for thousands of years, plus the healthful restoration yoga breathwork creates. Though it is not beautiful, and can be harmful in fact, sometimes a "good fight" between two family members lets off steam, clears the air, moves out bottled words and feelings (especially in suppressed households). The key with fights is to be able to apologize and forgive and to never "name call" or say things so vile they can never be taken back because the venom and unkindness cuts forever. A loud, angry voice of authentic truth is one thing; a tyrannical rant of vicious, degrading comment creates wounds. Protective barriers, like deafness and a shielded heart, are put in place. That happy communion is broken.

Besides engaging in a personal healing practice involving breathwork or singing, finding ways to express often decades-old holding patterns, relationship scars, and childhood wounds is important to reclaim balance in chakra 5. We find the sinuses, lymph nodes, lungs, the thyroid and neck, eyes, ears, and shoulders in chakra 5. Lupus, Hashimoto's thyroiditis, Graves' disease, Bell's palsy, tinnitus, Lyme/bartonella, neck pains, and MS show us symptoms and imbalances in this area.

When we are tense, afraid, sad, or lonely, we do not breathe deeply or fully. Our chest space deflates and narrows. I am certain many of you feel the hollowness, the sense of deflation in your chest. Lyme disease in particular very much correlates with this emptiness in chakra 5. With so much loss instigated by chronic illness, we easily become defeated, lose joy, and slip into isolation—a terrible insult to an already wounded body and soul.

Let us practice breathwork to shift the blockage in chakra 5 and generate fresh energy for emotional and cellular change. This is easy, and you can begin even when bedridden.

CHAKRA 5 EXERCISE: BREATHWORK

Breathe slowly and fully, all the way, moving air deeply into your lungs. Draw your breath totally in, expanding your chest, pushing your shoulders back and consciously pressing your diaphragm muscle and stomach outward.

Then exhale and see your breath, in your mind's eye, moving up and out of your body. Exhale it all out through your open mouth. Repeat this breathing pattern at least ten times. Add mindfulness to the equation: on each exhale imagine what you want to release, whether it is disease, sorrow, neck pain, feeling stuck. Imagine it all floating away from you in a hot-air balloon out into the universe. Say good-bye or wave it farewell.

On the inhale, draw in fresh, clean energy and new images—see yourself dancing, at the beach, playing with puppies, anything that brings you joy. Sense if a smile comes to your face. I feel one on mine!

Practice this breathwork daily and repeatedly. Be conscious of mending your fifth chakra. Say good-bye to the symptoms here, the old holding patterns, the shadow of you. Welcome in your most authentic self, the fullest expression of you! Be bold. Be brave. Be beautiful.

CHAKRA 6 (THIRD EYE CHAKRA): OPENNESS

The sixth chakra houses our vision keeper. Our third eye sits in the center of the brain, called the pineal gland. One of the key players in the symphony of the delicately orchestrated endocrine system, comprised of nine glands, this energy network metaphysically reminds us to stay "attuned." Our pineal gland, the conductor of our orchestra, is your vision-keeper, the wise ruler in your unique personal temple of body and mind, the spirit.

As a homeopath, I developed my "third eye" powers without even knowing, by perceiving my clients' nonverbal body language, taking in their visage, listening to their stories and symptom nuances, all in a nonjudgmental way, knowing judgment would interfere with my ability to select the proper remedy. I could note an individual with a quick switch to anger as a guiding characteristic, but not react to him or her positively or negatively about such. "Assess but do not judge" is a homeopath's position. Stay open to perceiving what a being projects. My role was to attune and pay close attention.

In this position as a respected healer, I allowed myself to remain in a posture of openness, of clarity, my third eye receiving information and a person's essence, the message of their soul. Little did I realize I was balancing and tending to my own sixth chakra with my daily work. I would find the client's remedy, and the croup would clear up, or ten years of asthma would disappear, and every chronic childhood ear infection case was cured, never to occur again. My clients' discomforts were gone, their energy renewed, and their moods more joyful. I treasured every day as a practicing homeopath. Its riches gleamed like jewels in my treasure chest of life. My clients and I loved each other greatly. These were purposeful and emotionally prosperous years. What a privilege this era was for me.

I share this twenty-year passage in my life here because it is a profound living example of allowing the open receptivity and the power of intuition—the key functions of the sixth chakra—to shine. Chakra 6 asks us to keep tempo with our inner guide, that sensing, intuitive, observing right hemisphere of our brain, led by the symphony orchestrator, the pineal gland, and in turn harmonizing the entire endocrine system. Quietly, behind the scenes, the endocrine system finesses us through myriad daily ups and downs, and acts as a screening device of emotional interplay between mind and body.

Physiologically, the pineal gland is known to regulate sleep cycles by producing melatonin, and correlates to time and light changes of day and night, as well as controls sex drive, hunger, thirst, and the body's aging process, in tandem with the hypothalamus.

Metaphysically, the pineal gland, our vision-keeper, asks us to receive guidance from "above"—God, our seat of higher consciousness. Overmentalizing our way through life pushes the reactionary sympathetic nervous system into high gear. We oversecrete cortisol, which revs up the adrenals and triggers the thyroid, pituitary, thymus, and other endocrine glands to overproduce hormones. The orchestra conductor has picked up the tempo too fiercely! Our body and mind get into a "fret" when we live at such a didactic, analytical-only, hopped-up tempo.

Tensions mount, moods swing, we crave bad substances. We live in reaction and overdrive, and after too many months or years, symptoms, syndromes, and autoimmune-style illnesses manifest. Our endocrine system and sympathetic-dominant stressed nervous system are root cords to the vastly exploding autoimmune-style illness states. It does not need to be this way. We can change the dynamic. You have the power to help your own self here, even if medications and/or nutritive supplements are required for a while. Understanding that you can gain inner control is the first step.

Meditation is one of the most influential energy forms we humans bear. Yet most of us (in Western cultures) were never trained in childhood, and as adults some of us have attempted learning this skill, yet quickly become discouraged and dumped the practice as malarkey. Hear me out, please. I want you to be well and happy and heal. Meditation is a natural energy state born to all mammals. It is enriching, restorative, and enhances wisdom.

Any of you with a cat or dog witness these creatures loll and be still. They let down after their backyard squirrel chases, hours of shepherding, and nighttime forays of sofa surfing, and just "chill." If you watch any wildlife, you will witness something similar—a lion lounging on a high limb on the African plain, or a turtle sunbathing on an emergent rock. I cannot vouch for the thoughts or non-thoughts these critters may be having, but my keen skills of observation show me they are resting in a posture of receptivity, akin to that of meditation. Like a monk in his sarfu, the mind has gone slack, allowing the parasympathetic "calming" side to predominate. At the energetic and metaphysical levels, the circuitry between body and mind are able to harmonize. Neither one overdominates the other.

Meditation is thousands of years old. All ancient and indigenous cultures revere their wisest elders—those who know how to maintain a reflective, still posture. This position or state of openness differs from prayer. Both are invaluable, and like the left hand and right, the night and day, the Yin and the Yang, they balance us and help us attain health and wisdom. Meditation practices can take many forms dependent upon the guidance and teachings of worldwide masters; whether it be Sufis or Buddhists, Quakers or Mayans, all are essentially directing the individual to a similar mental-emotional-spiritual-physical state, that of being and receiving.

In this act of clearing away our busy, analytical, even creative mind, we are learning how to still the thought process and center our mind's eye. When we leave behind the overdrive workings of the mental plane and allow ourselves to settle, to breathe deeply, to attune to our own heartbeat and breathing, something gracious happens—we connect to our authentic self and slowly, over time, or occasionally in miraculous moments and breakthrough realizations, we find our way home. Home to the essence of our unique spirit's true life purpose. This process does not necessarily happen quickly. We are referring to a multimonth or multiyear evolution for the majority of us. This is okay.

It takes twenty-five years for the human brain and nervous system to fully mature. Developing the true channel of receptivity and higher guidance for most of us will require practice, dedication, and ultimately success. For, when we attain those moments of bliss, the magic of a divine message, a true knowing that is undoubtable, well, there is no going back to the "old way." Such a place of richness will only want to be cultivated, not trampled by the overwrought thought process.

Meditation is the act of emptying our mind, allowing our channel to higher knowledge to remain open and simply receive. This is the left hand of life. Prayer is the right hand. It is possible to meditate with a visualization or affirmation held as intention, which makes this inner power tool even more potent. For starters we will commence with the simplest, purest meditation form of receiving and remaining open to divine source with the use of our breath and our vision-keeper.

Many of you may naturally drift into meditative moments. Staring at the ocean's horizon line while at the beach or out the window, eyes slightly unfocused, at a nearby tree, are examples. This is wonderful! You are innately intuiting, allowing perception to gestate and the calming parasympathetic nervous system to override the "junkie"-style sympathetic side.

Daydreaming children are naturally calibrating in such moments. Imaginary playmates, babies dozing in strollers, are all still attuned. Many of us do follow gut hunches or sudden visions. These are prime examples of intuition and the gifts of our "vision-keeper" at hand. Do not deny or question these moments. This is your inner wisdom speaking. It is when we adults start scheduling little ones with numerous after-school lessons, premature education, or electronic entertainment (with its visual and kinesthetic addictive aspects) that we unravel the inborn track of quiet stillness and the brain wave balancing that the human being needs for optimal health and well-being.

My personal opinion is that the majority of chronic autoimmune illness and Lyme disease states are not "accidental." They are merely by-products of the imbalance our culture has allowed us to slide into. Sadly, we live within our own bodies and psyches with such disharmony. Like the ancient yogi told me decades ago, "Every hour of mental concentration requires the same amount of physical and spiritual use in your day." These words were never more true!

So often we push aside the image that popped up in our mind's eye, or dismiss that job description we read that piqued our interest, or sadly disregard your child's impression of a new person you just met. We all too easily downplay intuitive impressions or messages as folly or non-rational. They really are valuable messages generated by a different portion of our brain than the left hemisphere and frontal lobe we have come to train and focus on greatly over the last hundred years. It is never too late to reactivate your vision-keeper and balance the delicate endocrine system with the graceful energy of meditation.

Our pineal gland was commonly referred to as our "sixth sense" for centuries, and is still revered by many cultures when an individual shows strong energy in the form of intuitions, perceptions, or prophetic dreams. You can tap into this wellspring. In all honesty, strengthening **chakra 6** is one of the most important factors in balancing the body and prompting healing from Lyme and autoimmune diseases. The endocrine system is severely impacted by infectious organisms, heavy metal accumulation, candida and estrogen dominance, toxic synthetics, and endotoxins created internally. Our emotions, when ramped up to negative high wattage (anger, fear, grief, greed, abandonment), wallop the delicate glandular hormonal production. Stress ransacks the endocrine system.

The pituitary gland, adrenals, and thyroid all control functions we do not think about, such as metabolism, production of sex hormones, and temperature regulation. This fascinating network needs ample nutritive support and true metaphysical attention. Every autoimmune disease and Lyme disease have endocrine imbalances: CFS/ME, MS, RA, lupus, IBS/Crohn's, fibro, IC, and more.

I cannot emphasize enough how very essential balancing and tending to your endocrine system with herbal, homeopathic, and nutritive supplements is, alongside your ability to soothe and harmonize this system with continual practices of meditation and visualization. Let us craft a personal practice to use this inner healing tool now.

Try and believe me when I say, your spirit needs just as much mending as your body. With this in mind, I suggest you take the opportunity every morning to spend twenty minutes in silent meditation. The practice of quieting our busy minds, of allowing our selves to draw down into our cores, to our heartspaces and bellies, pulls us away from the chatter of the left brain hemisphere and permits us to open to the receptivity and creativity of the sensing right brain hemisphere. In this posture of receptivity, we are allowing our yin energy to flourish. Yin permits nurturance and nourishment, which are healing energy states for us, allowing the parasympathetic portion of the nervous system to gain ground versus the hyper-reflexive sympathetic portion of the nervous system, which becomes high-wired by Lyme and coinfections, viruses, faulty diet, and electromagnetic bombardment.

Chronic disease insists that we nurture our own self. We must honor our unique beauty, our innate gifts, and love our own self from within, not just be propped up, medicated, or fed from outside sources. I honor your courageous spirit, which has invited you to read this book. It is not a whim or an accident you have found your way into these chapters, but an act of both curiosity and commitment to your healing and personal growth.

CHAKRA 6 EXERCISES: MEDITATION

Let us practice your meditation. If you are new to this do not be harsh with yourself if sitting still makes you fidgety or your mind wanders off. That is normal and a matter of conditioning to learn to focus inwardly. Our goal is twenty minutes, but if five or six is all you can manage at first, start there. Here is the simplest method.

Sit upright, shoulders square, feet flat on the floor if you can comfortably. Allow your hands to lie, palms upward and open, in your lap in a posture of receptivity. Close your eyes. Imagine a cocoon of white light bathing you, protecting and reviving you. Bring your mental focus and mind's eye to focus in your forehead. Open your eyes the slightest bit so you barely gaze down at your feet or ahead at a lit candle. Keep your gaze unfocused. Breathe slowly and deeply into your core. Just follow your breathing in and out with each inhale and exhale. That is all you need to do for twenty minutes. If a random thought or to-do item pops in your mind, just gently push it out to the sky and return your attention to your breathing. Keep breathing. Follow the inhale and exhale with your mind's eye.

If you feel too restless, add a sound or humming. OM is the universal chant. Just keep repeating this with each exhale and feel the resonance in your chest and throat. Stay with it. Soon you will get more comfortable and eventually crave your stillness and meditation time. I find that keeping a notebook at my side is lovely, as afterward I spend twenty minutes journaling—the most amazing discoveries rush onto my paper!

You can add a mantra, which is a positive statement to your chanting. Many other extensive chants exist. Websites, yoga classes, chanting CDs abound. Or you can craft one that is your own deep essence. "I am love." Or: "Let me be guided and protected now in these minutes and throughout the hours of my life." "Let only the highest good work through me. I am open to receiving love and healing."

By meditating you are opening the "third eye," the sixth chakra in our forehead, our wise vision-keeper and conductor of our endocrine system. Meditation is healing, restorative, and helps us align with higher Source. The act of remaining open in life creates luminosity and eventually enlightenment.

CHAKRA 7 (CROWN CHAKRA): CROWN OF DIVINITY

"Divine love has met and will always meet every human need."
—Mary Baker Eddy, *Science of Mind*

The above quote has been my mantra for more than twenty-five years. It soothes me to my core. The message reminds me to let go of the internal chatter, the worrier, the controller, and to trust in the fluidity of our spirit and mind to connect with the higher plane, that of divinity.

Some use the word or image of a figure—God, Buddha, Allah. These spiritual leaders refer to the higher source, the energy channel, as "divine love." Divine love asks us to accept and acknowledge that there is an energy bigger than us, outside our physical body, and of a higher dimension or vibration. The divine is what encapsulates so many religions of the world. Divinity scriptures often embrace endless structure, rules, and figureheads, as in Catholicism, Orthodoxy, even Mormons, Muslims, and others. The Quakers simplify to the "inner light" of stillness and contemplation. The Buddhists connect to the innate wisdom of clarity, emptiness, non-ego, and simplicity. Many indigenous cultures align to nature as their channels of divine connection—plant and animal spirits guiding with messages. Each of us is actually a reflection of divinity. Coming to accept and embrace this purity is one of life's deepest lessons.

Mary Baker Eddy found divinity's presence in her life when prayer and contemplation after a catastrophic paralytic accident and illness brought her into silence, reflection, and surrender. I also walked a similar path. Lyme disease ripped me from my formerly active, structured, busy, successful lifestyle. It slammed me into invalid status. I was forced into stillness, isolation, retreat, and contemplation. My mind and heart were racked with chaotic currents of fear, worry, sadness, shock, disappointment, confusion, frustration, anger, vulnerability, and loss. Physically, I was in dire pain, horrifically weak, infected with a raging systemic infection of duration. I was close to death's door. The knock was palpable and real. I contemplated suicide. My father coaxed me to "stay here." The death call reverberated.

My journey to recovery was one of profound discoveries and lessons. An individual of spiritual orientation, I had believed in God energy, the awareness of spiritual companionship, and my temple was the great forests and sweeping tableau of nature. Not a regular churchgoer, I was not a good "follower" of traditional sermons, scriptures, confessionals, sin-based theology. My Quaker upbringing and ecumenical exposure helped me assimilate divinity as a personal experience. Mary Baker Eddy's works and writings captivated me for a decade in my twenties. I found her orientation to clearing the mind of chatter and negative thoughts, and a need for external "matter," or "error" as she frames it all (drugs to correct, heal, or soothe a being, and negative mind-sets as impediments), to be very true in many ways. She was a spiritual purist. She had personally experienced complete healing through prayer, simplicity, a positive mind-body path, and an open channel at her seventh chakra to divine love or "God." She taught the masses and they loved her work and message for decades. They came to her sermons and talks, standing before her to the tune of 20,000 at a gathering.

I learned, however, that her beautiful philosophy and lifestyle were not easily lived in twenty-first-century laser-speed tempo, electronic swarm, chemically laced foods, and consumer-based society. The madcap frenzy and demands pull a being off their "center" of balance and clarity very quickly. The vibrations disconnect your heart-mind-spirit alignment. If one can live quietly in the countryside, homeschool their children, ban TV and electronic media, eat organic whole foods, and work in the outdoors, well then Mary Baker Eddy's philosophy is attainable. Modern USA is a far reach from this pace and purity of the 1880s, though. The accelerated race, the stress levels, and toxic accumulation in air, water, and food products turn us into a stew of disharmonies, and a bloodstream of cluttered particles, residues, and toxins. Of course a tick-borne organism or virus and toxins could multiply and thrive in our acidic pH, or a cancer could grow, or our heart could cramp up in a vise of overwork in "attack."

When I lay in collapse, year eight in my illness, during a particularly vulnerable spell, I had been praying for weeks for divine guidance on how I could heal. I called God, angels, and spirits for assistance. A "voice of God" never spoke to me nor delivered great solace. I felt abandoned spiritually on many occasions trying to "pray" as I was taught as a child. It did not work for me.

Yet, in this very fragile time, as I basically "let go" of all my holding on to certain coping mechanisms and expectations, I surrendered to the idea that I was dying and that though I would miss my ten-year-old son beyond imagining, I was okay with my death as a possibility. I trusted he would be cared for. In these moments, I prayed for guidance and protection, as usual, but in deep need. I opened my eyes from bed, peering out the window on a late summer's day, glimpsing the distant peak of a neighboring mountain. I suddenly felt this odd internal sensation, a humming of a gentle sort. Something was "shifting" in my own self. I closed my eyes. I saw an image in my mind's eye of a column of golden light streaming from the skies above the mountaintop, to the peak, then through the top of my head and into my body. Simultaneously, I felt a warmth trickling down through me. Words fluttered in my head.

"An open channel to divinity is available to you. Divine love is present. Be open and you will receive," rumbled through my mind. What was this? Momentarily confused, I allowed myself to absorb the feelings and images. Then, suddenly, I got it! By surrendering my old structures, coping mechanisms, and fears, and "letting go" into a state of nothingness, in my truly raw vulnerability, divinity presented its powers to me with this image and a warming channel. I stayed stock-still, eyes closed, sensing the feelings. A calm and comfort remained. Deep in my core I understood: divinity had reached me.

Soon I wrote it all down, so I would not forget the details of such a profound moment. It stayed intact. I continued my prayer, meditations, affirmations, and writings. Seven years later now, my seventh chakra and divinity's higher knowledge are ever-present. I take nothing for granted, offering my gratitude and blessings daily, most exquisitely floating on my back, with arms and palms opened skyward, at the end of my open water swim at the local pond. My reverence is very real for the great mastery of my own life and all of us on the planet. I move with respect for my second chance, and lend my compassion to help others. For as vulnerable, fragile, unsafe, and disoriented as I was during my many treacherous years struggling with chronic autoimmune-style illness and misdiagnosed chronic neurological Lyme disease and coinfections, it was belief, and a tiny ember of hope that made me hold on.

I turned away from orthodox medical authorities, and it was my own inner wisdom, faith, and a savvy clinical nutritionist, an integrative medical doctor, a fourth-generation acupuncturist, a gifted spiritual healer, and homeopathic remedies that helped me heal 100 percent.

"Divine love has met and always will meet every human need."

Ultimately, my spiritual practice became a cornerstone for recovery. Building a faithful practice of meditation and prayer brought me a new form of guidance, and nurturance. Now, I am here to help you open your own personal channel.

The seventh energy chakra resides on top of your head. The clergy wear tall, domed papal hats or bishop-style ones, drawing energy from the above downward, splaying upon their crown chakra. Royalty, formerly the most intelligent and articulate, had the finest upbringing and dignity. They wore tiaras; jeweled crowns encircling their seventh chakra. Older customs throughout the world place wreaths upon a bride's and groom's heads in ceremony; circling their crown chakras, sometimes tethering or uniting the two with a ribbon or vine, as they weave together a spiritual union. We depict saints and angels with halos—an energy form glowing around their head, again, the seventh chakra.

My favorite metaphor comes from the Wizard of Oz, when Dorothy so desperately longs to return home to Kansas, Glinda, the glittering Good Witch, circles her magic wand three times over Dorothy's crown chakra, opening it up energetically as Dorothy closes her eyes, clicks her heels, and recites three times, "There's no place like home."

In a poof Dorothy was back in her dusty country homestead in rural Kansas. The message so aptly conveyed that using your mind and heart in unison with conviction to belief, intention, and prayer can literally cause shape-shifting. Returning to "home" was more than Dorothy's rural homestead, but to her inner faith and heart, for there lay her loved ones and security, not the outside source of a wizard or someone else's powers, but her very personal gifts of vision, intention, belief, will, and love.

Chakra 7 governs the brain and the nervous system, linking together the marvel of our conscious and unconscious minds in concert with the circuitry of all our bodily systems. Emotionally, we seek protection and nurturance from the wise counselor of our inner self, the divine.

As we have worked our way through the entire body, the chakras and the companion emotional and physical states, we have come to understand that physical symptoms or emotional reflexes are not happenstance, but actually interplay in congruence. Just as diabetes, an inflammation at the islets of Langerhans in the pancreas, induces insulin insufficiency, we learn that metaphysically this individual is lacking "sweetness" in their life or spiritual state, their emotions and physiology interplay to cellular pathology (alongside a strong influence of stress or infectious microbes).

With the nervous system, we can find an enormous array of discomforts, diseases, and mental-emotional states, from palsies and headaches to Tourette's syndrome and dementia. The spectrum is enormous, with hundreds of diagnosed conditions and mysterious symptoms: MS, ALS, Lyme and coinfections, depression, anxiety, bipolar, neuropathy, migraines, neuralgias, etc. And all the conditions interweave within the domain of linking our conscious and unconscious mind to higher power, what we refer to as divinity, and what so many ego-centered people get tangled up in—a quotient known as authority.

Somewhere inside of you, all the answers lie. If you have not sensed those answers yet, your job is to learn how to access them. How do we get there? The simplest way is prayer. Prayer is centuries old and practiced throughout the world in all sorts of degrees, within households, on ship decks, in minefields, under open night skies and in squalid back kitchens. Prayer is universal, it is free, and it opens the channel of the seventh chakra. Prayer connects you to divine love and helps bring you answers and protection.

Prayer soothes the nervous system. It quiets the overactive mind and quells the runaway heart. Most importantly, prayer opens us up. Because when we utter a prayer, out loud or internally, we are asking for something:

Please heal me.

Please help my son.

Get my husband a better job.

Keep me safe.

Bless me.

In this gesture of request, we reach outside ourselves. When praying to God, or the Universe, or Jesus, we are seeking and opening our crown chakra upward like Dorothy and Glinda did, and we need to bring the message we receive back home to our very Self, because that is when we get empowered and can shape-shift, or heal a wound, or draw in a new job, or ignite the mind-body healing pathway. The magic and power of receiving a message, or intuition, an image or words heard, is very powerful. I myself dismissed these "hunches" for decades, and got myself into very big trouble—a horseback riding accident, a painful divorce, a poor and demeaning job choice, because I did not honor Divinity's words. Instead, I should have been listening with more authenticity and honoring God's guidance when subtle messages drifted through my gut. Many years later, I finally "woke up," and once I saw that vivid, golden channel, my awareness shifted dramatically. Certainly, some of you can relate to having ignored similar messages or instincts.

All of you have access to this higher knowledge, with prayers as the conduit. A simple prayer is easy to create. A one-line sentence is all that is needed. A focal point is required. Being still for even a few seconds and drawing your attention together in that moment of prayer is like a laser, an instant connection beyond your freestyle mind in orbit, but instead to a conscious intent.

Make yourself a crown, or find one at a costume store. Better yet, dig out a vintage one on eBay. This is a fun gesture, or a truly empowering one. Totems and props help us embody energy states. Wear your own authority in this way. You can be your own clergy and royalty, even when you feel so ill and wretched or bankrupt and disconnected. Because stirring the seventh chakra means you are giving credence to, or connecting, the wellspring of the divine to your own wisdom.

When we meditate we get very still, purge all thoughts, and quiet the mind. Meditation allows us to receive. Prayer in turn is the gesture of request. In asking for protection, guidance, comfort, blessing we are reaching upward above the crown chakra and opening our channel. These are two very different yet powerful and effective energetic stances. The ability to embrace both helps us calibrate our body, mind, and spirit. Both are healing and restorative, and very necessary. Attuning and empowering these energy chakras, their companion biological systems, and fostering balance within are in your grasp. You can master this. No one outside can do it for you. This is your power.

Prayer does not need to embody a religious tone. There is no one better way to pray than another. Some orthodoxies request certain prayer positions, such as kneeling. This is not imperative. What kneeling does is make you get still and helps control focus, which is key in drawing your mind's eye inward to the soul's center and heart. By unifying heart and mind with words of intention and request, you create a prayer.

Each of us can craft our own prayer. It does not need to be long stanzas like a psalm; a sentence or two is fine. I recall my parents teaching us how to create our bedtime prayer, which I continued to recite for fifteen years flawlessly. Then prayer vanished from my life, to return again first as gratitude. Then, in dire illness, a beseeching form of prayer surfaced for me. Prayer can have any tone. Most importantly, prayer must be true. Prayer is your very own sacred act of instilling power to your soul.

Feeding Spirit is a necessity if we want to remain happy and healthy. Most illnesses ask us to tend to our spirit. My personal belief is that illness brews from spiritual suffering, spiritual loneliness, spiritual sadness, and lack of spiritual nourishment. Our spirit is more powerful than our body. When our spirit is full and radiant and creative, we can take any moment, any condition, any disaster, any societal hardship, and help transform it. Spiritual energy and spiritual happiness are magnificent.

Let us learn how to use prayer as a means to shift blocks in the nervous system, help soothe woes, and start to shift symptom states, as well as enable you to create a stronger conduit to higher knowledge and divine love. Remember, you can attune to your own inner spiritual authority and maintain the nurturing caregiving of your own spirituality. For tending to the spirit means you can mend in so many amazing ways. Life is yours to live, recreate, and flourish within.

Now let us open that channel of love you bear. Let us create your prayer.

CHAKRA 7 EXERCISE: PRAYER

What are one or two most imperative pieces you need guidance or assistance with? A better-qualified healthcare practitioner? A new job? Help to manage your daily self-care? To gain confidence? Get very clear on what you need guidance or help with. Write this word or sentence down.

Now, we will resume our traditional practice of tuning in to the heart. Close your eyes, center your mind'e eye on your lovely heart. Place your hands over it. Take three or four long, slow, deep breaths, thanking this mighty organ for its love and steady work.

Now, in concert with your heart energy, we will create a simple prayer.

"Please guide and protect me and my loved ones." Then, fill in your sentence, e.g., "Help me find the healthcare practitioner who has the skills to help me heal." (Or whatever is appropriate.) "I believe in my better future."

Make sure you believe your own words in this prayer. Belief activates the mind and ignites the chemistry of our neurotransmitters. Belief is a very potent medicine. Belief is intrinsic to prayer and is the foundation of any faith. Belief enables you to see and feel beyond the difficulty into a more optimal tomorrow. Your ability to believe in your Self, in a guiding God or loving guardian, and the powers of your own resurrection are as intrinsic to healing, and more importantly transformation, than a runaway autoimmune illness or collapsed lung.

Your belief system is very powerful. This entire chakra circulates around belief and authority. Do not allow an external authority to override your very blessed and loving personal one. Many of us are lost. We are seeking. We are on a quest, journeying through the deep, treacherous pitfalls of disease, and we can find our own "holy grail," our place of safety and surrender, and ultimately, inner love and true healing.

Prayer is powerful and never-ending. Use it often and with respect. You can change your prayer as your condition improves or alters. But keep the prayers going. You will reinforce that upward extension of your seventh chakra and open your channel to divine source. Anything is possible. Believe in your true self-worth and your vibrant future. Know that "divine love has met and always will meet every human need."

In Closing

THE SEEKER

A quest. What is that catalyst, the yearning, the pull that draws some of us from the robotics of daily living, the humdrum of tedium, chores, labor, traditions, out and away from the practices of conditioned societal ways? Why do some of us stretch beyond conventions, reach for intangibles, try to find solace or enlightenment or this very word, truth?

We are born into a physical body. It senses and moves, responds, propels us. Our bodies are miraculous, thriving, striving, transporting us on many levels. The heart bears our emotion, our passions and compassions, as well as our sorrows. It is from our hearts that our life stories are written and in turn we possess a mind—a brain capable of thoughts, analysis, creations, inquiry. This mind is a powerful ally, helping us to navigate the world, communicate, and destroy.

Behind it all is the spirit, a mighty conduit of powers, expressions, synthesis, and knowing. Spirit is essence.

The Seeker, the one ordained to comprehend "truth," has hopscotched beyond the physical, emotional, and mental fabric, knitting for years even decades his or her life experiences together in such a fashion that the given, palpable reality no longer holds fascination or marvel or real pleasure. The material plane, the basic essentials, even the extreme pleasures no longer capture or hold one's attention or achieve satisfaction. They are merely temporal.

What manifests is a journey, a quest for something more meaningful, profound, and ultimately more pure. Truth. What is truth?

Truth is an awareness. A place of complete acceptance. No façades, barriers, gates, or mechanizations. Pure and crystalline, truth shows complete acceptance by being in inner repose—a calmness, a serene knowing. Emotions and mental thought processes do not clutter truth. Those extensions have found their reservoir pools of holding, or better yet have fluidly passed by, not trapping a being or steering the journey. Instead, one is emptied of such reflexes, defensive postures of control, and clever conditionings.

Truth asks for clarity within. An open channel to source. Truth asks for composure, listening, and most profoundly, a core belief that all is well. Wellness embodies faith. Faith is one's capabilities, their inner understanding that all the right people and circumstances are available as needed, and only as needed. Not based from greedy, fearful, or egocentric needs, but basic, simple, life-path needs. The need of each unique soul's centered life's work.

When such clarity, simplicity, austere commitment to a spiritual life is based in truth, shifts happen. It is not the chaotic, unsure, dramatic chaos, but the powerfully aligned creative-force energies seeking to achieve life purpose, lived with heart and authenticity and commitment. From there, all falls into place. Source aligns, magic is real, and truth flows from above down and within, like a prismatic moonbeam. We become filled with light, with abundant powers, with vivid insight, with immediate perception and, most beautifully, the inability to turn back into the "old" ways of being and living.

Once a Seeker summits their mountain peak, has traversed the craggy rock face, endured the slogging muddy low points, looked death in the eye, and brazenly call out for guidance, this voyager cannot fail. Instead, a place of divinity awaits. And there, bathed in beauty and anointed with self-trust, an angel appears. An angel of mercy who will guide this brave warrior, this patient lover, the open being to the throne of truth.

This passage is not for all. It is the most courageous, the most valiant seekers who climb above the mountain of conditioning, out of illness and trauma and externalized grasping hysteria, to instead follow the call of Spirit, the wisdom of the eternities. For only here, in quiet repose, in a space of love and serenity will truth show its wise face. Once received, we are forever altered, forever graced. Love prevails. Embrace your journey, you will be rewarded.

YOUR GIFT

Each and every one of us was born into this lifetime with a gift. Let me ask you this question: What is your gift?

Throughout the many pages of this book we have explored various aspects of the body and how it functions, the role of your emotions in your daily life and as pertains to illness and mending, and of course the absolutely magnificent components of your spirituality. By now you realize how intricate your being is and how miraculous every day of your life can be when we recognize the myriad of functions your body is performing for you just to keep you alive. How complex we are, yet simultaneously rather simple in our basic needs for love, comfort, safety, and fulfillment.

I hope you have come to understand that internally we bear enormous powers. The fact that many of us have glossed over aspects of our creativity or our ability to have vision or ignite the mind-body healing pathway need not be either an impediment or a deficit. Mending has served as kaleidoscope into the multidimensional facets of our internal being that unite in concert with what we actually exhibit or manifest at the external level and display to the world.

Each of us is unique and graced with many lovely qualities and aptitudes. Western society applauds us for the efforts of achievement and success on the material plane. Yet, my belief is the inner riches you bear are far more precious and life-giving than what society has deemed to be valued. This is not to say that being responsible about maintaining your job or taking care of your home or having money put aside for emergencies is not right or important. These skills and matters of intention are definitely essential to keep us functioning in our culture.

Having said that, though, I still want to remind you of that precious gift that you were born with that really makes you shine. Some of us have been graced with more than one gift. This is an extra dose of grace for you to in turn share with others.

All of us have been blessed with the great gift of love, to open our hearts and love those in our family, our friends who are meaningful to us, or even complete strangers who touch us in some way. Love is a very beautiful and powerful energy that never ends. By loving we keep ourselves alive and by loving we give to others. In turn, love is returned to us in so many unsuspected ways. Love remembers. Love builds. Love heals. Love glows. Love never dies. For our spirit is eternal and love gives it wings.

I want you to think about the gift that you were born with. Throughout the exercises in this book you have touched into your wise counselor and the deepest parts of your soul. You have thought about aspects of yourself that perhaps you never quite examined so closely before. Or if you did, perhaps now you have a more complete perspective on your being. What comes to my mind, however, is the truth that you are very precious and you are very wise and you are capable of creating most anything in your life that you choose. That is, if you get very clear in your conscious mind, if you honor your heart's calling, and you make your choices based on love, not greed or envy or malice.

Please think about your gift. Are you using your gift to the best of your ability? If not, why not? If so, I am sure it fills you up. If someone is taking advantage of your gift, then that must stop! Please honor your gift.

My final parting gesture to you is to create a small altar. It does not have to be anything more than a corner of a tabletop or a spot on the windowsill. Make this a special spot of reverence or a large display, one that reflects your gift and what you value. My altar has pieces of nature there: shells, stray bird feathers, a miniature pinecone, a Brazilian quartz, as my connection to the kingdom of God is through nature as my temple. My gift is healing, and staying close to nature helps my healing powers stay strong.

Intuitively, you will know what you want to put on your altar. You may find a photo or two or small animal totems, an image of Jesus, or flowers, or a sketch you have done. None of the specifics matter, except to you. It is about what you connect with. I want you to write your gift down on a piece of paper and put that on the altar. Put something special with it—a candle or a star or a piece of jewelry. Take a moment every day or night and stand at your altar. Feel your relationship to the energy forms there and know that you are imbuing yourself with reinforcement. All of this is good. Allowing the beauty in your spirit to grow and express itself in full glory is your right.

Thank you for spending the time with me in these pages and working so intimately on your mending. It has been a great privilege to share my thirty-five years of healing experience and knowledge with you. We are all entwined together in the cosmos of life. May you be forever blessed. May your healing be full and may your spirit touch the lives of others. And may my words bring you comfort and guidance as you find your way home to your very own precious deep heart. May my spirit touch yours.

Namaste,
Katina I. Makris, CCH, CIH
New Hampshire, USA
Spring 2015

PATIENT CASE STORIES

RHEUMATOID ARTHRITIS, FIBROMYALGIA, CFS EXPOSED

As a Cape Cod child running the beach dunes to climbing trees, I was exposed to hundreds of ticks over twenty-five years.

At age eight I had growing pains every night for approximately 1.5 years. The doctor never tested anything, but instead just said "growing pains . . . take Tylenol or Motrin." My mother and I would walk the halls every night until the medicine kicked in.

I was a very active child in sports—first pick for teams always. They moved me into boys' leagues as a youngster and by eighth grade scouted me out in basketball and softball and high school varsity. So you can imagine why "growing pains" made sense.

No one ever knew the trauma going on behind the doors from ages four to twenty-five. I'm not here right now to get into that, but knowing this I feel is very important. My stress level was extraordinary as a child, but I kept it to myself. Unconsciously, I kept swallowing and holding my breath. By high school freshman, sophomore, junior, and senior years, I had been in and out of the ER for my neck at least ten times. No one ever truly looked at my neck, but would instead merely ask, "Can you move it this way? How about this way?" No one ever took an x-ray, nor a blood test. I was always just sent home with a soft collar to heal, and after a few days I would. My annual doctor appointments never really addressed much and I was never referred anywhere.

After high school I was on my own and working as a financial advisor for Fidelity Investments. You can imagine the kind of stress that was for a nineteen-year-old working alongside salesmen with fancy college degrees who did not respect my accomplishments. Still, I was number one in sales and still battling my neck pain, but no longer going to the ER as most people would. I dealt with pain at that point by myself.

I decided to take time off for once in my life at about twenty-two years old, and moved up north to NH, but my one requirement was that my primary please get me an MRI of my neck before I left my big job, that I already had given my notice to. She finally agreed. Within a very short amount of time I found myself in the operating room with a neurosurgeon removing my herniated disc that had been lodged inside my spinal cord!

Finally, some relief after healing from that. I finally had a break from pain as I worked at a ski resort. The doctor had said to take it easy because my discs above looked awful and he did not want me to end up back in surgery.

After an amazing year of enjoying the earth elements and pushing my usual sporting fun like skiing, snowboarding, rock climbing, ice climbing, kayaking, hiking the Presidential Range, the black flies shooed me away, back to making money so I could travel. So, off I went back to the financial industry where I could afford life again and also pursue a dream of cosmetology school at night.

Again, my stress level grew, and unconsciously I was breathing shallowly and the pain returned. I tried everything to stretch and again the doctor did an MRI. Another cervical disc had ruptured, this time into my right arm root, which would cause damage if it was not removed. Back into surgery I went. I was hoping for the same pain-free outcome but soon realized this wouldn't be the case.

I went from doctor to doctor trying to find relief. RA positive, "systemic arthritis," fibromyalgia, chronic fatigue syndrome, and macular degeneration were my assorted diagnoses. Then came the cervical epidural injections, steroids after steroids. There were injections shot directly into my head for what the doctor called a diffused headache (I had no headache, just my eye was sagging and there was lots of pressure). My skin hurt, I had numb spots on my feet. The list just goes on.

I thought starting a family would cure my hopelessness, which it did for some time. I married and we had a daughter and then I thought, let's move closer to family and I can start my salon business with support. I was then pregnant with my second child. We moved back to the Cape for family and bought a new house and I still was not feeling great, but who does when you are simultaneously pregnant, selling a home, buying a new home, and preparing to start a business? Approximately six to seven months pregnant, I looked down on my belly to find a bull's-eye rash with tick still embedded! I knew enough to go to the walk-in clinic, give them the tick and get tested ASAP. Doctors advised me to wait until the test came back, because I was pregnant and "we don't want to give medicine for no reason," and I agreed ignorantly. Two days later I thought I was free, as I had tested negative on the standard ELISA Lyme disease test.

About a month later I began feeling really crappy. I began to have unwanted contractions. I was only eight months pregnant, so in to the hospital I went. The doctors gave me some labor preventive medication, but still about every other day for a month preterm labor contractions would trigger. Again, no one ever looked into anything.

My second daughter came a little early, actually the exact same as my first thirty-seven-week pregnancy, and they both weighed in at 6 lbs. 14 oz. However, my second had to be transported to Children's Hospital, Boston, because she had a collapsed lung. I'll never forget holding her for the first time and within thirty seconds me screaming for help and the doctors kind of reassuring me that "everything is okay, you are just traumatized by all you have been though, she is fine." I finally screamed loud enough that the nurse said, "I think Mom needs to rest." They came over to see my daughter turning blue and frothing at the mouth and called a code and stat and every other emergency word you can say. They soon realized that I was sensitive, not "reactive." My baby daughter left me overnight and came back perfectly healthy, thank God! I successfully breastfed as I did my first, and we went home happy and healthy, except she was a bit colicky. Nothing I couldn't handle.

Life moved on and my business and my children were growing. Little things happened, like my youngest was allergic to Amoxicillin. But, all in all the kids were healthy and I just had severe chronic neck pain with arthritis and my immune system was kind of messy. Doctors insisted my neck arthritis was to blame, even for my leg pains (growing pains again?), and they said the night sweats were from medicine and stress. I was sleep deprived too, as a mother, housewife, and business owner. I didn't drink alcohol because it made me feel horrible. I thought the horrible leg spasms were so bad because I stood on my feet hairdressing and my arms fell asleep due to carpal tunnel syndrome onset.

My home life to me felt horribly wrong. My body kept telling me I was dying. I told my doctors, my mother-in-law, my husband that my body couldn't sustain itself, I needed help! But everyone seemed to think I was just dramatic, so I believed this too after a while, telling myself, *Bethany, this is all in your head.*

I decided I had to change things or I would die. I asked my husband to please make some changes. No matter what I asked for, nothing was helping my body from dying. I turned to therapy. I begged for a while for us to both go, then finally went myself. As you can tell, by then we were not even in the same game of life anymore. Me, in survival mode starving for help, and him unaware and ignorant to anything I had expressed. So, our marriage failed.

During this time of divorce with two children and me feeling as though I couldn't make it, I actually finally hit the deck! Encephalitis, spinal meningitis, old Lyme, new Lyme, CDC positive, Bell's palsy, mono, and a few others. I can't remember all the diagnoses. In the hospital for about a week, I could not open my eyes or deal with any sound. My legs were numb from my waist down and the pain in the rest of my body I can't begin to explain. They put me on IV Rocephin, then sent me home with Doxycycline for twenty-one days. That was the beginning of my understanding of what "Lyme" even meant.

Every pain I have ever had in my living years was magnified tenfold. *No* medicine could help me, no one could help me. My veil was so thin I knew I could choose life here or move on. All I had to do was give up. Every day my children gave me one reason to make it to the next day. I thank God they chose me as their mother, for without them I would have chosen to leave my body.

Ten months I lay in my bed or on the recliner. No music, no TV, just pain and researching. My primary of seven years asked me to leave because she said, "If I were you, I would leave with the treatment you have received." What do you feel about that? When your own doctor asks you to leave her practice? I felt so abandoned. She gave me all the referrals I asked for until I found a new primary care. The big hospital in Boston I was referred to had the top doctor in neuro-infectious disease, directly under Dr. Steer. They thought I should have had a PICC line placed, though that at this point they would not treat me. I couldn't even walk, yet.

I did get an LLMD, after more research, and began Western medicine because that was his protocol, which later I learned is inhumane with the amount of bacteria I was holding and trying to kill off with his method. It crippled me. I researched more and had friends lead me to a Chinese doctor in China who said via email as a friend, "Please, please have faith in God and find a way to get IV vitamin C and glutathione ASAP." So, I did. This is where I am currently. I am finally being treated for Lyme disease and coinfections with Eastern and Western medicine integrated; we are treating the physical body, the emotional body, the chemistry body, the outer and inner energetic being, and the spiritual person inside.

After realizing that antibiotics can cause such horrible pain and suffering I reflected pretty quickly on my daughter and her allergy to Amoxicillin at age one. She had bruised on all her joints and they also swelled when taking Amoxicillin, one of the primary antibiotics to kill Lyme bacteria. She had a rash with fever that all occurred the day after the last day of treatment. I thought, "Ohhh wow . . . autoimmune response to die-off from Lyme." That's typical of Lyme disease sufferers, but we never knew about that back then!

I quickly had both of my children tested. My first daughter was negative on both ELISA and Western blot tests, and my second daughter was positive on ELISA and CDC negative on Western blot BAND 41 (both tested in a healthy status at the time). As you know, ELISA positive means quite a bit, but was not acceptable in the world of Massachusetts medicine, yet. My second daughter had always reacted poorly to antibiotics, usually with hives. She also gets hives and stomachaches when run-down or emotionally taxed.

Though generally she is very healthy, this past month she ended up with pneumonia, from a virus, and was treated on a Z-Pak. She was on the antibiotic pills, and then it stays in your system another five days. On the sixth day she got a low fever of one hundred. It didn't last long but she was out of her character and very lethargic. Three days later I was watching these episodes that were like tiny seizures, coming and going. I told my boyfriend and he agreed. I got nervous and messaged my doctor, but held back a bit because I also had this feeling that I was projecting my illness onto her. (I too had mini-like seizure episodes.) I doubted myself. Then it turned into a full-blown huge seizure, with a 911 call, lasting longer than a mother will ever want to see!

She had her EEG and the neurologist wanted to treat her as if she had epilepsy due to the fact that her seizure activity was too high when sleeping or awake. I asked if there was any relationship between a low immune system and the seizure and they said no, that was not a possibility. The neurologist did state that dehydration, overtiredness, or an infection could cause the kind of seizure she had; hereditary seizures.

The autoimmune doctor, however, stated there is no relation whatsoever. So, I asked if, instead of focusing on the seizures, we could figure out why she gets these hives and IBS symptoms, etc. He said there really was nothing he could do. I asked about diet, nutrition, exercise, mold toxins, allergies to food, environment, etc. He said, "No." Mind you, these are the best doctors in the world at Children's Hospital.

I would like to finish this story, but today is where I leave off. I can say this, I am stronger than anyone will ever know and I promise this one thing: my kids will never endure what I have as a human, and I guess that is what every parent says. When I finally finish my story the end will be a success. My healing will have come and also a full healing from my daughter.

Bethany
Stylist, HBO Productions

TWENTY-SIX YEARS OF CHRONIC ILLNESS: LYME DISEASE IN TENNESSEE

I was healthy and canoeing a river when I got a tick bite in July 1989. Within a week I felt run over by a truck! Doctors diagnosed me with thyroid, MS, lupus, brain tumor, fibromyalgia, rheumatoid arthritis, and other conditions. Doctors also thought perhaps I was a case of psychological affliction or "bored housewife" syndrome.

In truth, It was the infection of the spirochete corkscrew-shaped bacteria called *Borellia burgdorferi* that caused such disability, also known as "Lyme disease."

Today four of my neighbors have official Lyme disease infections confirmed by positive blood tests. But twenty-four years ago the tests were not given and they were even less reliable back then.

As advised after countless MS tests, CAT scans, and spinal taps, etc., I contacted the researcher in Missouri who was a leading physician battling Lyme named Dr. Edwin Masters. He helped treat me.

But the first large dose of Doxycycline from my Nashville doctor who was finally agreeing to treat for Lyme (which came two and a half years into the infection) caused a massive inflammatory reaction that resulted in a stroke. Such events are not uncommon with late untreated Lyme. That put me into a very vulnerable state at only age thirty-four.

I was bedridden for a long time and read a medical student's library I had purchased at auction for $2. I had nothing but time on my hands in bed. My story is regrettably too typical for late-stage untreated Lyme disease. I know one child stricken at age thirteen still bedridden now at age thirty! Becoming bedridden is common with severe Lyme.

I also had other tick-borne infections including one called babesiosis that is a cousin of malaria and caused fevers of 102 for weeks on end. Doctors could not agree that these diseases existed in Tennessee. It cost much out of pocket for me to keep searching for help. My songwriting career kept going, as I could write while sick, but I couldn't physically keep up with eighteen to twenty hours in recording studios as I had done in the past.

I was neurologically impaired and weak on the left side. I could not take baths. I had to pour witch hazel over my long hair and towel it off to have clean hair. Even though this is a long story of suffering, mine is also one of learning.

By God's grace alone I rehabilitated myself with walker, canes, and limped onto a plane to Dallas and later NYC to see specialists who formally diagnosed me as having Lyme and other microbial infections with DNA and other testing.

I ended up meeting the German scientist, Willy Burgdorfer, who isolated the germ, and it was named in his honor. That happened in 1999 at an International Tick-Borne Diseases Medical Conference in NYC. I am a very lucky survivor so far. I am not a quitter. I received years of mixed oral antibiotics, then intravenous Rocephin, then Chinese herbs. I am not cured, however. I am still prone to relapsing.

What many do not know is that "Lyme" is not just a word, but an infectious illness "state" that actually represents one to twenty and more mixed bacterial, fungal, and viral pathogens! In reality it is not one disease, but instead a many-headed dragon, mimicking assorted auto-immune illnesses and other disorders.

Complex infections are extremely hard to diagnose and prove to insurance companies. Insurance companies have death on their side, because with no diagnosis, they do not have to pay for expensive treatments, whether they are experimental or officially sanctioned by the Infectious Disease Society of America.

The IDSA controls the AMA physician-approved protocols for diseases. The IDSA is a political group and they are currently not supporting the handful of honorable physicians who treat Lyme disease and the coinfections. Medical politics is very real and diseases that get stigmatized are in a throwaway kind of place until enough approved studies are done.

These complex parasitical-microbial infections such as Lyme, babesiosis, anaplasmosis, Heartland virus, ehrlichiosis, leptospirosis, mycoplasma, etc., are also in mosquitoes and fleas—not just ticks! So many people are sick shut-ins and they have no clue their condition came from a tiny, unseeable insect bite. They are suffering and little help or hope awaits.

And as for the famous diagnostic "bull's-eye rash" of an early acute Lyme disease infection, only some cases have it. Many recall no rash. A purple spot in the scalp where a tick once attached and fed is rarely seen! I had a red hives rash behind both knees after tick bites. I later had a bull's-eye rash surface under my armpit after being given Amoxicillin.

My story is indeed a long one. I am betting there are others in the hoarding/clutterers support group online with late Lyme, MS, and other conditions. These diseases, which are brain and central nervous system infections, do strange things to behavior. Once the microbes hit the spinal fluid, nervous system, and brain, all sorts of imbalances and emotional feelings and problems arise. People are not "imagining" their anxiety or depression or strange symptoms.

After twenty-six years of chronic illness from that initial tick bite and more to come, in the southern region of the United States, I know how real and rampant this infectious illness is and how seriously ill someone can get. The doctors of the world need to be educated on diagnosing and treating all stages of the illness. I hope that we will see these medical mysteries unraveled and cures found soon.

Bonnie Huntsinger
Nashville Lyme Disease Support Group

THE GREAT SURRENDER: DEATH, REBIRTH, AND CREATIVITY

Many people who are very ill with Lyme have been told that their symptoms are psychosomatic, all "in their heads." So, one thing about my case that makes it useful, I think, is that I can offer an example of what it might look like to accept that theory and run with it.

Until six years ago I could control my health through mental strength; by strong-arming myself into working harder, pushing my body, making myself try to focus on having a positive attitude, focusing on positive thinking, all that "New Age" mythology. I really tried very hard to apply it. If my sickness was just in my head I certainly would have mastered control over it! But, the bottom kept falling out, no matter how hard I tried.

Like many people, I actually experienced a sort of shame about being sick, so I didn't complain. I believed I wasn't doing something right to earn good health or maintain it or manifest it. Eventually, I hit rock bottom, too sick to do anything besides surrender. By then, I felt tipsy and mildly carsick most of the time. I could forget my phone number while dialing it, trip walking up my stairs, react with panic if startled by a sudden loud, violent noise such as dropping a fork on the kitchen floor! I felt too overwhelmed to think straight while grocery shopping and sometimes just drove home. The nerve, joint, bone, and muscle pain was excruciating. I was so fatigued that holding onto a phone for a short call made my arm burn like holding a tough yoga pose. I frequently felt stupid and anxious, unable to follow conversations and verbal instructions well, since my short-term memory was severely impaired.

I resigned from my work as a grade school teacher, but continued to tutor and teach art from home. Eventually I stopped being able to remember the names of everyone around my dining room table, so I even quit that and gave away most of my art supplies. Being an artist had always been a part of my identity. I have albums going back to early childhood. But, when I was ill for so many years, I gradually lost the drive and urge and energy to make art.

When I finally acknowledged an inner urge—and worthiness—to reach out for help, one of the first things that happened was seeing a book at my local library about Lyme disease. I got the idea, for the first time, that maybe what I had was actually a *disease*. I realized I had probably had it for many years, and that if I didn't get on with dealing with it I could actually die from it.

Another shift in this period was a shift from feeling as if I were guilty of failing; failing to earn much money, failing to be able to work regularly, failing to maintain being a calm, focused communicator, and more. Instead, I felt a tiny sense of worthiness to look into being *helped*.

It took some time to amass a written health history, to petition for more attention, and share facts about chronic Lyme disease with other people, but eventually I was given great care by a very understanding doctor. I also began learning more about self-care. I had to learn that it actually included taking responsibility for myself to rest more, to feed myself more carefully, to stop expecting so much from myself and putting my body in harm's way.

I learned a lot about chemical sensitivities, to avoid environments that added more burden to my immune system, to avoid foods that I had sensitivities to, and to acknowledge my intense energetic sensitivity. I learned that some of my sensitivities could actually be considered gifts. I just needed to honor myself by changing many things about how I was living, to say it's okay that I am actually this sensitive. Instead of feeling like a social, professional, and financial dropout who had gotten too sick to work outside the home and have clear conversations with people, I began practicing accepting that what I was experiencing was literally a state of "health emergency."

Even months into my treatment it was impossible to return to my old life, and impossible to predict if or when I would get better and what my life would be like then. I know it seems counterintuitive to say that giving up having goals and dreams can be a good thing, but in my case it was actually a relief to just let go of having a future, to stop trying to get somewhere, to stop trying to choreograph where my life was going—instead, to just be present with the pain and the disability and the unknown, in a liminal state, like a caterpillar melting apart inside a cocoon.

Meanwhile, I was in touch with my doctor regularly, trying to describe what I was feeling and how symptoms were changing. I kept using visual metaphors since that way of perceiving comes naturally to me. I kept getting very clear images in my imagination of how one might illustrate a certain symptom. Several months into treatment I still felt too tired and sick to want to paint landscapes or portraits, those things requiring looking outward and making something accurate. But eventually the urge to paint these Lyme symptoms got stronger. I felt a new sort of inner motivation to paint them, a sort of effortlessness, like I didn't have to personally figure it out. I just needed to sit at my desk and show up and see what came out.

It was an amazing process. Within three months I had enough artwork for an exhibit, *In the Lyme-Light: Portraits of Illness and Healing.* When that show went up a whole lot of people resonated with it. I shared an insider's perspective of the disease and how it changes your life. I felt inspired to write some descriptions as well. A year later I self-published the collection as a book, and it became a communication device that helped many people explain what they were going through to their family, friends, doctors, and therapists.

I recently published an updated edition, *In the Lyme-Light II.* This project came out of the suffering and also helped transform it. It resulted from a stance of being in a quiet reflective mode, humbly waiting and listening for guidance by a sort of universal inspiration or divine will. Though I had certainly worked on honing artistic techniques for years, and considered myself to be a good artist already, this work really came from a whole different attitude than my former work. Through this project I gained much more trust in intuition. Not as a special rare thing inside of me that others didn't have, not as something that I personally was succeeding at, more like uplinking to an inspiring creative intelligence, being flowed through me and held within it.

As I was healing more and more, I found that my life was being transformed. I used to navigate with very mental, head-based energy. That only took me so far. I developed a lot of self-discipline and drive, but that way of operating had its limits. In order to heal from Lyme I had to let go of a lot of beliefs that were no longer serving me, do some healing of old wounds, touch into some deeply buried grief, access some other realms of intelligence and of feeling that could not be dealt with through mental control. Now there is so much more living from the heart and the gut. The healing process was not easy and it still continues, but as I have surrendered to where healing is taking me, I continue to deepen in my sense of connectedness with everything. Though I can still be very practical and function in daily life (I'm still living as a single parent, still responsible for a young one at home), I rely more and more on a sort of soft-focused presence rather than trying to mentally figure out what to do when and how. It is a more restful way to be. Now, I actually see my struggles with Lyme as a catalyst for awakening. I am grateful for this new form of living, receiving, giving, and birthing in creativity. Lyme has helped me evolve and the access to creativity is one of the healing passageways.

Emily Bracale
Author, *In the Lyme-Light*

HEALING FROM CHRONIC DISEASE ON THE SPIRITUAL LEVEL: A HEALING JOURNEY

In November of 1999, my wife and I moved from the Philadelphia area to southwestern Connecticut to start a new life and raise a family. Within three years of moving into our new house, I began noticing some strange symptoms that were not "classic" to Lyme disease or any other illness that I knew of. At the time I was in very good physical condition and I had been going to the gym three times a week working on bodybuilding. However, I was feeling fatigued and foggy every time I ate a meal.

After two more years of bouncing from doctor to doctor, I still had no answers. On two separate occasions, I had MDs tell me, "Your symptoms aren't life-threatening, so maybe you should learn to live with them." I was shocked at their lack of curiosity, and since I was paying them for a service that I wasn't satisfied with, I "fired" them. In the meantime, I was feeling worse and getting worried.

Finally in 2005, I visited a holistic doctor who asked me to chronicle my symptoms in a journal for one week. The day I visited her, she read my journal and immediately said, "You have Lyme disease. I can test you to be sure, but I can start you on a round of antibiotics right away."

I was relieved that the mystery illness now had an identity, and I was hell-bent on disinfecting my body and getting rid of it as soon as possible. I began taking oral Doxycycline and immediately began to feel worse.

I visited my holistic doctor a week later and she asked me how I felt. "Terrible!" I said. "Good!" she responded. "It means the antibiotics are working. They're breaking down the cell walls of the bacteria and releasing toxins in your bloodstream. That's why you feel so bad."

The funny thing is, she never gave me much advice on how to rid myself of these toxins, so I continued to feel worse. It would be years until I would learn how to diminish and avoid the Jarrish Herxheimer reaction, or "herx" as all the "Lymies" were calling it online.

I also learned about something called a PICC line during my daily quest for research online, and I asked my doctor about that. To me, this seemed like the "nuclear option," which involved a port installed in your arm so you could administer your own daily dose of antibiotics, directly into your bloodstream. This appealed to my idea of disinfecting my body.

But my doctor thought the PICC-line route was too harsh and risky and would not agree to sign off on it. So I found another doctor who would, and within weeks I had an appointment scheduled at a local hospital for the procedure. I have to admit, I was not prepared for what the PICC line was all about. I thought it was a simple prick of the arm and easy insertion of the port, but it was a full-on surgical procedure. I was laid on an operating table with an x-ray machine above my chest and three attendants helping the doctor. During the procedure, the doctor ran a wire lead to route the line close to my aorta and he went too far and jabbed my heart. My blood pressure began to drop and I began to feel like I would pass out while lying on the table. Everyone got worried, but I managed to pull through and they wheeled me on a gurney into the hallway, fed me some lunch, and kept me for observation for a few hours.

I ended up driving myself home from the hospital and I felt okay until I went to sleep that night. While in deep sleep, I rolled over on my left side and apparently the PICC line jabbed my heart farther because wild palpitations and pain woke me from my sleep. I didn't know what to do, so I went downstairs and lay on the couch to see if I would die or make it through the night.

When the first rays of sunlight broke through my living room curtains, I called the emergency line at the hospital and talked to the doctor on call. His advice surprised me. "You've been through the worst of it," he said. "Do you think you can tough it out and keep it in for a few weeks and try the antibiotics?"

I was so intent on ridding myself of the disease that I took the doctor's advice and tried to tough it out. As I administered my own antibiotics each day, I began to spiral downward. I developed a severe intestinal infection, strong headaches, and paralyzing depression. I felt like a walking zombie and began to feel detached from the world.

When the PICC line was finally removed, I felt slightly better for about three months but then backslid into worse symptoms and actually had a second PICC line inserted, this time with no anesthesia and no x-ray. The procedure felt like someone jabbing a ballpoint pen in my bicep for forty-five minutes.

Unfortunately, this PICC experience was no different than the first with the added aggravation of having this second line broken during a routine weekly cleaning by a visiting nurse. I had to have the line reinstalled again, making it three surgical procedures in one year. I had never been to a doctor for anything more than a plantar wart removal prior to this and I was losing hope after the symptoms returned three months later.

I began seeing a new Lyme-literate doctor in NYC who did further testing and found I had several coinfections; other bacteria besides the *Borrelia burgdorferi* (Lyme bacteria). He prescribed multiple antibiotics simultaneously. I felt slightly better than I had with the PICC line but I was far from feeling "disinfected."

I'm a musician, and one night during a performance I almost passed out on stage for no apparent reason, and I instinctively felt the need to get off of all antibiotics. I discovered another doctor in Manhattan who prescribed a combination of herbs instead of synthetic meds. After starting his protocol, I experienced stronger herx reactions than I had with the PICC line and he recommended I scale back my dosage until I felt better.

I remained on this protocol for a few years but felt my quality of life was only a fraction of where I wanted it to be. I continued to do research online and during my travels I stumbled upon a video episode of Oprah Winfrey, featuring a healer from Brazil named John of God.

Something about this episode appealed to me. The fact that thousands of people traveled to meet this man who healed them through energy, love, and faith, and trained doctors who had been sent to debunk him couldn't. In fact, many of them had spiritual experiences that showed on their faces. I was intrigued enough to book the ten-hour plane flight and take the pilgrimage.

On the day I arrived, two counselors sat down with me to find out why I had made the journey and to translate my healing intention to John of God, who only speaks Portuguese. When I told them I was there to be healed from Lyme disease, they looked up from their notes and said, "And what else?"

I laughed, "Do I get three wishes?" to which one of them asked, "Why stop at three?" I could see they were serious, so I told them I'm a musician and I would like to heal people with the music I write and perform.

The next day, I went with a group of people to see John of God to be "diagnosed." Several hundred of us gathered in an open-air room called "The Casa" where João Teixeira de Faria (John of God, as he is called by the local Brazilians) took to a small stage and began speaking in Portuguese. Later, I was told that he had said that he wasn't the one doing the healing but that God did all of it. Soon after his speech, he dropped the microphone and a shudder ran through his body. His appearance began to change instantly, and his body seemed to swell and his eye color changed. He stumbled for a second and then attendants brought surgical instruments to him and he turned to a woman who was standing as if in a trance onstage. I was standing a mere six feet away and I grabbed my camera phone and started filming him cutting into her abdomen while she neither flinched nor bled. The energy in the room made me feel as if I would pass out and one of the attendants actually did so and dropped a container of rubbing alcohol. The woman was wheeled away in a wheelchair, and several days later I saw her on the street and she lifted her shirt to show she barely had a scar from the whole experience.

Many of the people in my group later waited in line to go up in front of John of God, who had retreated to a large meditation room in the back of the Casa. We all went before him silently, while a few hundred people meditated in nearby benches that reminded me of church pews. As we all touched his hand, he told us our next step, and mine was to have "spiritual surgery." I was told to return in the afternoon and meet a few dozen others in a private meditation room where we were asked to meditate and keep our eyes closed. After sitting in silence for about fifteen minutes, we could hear John of God enter the room and offer a blessing in a booming voice. I felt electrical sensations all over my body and several members of my group confessed they had felt shoved forward or to the side when there was no person there to physically do this.

When the session ended, we were met by our group leader who put each of us in a taxi to make the block-and-a-half ride to our hotel. We were told to immediately go to bed even though it was in the early afternoon. I lay there with my eyes wide open and wondered how I would be able to sleep, and then I woke up sixteen hours later, feeling as if I had been hit by a truck.

We each went through this experience again later in the week and one day, I looked in the mirror in my bathroom and burst into laughter. The face that stared back at me looked ten years younger. I grabbed my phone to video chat with my wife and the first thing she said to me was, "What happened? You look different!"

I choked back tears and said, "I'm healed!" and I could feel that every symptom I had ever had simply vanished. All of this had occurred through the energy John of God had brought forth but it was held in place by my faith and positive thinking, as the counselors had instructed us. Some in my group had even more dramatic experiences but I noticed that the ones who didn't were struggling with their own limiting thoughts and internal "demons."

When I returned home, I also experienced a surge of songs and lyrics that seemed to come from nowhere. I've since recorded two CDs full of music that I never would have written had it not been for my experiences in Brazil. I have returned to the Casa five times since, more for my own spiritual evolution than for healing purposes, and I have begun devoting my life to helping others stricken with Lyme and tick-borne illnesses through the music I create and the Lyme disease benefit concert series I've created called the Ticked Off Music Fest: www.tickedoffmusicfest.com. The funds we generate from the concerts go to research and patient funds, and I've begun doing motivational speaking to help others struggling with chronic illnesses.

Gregg Kirk
The Zen Engines
Founder of the Ticked Off Music Fest series

OUR LIFE PURPOSE

Working with a spiritual teacher evolves our unconditional trust and love. The spiritual relationship encourages us to trust our basic wisdom. We must become internally steadfast and learn to not question our Self. Developing trust of our own Self is critical so that we don't always identify with our fears and neuroses. Fear is the basis of all limitations. Finding confidence in our innate intelligence and loving kindness are the gateways out of emotional, spiritual, and physical entrapment.

Daily life is rife with violence, meanness, beauty, acts of courage, interludes of tenderness. Moving through all these states of feelings and actions, we ultimately strive for living in our passion and finding our inner peace. Every person in our life is a teacher. Remaining open to the fact you are growing in awareness and expansion and ultimately enlightenment becomes empowering.

Can we allow ourselves to develop a vast open mind? To sit in our center (chakra one)? Dreams are born (chakra two) and we can bring them forward to our creative energies (chakra 3) and manifest our passion (chakra 4) to ignite with our authenticity (chakra 5) and keep attuned to intuition and vision of a future outcome (chakra 6) unified with the wisdom and belief of our mind and spirit (chakra 7) to live a fully conscious and transformational life.

Our life purpose is to ascend the morass of the earth plane's material tests and the demons of emotional trappings, in concert with the trickery of our mind's push and pulls. Ultimately, spirit calls us to bring forth the essence of our personal unique truth and hold an openness to the process of our evolution and contribution to mankind and those we touch.

Serious illness is a configuration of all these aspects, forcing us to put a magnifying glass on who we are and why we are here and how we can change to evolve into the purity of our highest self.

You are being offered a test, and more importantly a quest of personal transformation, through the journey of serious illness. As this guidebook so specifically defines, there are many toolboxes to reach for at the external level, as well as talented practitioners available, and the deepest, most profound work will be done on your own inside. When unifying all these facets, ultimately your rebirth and personal purpose in life will bloom anew.

God bless,

Katina

APPENDIX 1:

LYME DISEASE SYMPTOM CHART

There is a very strong possibility that tick-borne organisms could be part of your autoimmune disorder.Too much clinical evidence and newer research from the cutting-edge doctors and scientists are isolating the crossover from mycoplasma to rheumatoid arthritis, Lyme disease to multiple sclerosis and CFS/ME, fibromyalgia and even coinfections like bartonella to interstitial cystitis and many neurological issues. If you can determine that a "hidden" or misdiagnosed Lyme infection could be part of your autoimmune situation, then ridding the microbes from your system and rebuilding the depletions and imbalances as the Recovery Guide portion of this book has illustrated, then there is actual HOPE for restoring wellness and a better quality of life. Of course using state-of-the-art Lyme labs is essential (those indicated in the resources appendix), not a local commercial lab with a mere 30 to 40 percent accuracy rate!

This symptom questionnaire originally came from IGeneX Labs a few years ago and I added some other symptoms that we have since come to know are part of Lyme disease. If you find correlations to your condition it is well worth being tested at IGeneX, Clongen, or NeuroScience with their more refined and sensitive parameters. Please take this questionnaire.

LYME DISEASE SYMPTOM QUESTIONNAIRE CHECKLIST OF SYMPTOMOLOGY

Lyme disease can present with a broad array of symptomology. More than one system of the body may be affected. The format below clusters complaints referable to specific organ systems. If you note ten or more symptoms, especially moderate or severe, seeking professional help and testing is strongly encouraged.

Have you had any of the following? *refers to symptoms most unique to Lyme disease.

Tick bite	**Y**	**N**
Spotted rash over large area	**Y**	**N**

Bull's-eye rash (red circle with dot in center)	**Y**	**N**
Linear, red streaks	**Y**	**N**

	CURRENT SEVERITY			
SYMPTOM OR SIGN	**NONE**	**MILD**	**MODERATE**	**SEVERE**
Flu-like symptoms (fever, chills, cough, aching)				
Headache/stiff neck				
Meningitis				
General malaise				
Apathy and mental dullness				

Persistent swollen glands				
Sore throat				
Fevers				
Sore soles, especially in the a.m.				
*** Joint pain**				
Fingers, toes				
Ankles, wrists				
Knees, elbows				
Hips, shoulders				
Joint swelling				
Fingers, toes				
Ankles, wrists				
Knees, elbows				
Hips, shoulders				

Unexplained back pain or hip pain, lying on side produces hip pain				
Stiffness of the joints or back				
Muscle pain or cramps				
Obvious muscle weakness, legs feel unable to support, rising from seat laborious and painful				
Twitching or paralysis of the face or other muscles				
Tremors and/or jittery feeling				
Seizures				
Headache, including migraine				
Light sensitivity				
Sound sensitivity				

Vision: double, blurry, floaters, dry eyes				
Ear pain, prolonged or repeated episodes				
Hearing: buzzing, ringing, decreased hearing				
Increased motion sickness, vertigo, spinning				
Off balance, "tippy" feeling				

Tingling, numbness, burning, or stabbing sensations, shooting pains, skin hypersensitivity – worse on left side				
Facial paralysis – Bell's palsy				
Dental pain				

*** Neck creaks and cracks, stiffness, neck pain**				
*** Fatigue, tired, poor stamina, exhaustion, collapse**				
*** Insomnia, fractionated sleep, early awakening**				
Excessive nighttime sleep				
Napping during the day				
Unexplained weight gain				
Unexplained weight loss				
Unexplained hair loss				
Pain in genital area				
Unexplained menstrual irregularity				

Unexplained milk production, breast pain				
Irritable bladder or bladder dysfunction, repeated UTIs (urinary tract infections)				
Erectile dysfunction				
Loss of libido				
Queasy stomach or nausea				
Heartburn, stomach pain				
Constipation				
Diarrhea				
Low abdominal pain, cramps				
Heart murmur or valve prolapse				
Heart palpitations or skips, atrial fibrillation				
"Heart block" on EKG				

Chest wall pain or sore ribs, clutching sensation in ribs/ chest				
Head congestion				
Breathlessness, "air hunger," unexplained chronic cough				
Night sweats				
Exaggerated symptoms or worse hangover from alcohol				
*** Symptom flares every four weeks**				
Gray skin pallor				
Unexplained skin rash or eruption				
Elevated white blood count				
Elevated lymphocyte count				

Persistent yeast/ fungal infections				
Confusion, difficulty thinking				
Difficulty with concentration, reading, problem absorbing new information, brain fog				
Word search, name block				
Forgetfulness, poor short-term memory, poor attention				
Disorientation: getting lost, going to wrong places				
Speech errors: wrong word, misspeaking				
Mood swings, irritability, depression, suicidal feelings				

Anxiety, panic attacks, overreaction to news, even minor events					
Psychosis (hallucinations, delusions, paranoia, bipolar)					

APPENDIX 2:

PAIN MANAGEMENT & ANTIMICROBIALS FOR AUTOIMMUNE & LYME DISEASES

Pain is a chronic problem for those suffering with assorted autoimmune disorders and the array of tick-borne infections in Lyme disease. Within the world of complementary alternative medicine we have some helpful herbal and homeopathic aids that can help squelch pain, reduce inflammatory states, and even kill off the microbes connected to Lyme, the coinfections, RA or fibro, and more. This section is designed as a sort of "primer" to the topmost common remedies and for you to speak to your practitioner about integrating them into your protocol or perhaps you may elect to try weaning off of stronger pharmaceuticals that have side effects or no real aid for you. I cannot actually tell you what to take to get well, here as an author, but I can suggest these products as a pathway for you to explore and seek out help from qualified practitioners. The good news is that these all helped me to recover 100 percent. Integrative and functional medicine doctors, naturopaths, homeopaths, and clinical nutritionists will be skilled in these areas.

Here is a sampling of some of the common Lyme disease herbal protocols thousands of victims find success with regarding tick-borne infections. We blessedly have some wondrous plants with antimicrobial properties, as well as an assortment of other herbs to tackle the coinfections of babesia, bartonella, mycoplasma, Epstein-Barr virus, and more. Several decades into the Lyme crisis now, a handful of brilliant herbalists have established Lyme-specific herbal protocols for overcoming the infections, especially useful in chronic cases and dovetailing nicely with nutritional supportive aids and detoxification measures.

As one prominent seasoned Lyme-antibiotic-skilled medical doctor said to me:

"Katina, I tell all my patients all the time, there is more than one way to get well from this disease," alluding to my success without antibiotic therapy. Research coming from some cutting-edge scientists, such as Dr. Eva Sapi, University of New Haven, CT, is illustrating that the Samento and Banderol products are more stable and effective in chronic infections than long-term antibiotics. Talk to an integrative Lyme-literate physician for guidance treatments.

There are herbs known to address Lyme and coinfections. But please, REMEMBER: Lyme disease is not a self-help illness. You need a skilled practitioner to manage your care as symptoms shift, inflammation rages, and the bugs play hide-and-seek and mimic or trigger all too many autoimmune illnesses in hundreds of thousands of cases. You need their lens of perspective and nuances of "which herb when."

COMMON HERBALS

Cat's claw (Samento best, highest-quality-grade brand)
Banderol
Teasel root (excellent for European strains)
Artemisinin
Andrographis

Parsley
Garlic
Grapefruit seed extract
Lauric acid (retroviruses, yeast)

There are proven protocols that show significant success, when adhered to with persistence (months and years), to choose from. Please explore these practitioners' work.

- The Cowden Protocol; NutraMedix.com
  Samento, banderol, pinellia, etc.
- The Buhner Protocol;
  Artemisinin, etc.
- Byron-White Formulas;
  A-bart, A-bab, A-Lyme, etc.
- The Zhang Herbs;
  Chinese herbal formulas in masterful blends
- Pekana and Beyond Balance Formulas; BioResourceInc.com
  Homeopathic European superior-crafted formulas for detox, drainage, restoration, Lyme

I was on a modified version of the Cowden Protocol, meaning we administered the herbal formulas, but I never progressed to the maximum number of daily drops suggested. My system is so finely tuned that I made excellent progress at just half the amounts.

The product "Monolaurin" by Ecological Formulas (lauric acid) essentially "saved my life" by *finally* putting that relentless Epstein-Barr virus into dormancy—this is a highly effective aid for all retro-virus groups, herpes, shingles, etc.

Each of us is unique. Seeking a practitioner who is well versed in any of these noted protocols will be extremely therapeutic.

Pain can sideline us from activities, put us in bad moods, make us reach for NSAIDS or stronger meds, and actually put some of us in wheelchairs or on walkers. I relied heavily on homeopathic over-the-counter remedies in the 6c, 12c, and 30c potency range for symptom use in various "flare" stages and even long term, for anxiety, stiff necks, and headaches. Some of these remedies you can experiment with for self-help over a two- to three-week period. But, if no relief is coming, STOP the remedy and seek a certified classical homeopath (CCH) to get the laser-like right remedy match. Do not see someone who says they are a homeopath unless you see these CCH or RSHom initials. Many take a few weekend trainings on basics but are not certified practitioners. This is a finely tuned healing art requiring years of in-depth training of remedies, psyches, symptoms, body types, remedy potencies, and more.

Having said that, homeopathic remedies are still safe and have no side effects. They either are the right match and work or do not energetically match with your physiology and then are flushed out like a water-soluble vitamin. See the Homeopathic chapter earlier. The way to administer is to study your main three symptoms, complaints, and modalities (i.e., better when moving, worse in heat, etc.), and then take the matching remedy—two pellets dissolved under a clear tongue, at least twenty minutes away from food or drink, so no flavors negate them. 6c and 12c strengths are usually taken two to four doses per day until symptoms subside. A 30c strength is one to two doses per day. Let your body be your guide—when symptoms ease off stop the remedy. Overuse can make them lose effect.

Below are some common helpmates.

Ledum palustre: The "go-to" remedy for any tick bite, bull's-eye rash, early flu-like feelings, or achy pains. Another characteristic symptom is pain in the soles of the feet, especially the heels, often worse first steps on waking. Can feel like you are walking on pebbles. With a "fresh" tick bite three doses immediately in first twenty-four hours to potentially "abort" an infection while you seek medical help.

Bryonia alba: Right-sided body/joint pains, headaches, migraines. Worse with movement. Wants to lie still. Often irritable. Can have extra thirst. Favors formerly active, energetic, business-minded-type people. Fibromyalgia, rheumatoid arthritis, Lyme, bartonella, ehrlichia, constipation, neck pain, liver issues present.

Rhus toxidendron: Classic arthritic-type pains. Any joint can be involved. Worse in damp weather or aggravated by getting wet (even a bath). Pains are worse on first movement (mornings, rising from a chair) but ease off after up and about for a while, often to digress in the evening. Restless feelings in bed at night. Neck, shoulder pains common. Skin rashes, shingle-type burning pains too. Depression settles in over time commonly. RA, MS, CFS/ME, lupus, Lyme and coinfections, IC, fibromyalgia.

Eupatorium perf: A classic "flu" remedy where deep bone pains and upper back pain are persistent. Fevers or sweats can manifest. Deeply tired. Violent headaches. Strong liver cleanser. (A favorite Lyme remedy of mine.) Depressed. All autoimmune cases with a STRONG pain component of the upper body.

Kalmia: Wandering muscle and joint pains with true fatigue and malaise: fibromyalgia, CFS, arthritis, MS, thyroid, lupus, Lyme all are suspicious diagnosis. A heavy fatigue and brain fog. It is a rare "pain free" day with a Kalmia case.

Pulsatilla: Another migrating body pain remedy. Feel slight improvement getting outside, with fresh air or open windows. Company and consolation improve the weepy, sad, forlorn patient. Often a fearful, childlike helplessness is present. They crave warming comfort foods, dairy products. Many GI issues present; IBS, Crohn's, diarrhea, food allergies, bloating, leaky gut. I consider this one of the TOP fibromyalgia and MS remedies, as well as Lyme, thyroid, and early RA cases. Many cases that have bounced through the medical systems with no real healing success are forlorn, let down, feel betrayed, and are close to "giving up." I like this remedy a lot for those weary and needy and sad people.

Gelsemium: Another "flu-like" state with overall muscle versus bone pains. Back of the neck tension pains and occipital or frontal headache are common. Eyelids feel heavy. Drowsy, weak limbs. Occasional trembling. Irrational fear or anxiety, out of the blue. Clammy sweats. Diarrhea or IBS, Crohn's, colitis. VERY common MS, fibromyalgia remedy. Once fearless individual now feels weary and anxious. This remedy can have sterling help when it is the correct match!

Arsenicum album: A classic Lyme and coinfection remedy. Lots of burning pains anywhere. Skin, GI tract, joints, muscles, nerves. Very weak, tired yet restless. Cannot get away from the overwhelming pains. Insomnia. Pacing the floors or writhing in pain. Seizures, fits of rage, panic, fear. Suicidal thoughts. Oversensitive to "everything"—foods, medications, vitamins, weather, the wrong pillow, smells, etc. Nervous system feels fraught. Very useful for any form of neurological Lyme, coinfections, interstitial cystitis, lupus, fibro, CFS. Even helpful to ease apprehension of traveling to or visiting a doctor. Usually slim, spare frame, or are losing weight when ill. Start with 6c or 12c, as these are sensitive people and usually on delicate diets and need low potency and little to "rock their boat."

Kali phosphoricum: My favorite for CFS/ME, collapsed, bedridden cases. Completely drained, exhausted, hopeless states. Mental dullness/fog, depressed, forlorn, very weak, fragile. Insomnia. Strange nervous system sensations—buzzing, twitching, trembling. Tiring to "breathe." Homesick. Formerly responsible, usually hardworking types. Now cannot handle even a phone call, company, cooking. This is a wonder remedy for so many deteriorated Lyme disease cases, fibro, and MS that have slipped down the corridor of collapse. Again, often best results when 6c or 12c strengths are taken two to three times per day to slowly boost up electrolytes, adrenal fatigue, nervous system exhaustion, cellular function, mitochondria collapse.

Natrum muriaticum: Excellent for long-term chronic cases that have been misdiagnosed, malingering for years. Patient is weary, filled with grief over so much loss in their life. Trying to be stoic, yet spells of anxiety, insomnia, moodiness arise. Low back and neck pains, migraines prominent. Lyme disease, IBS, fibromyalgia, thyroid, MS, deep depression, hormonal issues common. This remedy helps stabilize many chronic cases so that herbal support, hormonal therapy, nutritional therapy can work better. My observation is that a large majority of chronic (i.e., advanced Lyme over five years' duration) benefit from several months on this remedy.

The list goes on rather extensively with how homeopathy is a VERY helpful tool in rectifying many, many symptoms of autoimmune illnesses and Lyme disease. Some cases will completely cure and many go into remission or find solid improvement. The key of course is finding the RIGHT homeopath to help you. Client-practitioner rapport is essential with this healing art, as very good skills are needed by your homeopath and a clear ability to be honest about yourself as a client helps weave together the insights enabling the homeopath to select from over 4,000 natural remedies to move your case in the healing directions we desire.

Websites:
http://www.CouncilForHomeopathicCertification.com

http://www.NationalCenterForHomeopathy.com

http://www.HomeopathicEducationalSystems.org

APPENDIX 3:

AUTOIMMUNE & LYME DISEASE-RELATED RESOURCES

There are many autoimmune illness and Lyme disease books, associations, support groups, blogs, and websites. Additionally, finding complementary alternative medicine practitioners can be sought by referral or some national websites. Please see my website, www.KatinaMakris.com, for a more complete listing as well as supply resources for herbs, homeopathic remedies, and recommended books.

Below are a few significant tick-borne-disease resources:

International Lyme and Associated Diseases Society; doctor training and info;
www.ilads.org

Tick-Borne Disease Alliance; awareness and fund-raising;
TBDAlliance.org

Global Lyme Alliance; fund-raising for research, awareness, and education; community support;
www.GlobalLymeAlliance.org

The Lyme Times Newsletter; major support group network;
www.lymedisease.org

The National Capitol Lyme and Tick-Borne Disease Association;
www.natcaplyme.org

The Lyme Light Foundation; financial assistance;
LymeLightFoundation.org

Lyme Disease Talk Radio; resources, practitioners, testimonials, inspiration;
LymeLightRadio.com

Lyme-Testing Laboratories;
IGeneX Labs, Palo Alto, CA;
www.IGeneX.com
Clongen Laboratories, Germantown, MD;
www.clongen.com
NeuroScience - the iSpot Test;
www.Neuroscience.com

Lyme-Literate Physicians;
ILADS.org
LymeDiseaseAssociation.org

COMPLEMENTARY MEDICINE RESOURCES

Acupuncture:
National Certification Commission for Acupuncture and Oriental Medicine;
www.nccaom.org

People's Organization of Community Acupuncture;
https://www.pocacoop.com

Classical Homeopathy:
National Center for Homeopathy, Arlington, VA;
www.nationalcenterforhomeopathy.org

Naturopathic Medicine:
www.Naturopathic.org

Clinical Nutrition:
American Society for Nutrition;
http://www.nutrition.org

Integrative/Functional Medicine:
Institute for Functional Medicine;
www.functionalmedicine.org

Metaphysical Training:
www.Stillpoint.org

AUTOIMMUNE ILLNESS RESOURCES

www.TheAutoImmuneSummit.com - series of educational video interviews with functional medicine physician Amy Myers, MD, and experts.

Lupus Foundations:
Lupus Foundation of America;
www.lupus.org
Lupus Foundation of Minnesota;
www.lupusmn.org
Lupus Colorado Foundation;
www.lupuscolorado.org

Rheumatoid Arthritis Foundations:
Arthritis Foundation;
http://www. arthritis.org

Rheumatoid Patient Foundation;
http://www.rheum4us.org

Multiple Sclerosis Foundations:
Multiple Sclerosis Foundation;
http://www.msfocus.org
National Multiple Sclerosis Society;
http://www.nationalmssociety.org
Multiple Sclerosis Association of America;
http://www.mymsaa.org

Fibromyalgia Foundations:
National Fibromyalgia Association;
http://www.fmaware.org
National Fibromyalgia and Chronic Pain Association;
http://www.fmcpaware.org
National Fibromyalgia Research Association;
http://www. NFRA.net
American Fibromyalgia Syndrome Association;
http://www.afsafund.org
The Fibromyalgia Information Foundation;
http://www.myalgia.com/OFF_info/OFF_about_usB.htm

Chronic Fatigue Syndrome Foundations:
National CFIDS Foundation;
http://www.ncf-net.org
Workwell Foundation;
http://www.workwellfoundation.org
Autoimmunity Research Foundation;
http://autoimmunityresearch.org

Hashimoto's/Graves' Disease:
Thyroid Foundation;
http://www.thyroidfoundation.org

Graves' Disease and Thyroid Foundation;
http://www.gdatf.org

Crohn's Disease Foundations:
Crohn's and Colitis Foundation of America;
http://www.ccfa.org
Burrill B. Crohn Research Foundation;
http://crohnfoundation.org
The Crohn's Journey Foundation;
https://thecrohnsjourneyfoundation.org

Interstitial Cystitis Foundations:
Interstitial Cystitis Association;
http://www.ichelp.org
National Kidney Foundation;
https://www.kidney.org/atoz/content/interstitial
Cystitis and Overactive Bladder Foundation (UK);
http://www.cobfoundation.org

ADDITIONAL RESOURCES

Emotional Support Therapies:
http://www.EFTuniverse.com
http://www.EMDR.com

Herbal and Nutritive Supplement Suppliers:
http://www. BioResourceInc.com
http://www. MountainHealthProducts.com
http://www. NutraMedix.com
http://www. Boiron.com
http://www. StandardHomeopathics.com
http://www. PureEncapsulations.com

INDEX

A
Acceptance, 82, 96–97, 324
Acknowledgment, 93–94
Acupuncture
in China, 207
energy in, 208–209
licensing, 210
in Lyme disease, 209–210
meridians in, 208–209
needles in, 209
philosophy of, 207–208
Adaptation, 4
Addiction, 280–281
Additives, food, 11, 195, 263–264, 274–275
Adrenal acceleration, 241
Adrenal burnout, 245
Adrenal collapse, 238, 239
Adrenal glands
cortisol and, 238–239, 242
in fibromyalgia, 127–128
functions of, 237–238
in inflammation, 231
lupus and, 144
symptoms associated with, 240–241
testing, 241–242
Adrenaline, 231, 237, 238
Adrenal Reset Diet, The (Christenson and Gottfried), 242
Adrenal supplement, 96
Against All Grain (Walker), 266
Agartha: A Journey to the Stars (Young-Sowers), 223
Alcohol, 195, 235, 262
Allergies, food, 264–265, 276–277
Allopathic medicine, 34
drugs in, 78–79, 80
in history of homeopathy, 70
integrative medicine and, 215
natural medicine and, 73
Almond oil, 269
Altar, 404–405
Aluminum shielding, for bed, 289
Alzheimer disease, 159–160
American Homeopathic Association (AHA), 201
Amino acids
brain chemistry and, 280
dopamine and, 280
inflammation and, 234
in organic meat, 262
in paleo diet, 265
protein and, 279–280
Anderson, Wayne, 297
Anger, 8–9, 105, 314
Antibodies
dependency and, 80
in lupus, 137–139
in Lyme disease, 162
in rheumatoid arthritis, 164
tests for, 137–139
Antidepressants, 127
Antiganglioside antibodies, 162
Antimicrobials, 61, 63, 71, 80, 129, 439–445
Antinuclear antibodies, 138, 164
Antioxidant deficiencies, 52
Apathy, 33–34
Are You Tired and Wired? (Pick), 240
Arsenicum album, 444
"Art of Letting Go" exercise, 351–354
Aspartame, 263
Assessment, of wellness, 34
Attention, to symptoms, 36–37, 58
Authenticity, 96, 371–378
Ayurvedic medicine, 250

B
Babesia, 52, 147, 168, 180, 184
Bartonella, 52, 121, 134, 148, 162, 180, 183–184, 282
Basket of Gifts exercise, 342–343
Bedroom, 306
Beliefs, 309, 311
Betrayal, 330
Binders, 298
Birth control, 122, 129, 234, 244
Bladder. See Interstitial cystitis / bladder pain syndrome (IC/BPS)
Blebs, 162–163, 164–165
Blood-clotting time, 140–141
Blood tests
antibody, 137–139
in lupus, 137–141
in rheumatoid arthritis, 152–153
for thyroid, 155–157
Body
as ecosystem, 295
emotions and, 87
healing pathway and, 313–314
as miracle, 8
thoughts and, 310–311
Boericke, William, 201
Boiron, 205
Borage oil, 269, 282
Borrelia burgdorferi, 66, 162, 167–168, 177, 179–180. See also Lyme disease
Borrelia hermsii, 187
Borrelia miyamotoi, 165, 180, 187
Breathwork exercise, 377–378
Bridge of Belief, The (Lipton), 100–101
Bromelain, 248
Brown, Thomas McPherson, 153–154
Bryonia alba, 443
Buhner, Stephen Harold, 134
"Bulbs of Spring" exercise, 351–354
Busch, Bradley, 250
Butazolidin, 249

C
Cadmium, 233
Candida
fibromyalgia and, 129
interstitial cystitis and, 135
lupus and, 144
Case stories, 407–425
Cat-scratch fever. See Bartonella
Celiac disease, 252–253. See also Gluten
Cell phones, 5, 288
Ceres Nanotrap test, 181
Certified Clinical Nutritionist (CCN), 213. See also

Nutrition, clinical
Chakra(s)
first, 117, 131, 154, 322–323, 324, 337–343
second, 135, 322–323, 324, 345–354
third, 107–108, 117, 131, 150, 154, 176, 322–323, 324–325, 355–361, 379–386
fourth, 131, 135, 144–145, 150, 154, 158, 322–323, 325, 363–369
fifth, 131, 150, 158, 322–323, 325, 371–378
sixth, 158, 322–323, 326
seventh, 150, 322–323, 326, 387–396
in chronic fatigue syndrome, 117
energy and, 319–320
in fibromyalgia, 131
in interstitial cystitis / bladder pain syndrome, 135
in lupus, 144–145
in Lyme disease, 176
map, 322–326
in multiple sclerosis, 150
in rheumatoid arthritis, 154
in thyroid disease, 158
Change, 29, 30, 32, 95, 345–354
Chelation therapy. See also Heavy metal accumulation
in chronic fatigue syndrome, 115
inflammation and, 235
in lupus, 143
in multiple sclerosis, 149
Children
constitutions in, 287
health problems in, 15
Lyme disease in, 172–173
protein in diet of, 279
resiliency of, 93
China, 36, 207
Chlamydia pneumonia, 53, 116, 147, 149, 245
Choices, 5
Cholesterol, 268
Christenson, Alan, 242
Christian Science, 227
Chronic fatigue immune dysfunction syndrome (CFIDS), 113
Chronic fatigue syndrome (CFS)
case story, 407–413
chakras in, 117
fatigue in, 114
heavy metals and, 115
history of, 113–114
homeopathy and, 116
Lyme disease and, 66, 115
metaphysics in, 117
other names for, 113
quality of life in, 114–115
retroviruses and, 116
symptoms of, 114
Church, Dawson, 101
Cigarettes, 119, 256
Cimicifuga constitution, 202
Circulation, 45
Clarity, 400
Cling wrap, 283–285
Clot time tests, 140–141
Coconut oil, 259, 269
Cod liver oil, 271
Coffee, 53, 256
Colitis, triggers for, 120–121. See also Crohn's disease; Irritable bowel syndrome (IBS)
Colorado tick fever, 186
Commitment, 5
Compassion, 89–90
Complementary and alternative medicine (CAM), as term, 76
Complement proteins, 139–140
Confidence, 95–96
Constitutional types, 202–203, 287
Conventional medicine. See Allopathic medicine
Copper, 52, 233
Corn oil, 258
Corticosteroids, 141–142, 245
Cortisol, 238–239, 242
Costs, healthcare, 219
Cottonseed oil, 258
Cowden, Lee, 250
Coxiella burnetii, 187
Coxsackie, 53, 116
C-reactive protein (CRP), in lupus, 140
Creativity, 14, 17, 356, 416–420
Crohn's disease. See also Irritable bowel syndrome (IBS)
in allopathic medicine, 78
diet and, 122
gastroenteritis and, 119–120
gluten and, 120–121
history of, 119
metaphysics in, 122–123
risk factors for, 119
symptoms in, 120
Cupped Hands exercise, 367–369
Curcumin, 121, 250
Cure
directions of, 60–61
Hering's Law of, 59
Cytomegalia, 52, 116, 234

D
Dairy products, 260–261
Davis, William, 251, 252
DEHA, 284–285
de Meirleir, Kenny, 126
Denial, 93
Dental fillings, 52
Dependency, 80
Depression, 88, 226
Determination, 356–357
Detoxification. See also Toxins
binders for, 298
kidneys in, 298–299
lymphatic system in, 299–300
MTHFR marker and, 298
pushers for, 298
Didehydroepiandrosterone (DHEA), 244
Diet
additives in, 11, 195, 263–264, 274–275
alcohol in, 262
in clinical nutrition, 213–214
Crohn's disease and, 122
dairy products in, 260–261
fat in, 267–271
food labeling and, 273–274
food sensitivities and, 264–265
foods to eliminate from, 257–265
fried foods in, 270–271
gluten in, 252–253
GMOs in, 44, 53, 63
grains in, refined, 262–263
imbalance in, 44
inflammation and, 233, 235, 251–253
interstitial cystitis / bladder pain syndrome and, 134
irritable bowel syndrome and, 121, 122
meat in, 261–262, 270
organic foods in, 275–276
paleo, 265–266
processed foods in, 44, 52, 195, 251–252, 262–263, 268–269, 280
protein in, 280
red meat in, 261–262
resiliency and, 96
sugar in, 255–256, 257–258, 277
trans fats in, 259–260
vegetable oils in, 258–259
Diet Cure, The (Ross), 280
Dilution, in homeopathy, 200
Directions of cure, 60–61

Disconnect, 106–108
Disease. See also Illness
  defined, 39–40
  in functional medicine, 218
  language of, 41–42
Disorder, 40
Divine love, 387–391
DNA, double-stranded, antibodies to, 138, 164
Dopamine, 280
Double-stranded DNA antibodies, 138, 164
D-Phenylalinine, 281
Drugs
  in allopathic medicine, 78–79, 80
  antifungal, 293
  anti-inflammatory, 232, 249
  dependency on, 80
  for inflammation, 248
  for pain, 248
  reliance on, 66–67
Dry cleaning, 67, 233

E
Eddy, Mary Baker, 227, 387, 388–389
Education
  in clinical nutrition, 213
  in homeopathy, 203–204
  in naturopathic medicine, 193–194, 195–196
Eggs, 267
Ehrlichia, 168, 180, 184–185
Einstein, Albert, 329
Elderly, 87
Electric blankets, 289
Electromagnetic energy
  body meridians and, 208
  with cell phones, 288
  increase in exposure to, 287–288
  inflammation and, 53
  sleep and, 45
ELISPOT, 181
Emotions
  body and, 87
  energy and, 8–9, 16
  homeopathy and, 96–97
  immune system and, 88–89, 366–367
  metaphysical healing and, 226–227
  pituitary function and, 88
  power of, 82
  resiliency and, 94–96
  scars from, 346
  symptoms and, 105–106
Endocrine disruptors, 283–284
Endorphins, 280–281
Energy. See also Electromagnetic energy
  in acupuncture, 208–209
  aging and, 355–356
  cell phones and, 288
  chakras and, 319–320
  dark, 335
  electromagnetic fields and, 288–289
  emotions and, 8–9, 16
  in Feng Shui, 306
  of first chakra, 341–342
  healing, 330
  heart, 364–365
  meridians, 208–209
  of third chakra, 107–108
Enig, Mary, 267
Enlightenment, 332
Enzymes, proteolytic, 248–249
Epigenetics, 12, 100–101
Epstein-Barr, 52, 234, 245
  chronic fatigue syndrome and, 116
  lupus and, 142–143
Erectile dysfunction, 285
Erythrocyte sedimentation rate (ESR), in lupus, 140
Estrogen, 283–284
Eupatorium perf, 443
Europe, 36
Exercise, 41, 44–45, 240, 245–246, 298–299, 301–304

F
Faith, 103
Fallon, Sally, 251, 267
Family, extended, 333–334
Fat
  in diet, 267–271
  Lyme disease and, 160
  saturated, 267–268
  trans, 259–260
Fatigue, in chronic fatigue syndrome, 114
Fazden, Nicola, 251
Fear, 6, 16
Feng Shui, 306
Fibrinogen, in lupus, 141
Fibromyalgia
  adrenal glands in, 127–128
  antidepressants in, 127
  case story, 407–413
  gluten and, 128
  liver stagnation and, 130–131
  magnesium and, 129–130
  metaphysics in, 131
  mold and, 129
  predisposition to, 44
  symptoms of, 126–127
  thyroid in, 128
  vitamin D and, 130
  yeast and, 129
Ficin, 248
Fish, Durland, 165
Fish oils, 269, 282
Flaxseed oil, 269, 282
Flexner, Abraham, 71, 201
Fluoride, 233
Food and Drug Administration (FDA), 201
Food labels, 273–274, 276–277
Food sensitivity, 264–265, 276–277
Francisella tularensis, 187
Franklin, Benjamin, 356
Free radicals, 270–271
French diet, 268
Fruit, 258
Fruit juice, 258
Frying, 270–271
Fulfillment, 46–47, 356
Functional medicine, 5. See also Integrative medicine
  adrenal glands and, 243
  defined, 217–218
  disease in, 218

G
GABA, 281
Gastroenteritis, 119–120. See also Crohn's disease
Gelsemium, 444
Genes. See also Epigenetics
  Lyme disease course and, 164
  MTHFR marker and, 298
  in rheumatoid arthritis, 152
  thrivers and, 101
Genetically-modified organisms (GMOs)
  gluten and, 121
  in irritable bowel syndrome, 121
  naturopathic medicine and, 195
  nourishment and, 53
  nutritional imbalance and, 44
  organic foods and, 269
Genie in Your Genes, The (Church), 101
Gibran, Khalil, 97
Gluten, 52, 252–253
  fibromyalgia and, 128
  in irritable bowel syndrome, 120–121
  lupus and, 143
Glycine, 213, 281
Glycogen, 268
Glyphosate, 63, 67, 233
Goat milk, 260
Gottfried, Sara, 242

Grain Brain (Perlmutter), 251
Grains, refined, 262–263
Grapeseed oil, 259, 269
Graves' disease, 51, 158, 244
Gray, Bill, 204
Green, Susan, 178
Guilt, 330
Gulf War Syndrome, 184

H
Hahnemann, Samuel, 199–200
Hashimoto's thyroiditis, 51, 158, 162
Hay, Louise, 227
Healing crisis, 61
Healing energy, 330
Healing force, 99–100
Healing pathway, 313–315
"Healing rainbow," 331
Healing words, 27–28
Healthcare costs, 219
Health standard, in United States, 63
Heart center, 32
Heart's desire, 225, 363–369
Heavy metal accumulation, 52. See also Chelation therapy
  chronic fatigue syndrome and, 115
  inflammation and, 233
  lupus and, 143
  multiple sclerosis and, 149
Herbal medicine, Chinese, in Lyme disease, 210
Herbals, 440–441
"Hering's Law of Cure," 59, 60–61
Herxheimer reaction, 61, 297
Histamines, 231. See also Inflammation
Histone antibodies, 138
Holistic medicine
  allopathic vs., 78–79
  disciplines in, 76–77
Homeopathy
  in chronic fatigue syndrome, 116
  constitutional types in, 202–203
  education in, 203–204
  emotions and, 96–97
  Hahnemann in, 199–200
  Hering's Law of Cure in, 59
  history of, 199–201
  in history of American medicine, 70–72
  ideals in, 202
  inflammation and, 247
  Lyme disease and, 205
  lymphatic system in, 300
  overseas, 36
  remedies in, 205–206
  resurgence of, 204
  spread of, 200–201
  symptoms in, 57
Homeostasis, 194
Home space, 305–307
Horowitz, Richard, 142, 153, 160, 161 162, 164, 173, 174, 235
"Horse sense," 64, 67
Hydrogenation, 259, 267, 269–270
Hyman, Mark, 157, 250, 251

I
Illness. See also Disease
  circulation and, 45
  fulfillment and, 46–47
  nutritional imbalance in, 44
  personal transformation and, 83
  sleep and, 45
  stress and, 45–46
  structural factors in, 44–45
  toxins and, 46
Imbalance, 65
Immune system. See also Antibodies
  blebs and, 162
  emotions and, 88–89, 366–367
  healing force and, 99–100
  molecular mimicry and, 160, 165
  mycoplasma and, 186
  overactive, 232
  in rheumatoid arthritis, 152
Immunization. See Vaccines
Indigenous cultures, 225
Indocin, 249
Inflammation, 49, 50
  adrenal glands and, 231
  agents causing, 233–234
  benefits of, 232
  as common denominator, 231
  diet and, 233, 235, 251–253
  drugs for, 232
  fibromyalgia and, 128
  food sensitivity and, 264–265
  gluten and, 252–253
  gut flora and, 52
  heavy metals and, 233
  homeopathy and, 247
  Lyme disease and, 235
  pH and, 235
  physiology of, 231
  proteolytic enzymes and, 248–249
  reduction of, 247–253
  toxins and, 233–234
Inflamyar, 250
Inner tools, 330–333
Integrative medicine, 5, 33–34, 56
  allopathic medicine and, 215
  defined, 216
  principles of, 217
  rise of, 72–73
  Weil on, 216
Integrative Medicine Clinics, 81
Intention, 27, 310, 355–361
Interstitial cystitis / bladder pain syndrome (IC/BPS)
  defined, 131
  diet and, 134
  Lyme disease and, 134–135
  metaphysics in, 135
  symptoms of, 134
Inversion tables, 299–300
Iodine, 234
Irritable bowel syndrome (IBS). See also Crohn's disease
  diet and, 121–122
  gluten and, 120–121
  in Lyme disease, 51
  triggers for, 120–121
iSpot Lyme test, 181

J
Jernigan, David, 250, 296
Job displeasure, 34
Judgment, 364
Juice, fruit, 258

K
Kali phosphoricum, 444
Kalmia, 443
Kaprex, 250
Kefir, 260–261
Kent, James Tyler, 201
Kidneys, 298–299
Kilani, Ahmed, 179–180
Kindness, 365–366
Klinghardt, Dietrich, 288
Know Your Fats: The Complete Primer for Understanding Fats, Oils, and Cholesterol (Enig), 267
Krause, Peter, 165

L
La antibodies, 139
Labels, food, 273–274, 276–277
Laughter therapy, 90
Lauric acid, 116, 143
Lead, 52, 233
"Leaky gut syndrome," 52, 251–252
Ledum palustre, 442
"Letting go," 346–347

Lewis, C. S., 334
Liegner, Kenneth, 163, 166
Lifespan, 39, 221
"Like treats like," 203
Lipton, Bruce, 100–101
Liver
  fats and, 268
  food additives and, 274–275
  stagnation, fibromyalgia and, 130–131
Loneliness, 90
Love, 9, 30–31, 82, 89–90, 364–365, 404. See also Divine love; Self-love
Lupus. See Systemic lupus erythematosus (SLE)
Lyme disease
  acupuncture in, 209–210
  Alzheimer disease and, 159–160
  antibodies in, 162
  autoimmune involvement in, 164–165
  blebs in, 162–163, 164–165
  case story, 413–416
  in children, 172–173
  chronic, 20, 173
  chronic fatigue syndrome and, 66, 115
  co-infections, 167, 168, 183–189
  digestive tract in, 197
  as epidemic, 169–170
  fat and, 160
  genetic predispositions and, 164
  herbal Chinese medicine in, 210
  homeopathy and, 205
  inflammation and, 235
  inflammation in, 50
  interstitial cystitis / bladder pain syndrome and, 134–135
  "I's" of, 162
  metaphysics in, 176
  migraines in, 50–51
  multiple sclerosis and, 148–149, 160–162
  naturopathic medicine and, 196
  rash in, 170–171, 415
  sexual transmission of, 169
  spread of, 168
  symptoms of, 171–172, 429–438
  testing for, 148, 167, 168, 177–181
  ticks and, 170–171
  transmission of, 169
Lymphatic massage, 299
Lymphatic system, 299, 301–302

M
Macadamia oil, 259
MacDonald, Alan, 159–160, 161, 188
Magnesium
  fibromyalgia and, 129–130
  multiple sclerosis and, 150
Manganese deficiency, 52
Manners, David, 29
Massage, lymphatic, 299
McCammish, Susan, 250
Meat
  feedlot-raised, 261
  organic, 270
  red, 261–262
Medical condition, 40
Meditation, 96, 381–383, 385–386
Mending, 83–86
Menstruation, 284
Mental illness, 61
Mental patterns, negative, 225–226
Mercury, 52, 233
Meridians, energy, 208–209
Metaphysical healing
  emotions and, 226–227
  indigenous cultures and, 225
  negative mental patterns and, 225–226
Metaphysics
  in chronic fatigue syndrome, 117
  in Crohn's disease, 122–123
  in fibromyalgia, 131
  in interstitial cystitis / bladder pain syndrome, 135
  in lupus, 144–145
  in Lyme disease, 176
  multiple sclerosis and, 150
  in rheumatoid arthritis, 154
  in thyroid disease, 158
Microwaves, 44, 285, 289
Midwives, 69–70
Migraines, in Lyme disease, 50–51
Milk, 260–261
Mold
  adrenal burnout and, 244
  airing out for, 293–294
  chronic fatigue syndrome and, 115
  conditions for, 292
  fibromyalgia and, 129
  interstitial cystitis / bladder pain syndrome and, 135
  lupus and, 143
  natural aids for, 293
  as risk factor, 52
  symptoms of reaction to, 291–292
  testing, 292
Molecular mimicry, 160, 165
Molybdenum deficiency, 52
Monolaurin, 213, 441
Monosodium glutamate (MSG), 263
Moving with Intention exercise, 359–361
MTHFR, 234, 298
Multiple sclerosis (MS)
  diagnosis of, 147
  heavy metals and, 149
  Lyme disease and, 148–149, 160–162
  metaphysics in, 150
  MRI scans in, 147–148
  vitamin B12 and, 149
Multi-systemic infectious disease syndrome (MSIDS), 235
Music, 91
"My," 41–42
Myalgic encephalomyelitis (ME), 113. See also Chronic fatigue syndrome (CFS)
Mycoplasma, 52, 154, 162, 180, 186, 234, 296–297
Myers, Amy, 126, 152, 165

N
Natrum muriaticum, 444–445
"Natural" food label, 275
Natural medicine
  allopathic and, 73
  disciplines in, 75
  in history of American medicine, 71
Naturopathic medicine
  adrenal glands and, 243
  education in, 193–194, 195–196
  goal of, 194–195
  licensing in, 193, 195–196
  Lyme disease and, 196
  philosophy of, 194
  prevention in, 195
Naturopathic physician, 5
Needles, in acupuncture, 209
Negativity, 225–226
Nervous system, parasympathetic, 89
Neu5Gc, 261
Neurasthenia, 113. See also Chronic fatigue syndrome (CFS)
Nourishing Traditions (Fallon),

251, 267
Nourishment, 53
Nutramedix, 122
Nutrition, clinical
diet in, 213–214
education in, 213
Nutritional imbalance, 44
Nutritionist, 5, 213

O
Oils
fish, 269, 282
vegetable, 258–259
Olive oil, 259, 269
Omega-3 fatty acids, 258–259, 261, 269, 271
Omega-6 fatty acids, 116, 258–259, 261
Openness, 379–386
Opportunity, 30
"Organic" food label, 275–276
Organic meat, 270
Organic produce, 277–278
Outdoors, 338–339

P
Pace of living, 11, 66
Pain management, 247–248, 282, 439–445
Paleo diet, 265–266
Pancreas, 242–243
Papain, 248
Parasites, 52, 122, 148. See also specific parasites
Parasympathetic nervous system, 89
Partial thromboplastin time (PTT), 141
Patenting, 201
Pathway, healing, 313–315
Peale, Norman Vincent, 90
Penicillin, 71. See also Antimicrobials
Perlmutter, David, 165, 250, 251
Personal transformation, 22, 83
Pets, 87, 169
Pharmaceutical industry, 201–202. See also Drugs
pH imbalance, 53, 116, 233, 235, 257
Phospholipid antibodies, 138–139
Piazza, Laura, 251
Piazza, Paul, 251
Pick, Marcelle, 240
Pineal gland, 380, 383–384
Pituitary gland, 88, 242
Plastic
DEHA in, 284–285
as endocrine disruptor, 283–284
inflammation and, 234
Pneumonia. See Chlamydia pneumonia
Positive thinking, 90, 103
Post-Lyme syndrome, 179
Postural orthostatic tachycardia syndrome (POTS), 162
Posture, 45
Post-viral fatigue syndrome (PVFS), 113. See also Chronic fatigue syndrome (CFS)
Potassium deficiency, 234
Potentization, in homeopathy, 200
Powassan virus, 186–187
Practical Paleo, The (Sanfilippo), 251, 266
Prayer, 96, 320, 392–396
Predisease, 41
Probiotics, 56, 121, 135
Processed foods, 44, 52, 195, 251–252, 262–263, 268–269, 280
Protein(s)
amino acids and, 279–280
complement, 139–140
C-reactive, 140
in diet, 280
Proteolytic enzymes, 248–249
Prothrombin time (PT), 141
Pulsatilla, 443
Pushers, 298

Q
Q fever, 187
Quality of life
amino acids and, 281
in chronic fatigue syndrome, 114–115
in Crohn's disease, 120
in interstitial cystitis, 134

R
Rash, in Lyme disease, 170–171, 415
Rebirth, 333–336, 416–420
Rebounding, 299
Receiving, 337–340
Recipes for Repair (Piazza and Piazza), 251
Registered dietitian (RD), 213, 214
Reproductive system, 284
Resentment, 330
Resilience, 4, 7–8, 11–12, 93–97
Responsibility, 95
Rest, 102
Retreat, 23–24
Retroviruses, 116
Rheumatoid arthritis (RA)
antibodies in, 164
blood tests in, 152–153
case story, 407–413
in complementary and alternative medicine, 76
defined, 152
diagnosis of, 152–153
food additives and, 263
genetics in, 152
metaphysics in, 154
progression of, 151
symptoms of, 151
Rhus toxidendron, 443
Rhythms, 24
Rife machine, 288, 296, 298
RNP antibodies, 139
Ro antibodies, 139
Rocky Mountain spotted fever, 52, 168, 187
Ross, Julia, 280
Routine, 29

S
Sacred space
home as, 305–307
outdoor, 307
Safflower oil, 258
Saliva testing, 241, 285
Sanfilippo, Diane, 251, 266
Sapi, Eva, 169
Saturated fat, 267–270
Scammell, Henry, 153
Science, 9–10, 72. See also Allopathic medicine
Science of Mind (Eddy), 227, 387
Seasons, 25, 29
Seeker, 399–401
Selenium deficiency, 52, 234
Self-confidence, 95–96
Self-love, 102–103
Self-nurturance, 22–23
Serotonin, 281
Sesame oil, 259, 269
Sex, in Lyme disease transmission, 169
Shame, 330
Sheep milk, 260
Shock, 93
Shoemaker, Ritchie, 115, 294, 297–298
Silicea constitution, 202–203
Skall, Monte, 178
Skin, as "third kidney," 296
Skin brushing, 299
Slantboarding, 300
Sleep, 45, 169, 242, 288
Sm antibodies, 139
Smoking, 119, 256

Soda, 257
Soft drinks, 257
Solitude, 23–24
Soy oil, 258
Spirit, 222
Spontaneous Healing (Weil), 72
Stagnation, 29
Stillness, 24–25, 31
Stress, 45–46, 89, 120, 144, 238, 245, 384
Stricker, Ralph, 169
Structural factors, 44–45
Suffering, 333–336
Sugar, 255–256, 257–258, 277
Sugar Blues, The (Hyman), 251
Sunflower oil, 258
Support systems, 102
Surviving Mold (Shoemaker), 294
Susceptibility, 43–44
Swordfish, 52
Symptoms
  in allopathic medicine, 34
  attention to, 36–37, 58
  of chronic fatigue syndrome, 114
  of Crohn's disease, 120
  defined, 55
  emotions and, 105–106
  of fibromyalgia, 126–127
  in healing crisis, 61
  in Hering's Law of Cure, 59–60
  in homeopathy, 57
  in integrative medicine, 56, 57
  of interstitial cystitis / bladder pain syndrome, 134
  of lupus, 137
  of Lyme disease, 171–172, 429–438
  of mold exposure, 291–292
  mysterious, 63
  persistent, 57
  progression of, 59–60
  of rheumatoid arthritis, 151
Syndrome, 41, 112
Systemic lupus erythematosus (SLE)
  adrenal glands and, 144
  antibodies in, 137–139
  complement proteins in, 139–140
  C-reactive protein in, 140
  Epstein-Barr and, 142–143
  erythrocyte sedimentation rate in, 140
  fibrinogen in, 141
  metaphysics in, 144–145
  RNO antibodies in, 139
  symptoms of, 137
  urine testing in, 141

T
Tetrahydrochloride, 67
Third chakra, 107–108
Thoughts
  beliefs and, 309, 311
  body and, 310–311
  experiences and, 310
Thrivers, 90–91, 101
Thymus gland, 89
Thyroid
  adrenal glands and, 242
  in fibromyalgia, 128
  in Graves' disease, 158
  metaphysics in, 158
  sensitivity of, 155
  tests, 155–157
Tick-borne encephalitis (TBE), 186–187
Tick paralysis, 187
Ticks, 168, 170–171
Tick testing, 188–189
Toxins, 46, 195. See also Detoxification; Heavy metal accumulation; Mold
  emotional, 135
  enzymes and, 248
  in food, 251–252
  inflammation and, 233–234
  lupus and, 143
Trampolines, 299
Trans fats, 259–260
Truth, 400
Tularemia, 187
Tuna, 52

U
Urine testing, in lupus, 141

V
Vaccines, 10–11, 53, 63, 72
Vegetable oils, 258–259
Viral infections, 52–53. See also specific infections
Vitamin B12, multiple sclerosis and, 149
Vitamin D, 130, 271
Vitamin deficiencies, 52, 149
Vithoulkas, George, 204

W
Walker, Danielle, 266
Walking, 302–303
Wallach, Joel, 73, 122, 153, 154, 161
Water bottles, 285
Weight gain, 34
Weil, Andrew, 72, 215, 216
Wellness approach, 33–34
Wellness assessment, 34
Western medicine. See Allopathic medicine
Wheat, heirloom, 11, 33, 128
Wheat Belly (Davis), 251, 252
"(W)holistic," 34
Why Can't I Get Better? Solving the Mystery of Lyme & Chronic Disease (Horowitz), 142, 161–162, 174, 235
Will, 101, 355–361
Williams, Mara, 149, 189
Wisdom, 36
Wobezyme PS, 249–250
Words, healing, 27–28
Work environment, 34
World War II, 71

Y
Yeast
  fibromyalgia and, 129
  interstitial cystitis / bladder pain syndrome and, 135
  lupus and, 144
Young-Sowers, Meredith, 223, 315, 330, 331, 342

Z
Zinc deficiency, 52